P9-CRX-849

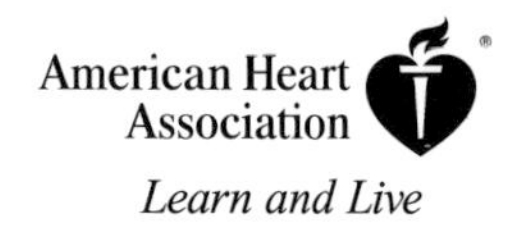

The AHA Clinical Series

SERIES EDITOR ELLIOTT ANTMAN

Cardiovascular Genetics and Genomics

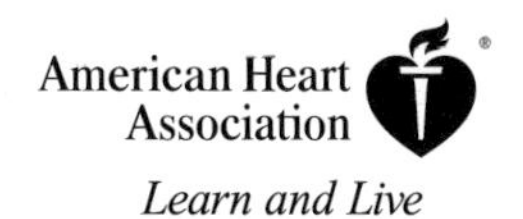

The AHA Clinical Series

SERIES EDITOR ELLIOTT ANTMAN

Cardiovascular Genetics and Genomics

EDITED BY

Dan Roden, MD

Professor of Medicine and Pharmacology
Director, Oates Institute for Experimental Therapeutics
Assistant Vice-Chancellor for Personalized Medicine
Vanderbilt University School of Medicine
Nashville, TN
USA

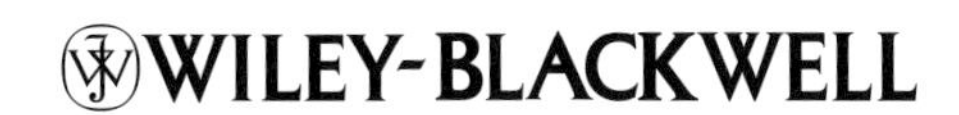

A John Wiley & Sons, Ltd., Publication

This edition first published 2009, © 2009 American Heart Association
American Heart Association National Center, 7272 Greenville Avenue, Dallas, TX 75231, USA
For further information on the American Heart Association:
www.americanheart.org

Blackwell Publishing was acquired by John Wiley & Sons in February 2007. Blackwell's publishing program has been merged with Wiley's global Scientific, Technical and Medical business to form Wiley-Blackwell.

Registered office: John Wiley & Sons Ltd, The Atrium, Southern Gate, Chichester, West Sussex, PO19 8SQ, UK
Editorial offices: 9600 Garsington Road, Oxford, OX4 2DQ, UK
The Atrium, Southern Gate, Chichester, West Sussex, PO19 8SQ, UK
111 River Street, Hoboken, NJ 07030-5774, USA

For details of our global editorial offices, for customer services and for information about how to apply for permission to reuse the copyright material in this book please see our website at www.wiley.com/wiley-blackwell

The right of the author to be identified as the author of this work has been asserted in accordance with the Copyright, Designs and Patents Act 1988.

All rights reserved. No part of this publication may be reproduced, stored in a retrieval system, or transmitted, in any form or by any means, electronic, mechanical, photocopying, recording or otherwise, except as permitted by the UK Copyright, Designs and Patents Act 1988, without the prior permission of the publisher.

Wiley also publishes its books in a variety of electronic formats. Some content that appears in print may not be available in electronic books.

Designations used by companies to distinguish their products are often claimed as trademarks. All brand names and product names used in this book are trade names, service marks, trademarks or registered trademarks of their respective owners. The publisher is not associated with any product or vendor mentioned in this book. This publication is designed to provide accurate and authoritative information in regard to the subject matter covered. It is sold on the understanding that the publisher is not engaged in rendering professional services. If professional advice or other expert assistance is required, the services of a competent professional should be sought.

The contents of this work are intended to further general scientific research, understanding, and discussion only and are not intended and should not be relied upon as recommending or promoting a specific method, diagnosis, or treatment by physicians for any particular patient. The publisher and the author make no representations or warranties with respect to the accuracy or completeness of the contents of this work and specifically disclaim all warranties, including without limitation any implied warranties of fitness for a particular purpose. In view of ongoing research, e+quipment modifications, changes in governmental regulations, and the constant flow of information relating to the use of medicines, equipment, and devices, the reader is urged to review and evaluate the information provided in the package insert or instructions for each medicine, equipment, or device for, among other things, any changes in the instructions or indication of usage and for added warnings and precautions. Readers should consult with a specialist where appropriate. The fact that an organization or Website is referred to in this work as a citation and/or a potential source of further information does not mean that the author or the publisher endorses the information the organization or Website may provide or recommendations it may make. Further, readers should be aware that Internet Websites listed in this work may have changed or disappeared between when this work was written and when it is read. No warranty may be created or extended by any promotional statements for this work. Neither the publisher nor the author shall be liable for any damages arising herefrom.

Library of Congress Cataloging-in-Publication Data
Cardiovascular genetics and genomics / edited by Dan Roden.
p. ; cm.
Includes bibliographical references.
ISBN 978-1-4051-7540-1
1. Cardiovascular system—Diseases—Genetic aspects. 2. Genomics. 3. Pharmacogenomics.
I. Roden, D. M. (Dan M.) II. American Heart Association.
[DNLM: 1. Heart Diseases—genetics. 2. Cardiovascular Diseases—genetics. 3. Cardiovascular Diseases—theraphy. 4. Genomics—methods. 5. Heart Diseases--therapy. 6. Pharmacogenetics. WG 210 C26843 2009]
RC669.C2853 2009
616.1'042—dc22

2008052143

ISBN: 978-1-4051-7540-1
A catalogue record for this book is available from the British Library.

Set in Palatino 9/12 by Macmillan Publishing Solutions
(www.macmillansolutions.com)
Printed and bound in Singapore by Fabulous Printers Pte Ltd
1 2009

Contents

Contributors

Editor

Dan Roden, MD
Professor of Medicine and Pharmacology
Director, Oates Institute for Experimental Therapeutics
Assistant Vice-Chancellor for Personalized Medicine
Vanderbilt University School of Medicine
Nashville, TN
USA

Contributors

Mark J. Alberts, MD
Professor of Neurology
Director, Stroke Program
Northwestern University Feinberg School of Medicine
Chicago, IL
USA

Donna K. Arnett, PhD, MSPH
Professor and Chair
Department of Epidemiology
School of Public Health University of Alabama at Birmingham
Birmingham, AL
USA

Richard Berg, MS
Department of Biostatistics
Marshfield Clinic Research Foundation
Marshfield, WI
USA

Michael D. Caldwell, MD, PhD
Department of Surgery
Marshfield Clinic
Marshfield, WI
USA

Dana C. Crawford, PhD
Assistant Professor, Department of Molecular Physiology and Biophysics
Investigator, Center for Human Genetics Research
Vanderbilt University
Nashville, TN
USA

Jacqueline S. Danik, MD, MPH
Assistant professor of Medicine
Harvard Medical School
Center for Cardiovascular Disease Prevention
Division of Preventive Medicine
Brigham and Women's Hospital
Boston, MA
USA

Dawood Darbar, MD
Associate Professor of Medicine
Direct, Vanelerbilt Arrhythnia Service
Vanderbilt University School of Medicine
Nashville, TN
USA

Jonas S.S.G. de Jong, MD
Cardiology Resident
Research Fellow
Academic Medical Center
Amsterdam
The Netherlands

Lukas R.C. Dekker, MD, PhD
Cardiologist
Catharina Hospital
Eindhoven
The Netherlands

Nauder Faraday, MD
Associate Professor of Anesthesiology/Critical Care Medicine and Surgery
Director, Perioperative Hemostasis and Thrombosis Research Laboratory

Director, Perioperative Gonomic Research
Johns Hopkins University School of Medicine
Baltimore, MD
USA

Jonathan L. Haines, PhD
Professor, Department of Molecular Physiology and Biophysics
T.H. Morgan Professor of Human Genetics
Director, Center for Human Genetics Research
Vanderbilt University Medical Center
Nashville, TN
USA

William Herzog, MD
Assistant professor
Johns Hopkins University School of Medicine
Baltimore, MD
USA

Carolyn Y. Ho, MD
Assistant Professor of Medicine, Haward Medical School
Cardiovascular Division
Brigham and Women's Hospital
Boston, MA
USA

Raymond Hreiche, PharmD, PhD
Faculty of Pharmacy
Université de Montréal
Montréal
Québec
Canada

Julie A. Johnson, PharmD
Department of Pharmacy Practice
Division of Cardiovascular Medicine
Colleges of Pharmacy and Medicine
Center for Pharmacogenomics
University of Florida
Gainesville, FL
USA

Yasmin Khan, MD
Maryland Endocrine, P.A.
Columbia, MD
USA

Calum A. MacRae, MD
Cardiovascular Division and Cardiovascular Research Center
Massachusetts General Hospital and Harvard Medical School
Boston, MA
USA

William J. McKenna, MD, DSc, FRCP
Professor, Cardiology in the Young
The Heart Hospital
London
UK

Ruth McPherson, MD, PhD, FRCPC
Director, Lipid Research Laboratory
University of Ottawa Heart Institute
Ottawa, Ontario
Canada

Veronique Michaud, BPharm, PhD
Faculty of Pharmacy
Université de Montréal
Montréal
Québec
Canada

Christopher Newton-Cheh, MD, MPH, FACC, FAHA
Assistant Professor of Medicine
Harvard Medical School
Broad Institute of Harvard and MIT
Massachusetts General Hospital
Boston, MA
USA

Michael A. Pacanowski, PharmD, MPH
Department of Pharmacy Practice
Center for Pharmacogenomics
University of Florida
Gainesville, FL
USA

Paul M. Ridker, MD, MPH
Eugene Braunwald Professor of Medicine
Harvard Medical School
Director, Center for Cardiovascular Disease Prevention
Brigham and Women's Hospital

Boston, MA
USA

Marylyn D. Ritchie, PhD
Assistant Professor, Department of Molecular Physiology and Biophysics
Investigator, Center for Human Genetics Research
Vanderbilt University
Nashville, TN
USA

Robert Roberts, MD, FRCPC, FACC
President and CEO
University of Ottawa Heart Institute
Ottawa, Ontario
Canada

Srijita Sen-Chowdhry, MBBS, MD, MRCP
Research Fellow in Cardiology
Inherited Cardiovascular Disease Group
The Heart Hospital
University College London
London
UK

Alan R. Shuldiner, MD
John A. Whitehurst Professor of Medicine
Director, Program in Genetics and Genomic Medicine
Head, Division of Endocrinology, Diabetes and Nutrition
University of Maryland School of Medicine
Baltimore, MD
USA

J. Gustav Smith, MD
Broad Institute of Harvard and MIT
Cambridge, MA
USA
Department of Clinical Sciences
Lund University
Sweden

Alexandre F.R. Stewart, BScH, MSc, PhD
Principal Investigator
The Ruddy Canadian Cardiovascular Genetics Centre
University of Ottawa Heart Institute
Ottawa, Ontario
Canada

Petros Syrris, PhD
Principal Research Fellow
Inherited Cardiovascular Disease Group
Department of Medicine
University College London
London
UK

Jeffrey A. Towbin, MD
Professor and Chief, Pediatric Cardiology
Executive Co-Director of the Heart Institute
Cincinnati Children's Hospital Medical Center
University of Cincinnati College of Medicine
Cincinnati, OH
USA

Jacques Turgeon, PhD
Faculty of Pharmacy
Université de Montréal
Montréal
Québec
Canada

Matteo Vatta, PhD
Department of Pediatrics (Cardiology)
Baylor College of Medicine
Houston, TX
USA

Arthur A.M. Wilde, MD, PhD, FAHA, FESC
Head of Department of Cardiology
Academic Medical Center
Amsterdam
The Netherlands

Issam Zineh, PharmD, MPH
Department of Pharmacy Practice
Division of Cardiovascular Medicine
Colleges of Pharmacy and Medicine
Center for Pharmacogenomics
University of Florida
Gainesville, FL
USA

Preface

Cardiovascular medicine is at a tipping point

The notion that risk for cardiovascular disease includes a genetic component has been ingrained into generations of practitioners. This idea has had two almost Janus-like faces: the rare patient with a seemingly exotic disease such as hypertrophic cardiomyopathy (HCM) or the long QT syndrome represents one "extreme." At the other end of the spectrum are patients with common diseases such as ischemic heart disease or atrial fibrillation. We have been taught that these conditions often include a genetic component, and, indeed if you ask, there is frequently a positive family history.

As interesting as bedside observations such as these might be, it has been very difficult to see how they made a whit of difference to the care of patients until the application of the tools of modern genetics and genomics began to unravel the disease genes and the underlying pathophysiologies. This new knowledge has, in turn, generated new approaches to risk stratification in the asymptomatic patient, management of the symptomatic patient, and development of new therapies. It is not possible for a practitioner, or even a member of the lay public, to be unaware of the tidal wave of new information in cardiovascular genetics and the promise that this information holds for improved prevention and therapy. However, the sheer volume of the information, and the very new tools being used to generate it, now presents a new series of problems to the practitioner, such as understanding new technologies and terminologies, and keeping track of which genetic variants cause disease, predispose to disease, protect from disease, or predispose to variability in drug responses.

The American Heart Association (AHA), recognizing these challenges, commissioned this monograph with the cardiovascular practitioner as the major target audience. The goal is to outline advances in gene discovery, and to describe how finding these genes might inform new approaches to practice and at the same time will certainly raise new and vexing issues with which the practice community is only now beginning to grapple. The first section presents principles, including discussions of varying approaches, statistical issues, and views of how this new knowledge will be incorporated into practice. The second section presents an overview of the current status of genetic and genomic knowledge in common cardiovascular diseases, and includes discussions of how genomic information may affect variability in drug responses. An Appendix provides simple definitions to help the practitioner make better sense of the concepts presented.

The evolution from genetics to genomics

The first major advance in cardiovascular genetics was the identification of disease genes by traditional linkage analysis in large well-phenotyped kindreds. Very rare DNA sequence variants in these genes usually alter the amino acid sequences of the proteins they encode and thereby cause disease. Many of these are discussed in disease-focused chapters in this monograph, and there are also striking conceptual commonalities across these syndromes. First, identification of disease genes for HCM or the long QT syndrome has shown that these entities are not as rare as previously thought. Patients who are asymptomatic or minimally symptomatic can now be identified, and the phenomenon of variable penetrance—differing extents of disease among mutation carriers within a kindred—is well recognized. Indeed, a major challenge in this field is to understand the mechanisms underlying such variable penetrance: environmental factors or coexisting common genetic variants seem reasonable possibilities. A second important lesson has been an emerging understanding of the underlying biology. Thus, for example, the long QT syndrome has been identified as a disease of ion channels; this understanding, in turn, led directly to identification of new genes—not necessarily encoding ion channels—whose function is to modulate ion channel activity and action potential durations. Similarly, hypertrophic cardiomyopathy has been viewed as a "disease of the sarcomere," but other HCM subtypes related to abnormal myocardial energetics are now being identified. The overlap among dilated cardiomyopathies and arrhythmogenic right ventricular dysplasia similarly is informing whole new areas of biology.

Progress in the area of monogenic diseases has also raised new questions. Genetic screening efforts may identify a previously unreported variant, and whether this actually causes disease or is irrelevant to the disease can be difficult to sort out. There seems little doubt that genetic testing has a role to play here and this will expand, especially as therapies individualized not simply to disease entities but to gene-specific or mutation-specific variants of those entities emerge. Nevertheless, the increasing appreciation that we all harbor thousands of possibly irrelevant DNA variants complicates interpretation of genetic testing.

The second great advance in cardiovascular genetics has been the sequencing of the human genome and the emerging understanding that common variation in this sequence can be used to identify genetic regions, and ultimately even single DNA variants, that confer risk for very common diseases such as atherosclerosis or atrial fibrillation. This approach has been extraordinarily productive, with the identification and validation of entirely new genomic regions associated with disease, and therefore representing great new opportunities for disease stratification, rational selection of available therapies, the development of new drugs, and ultimately effective prevention.

Thus, this field is expanding from focusing on single mutations causing rare diseases (genetics) to encompass the idea that common and rare variation across the whole genetic sequence of an individual (or a population) predisposes to variability in susceptibility to disease (genomics). This extends not simply to the development of disease, but to the tempo with which disease develops, the extent of disease, and variability in response to treatments. Much of this thinking centers around interactions among genetic variants, and the way in which our genomes determine how we respond to stressors in our environment: who develops ventricular fibrillation during an acute coronary occlusion or an unusual response during exposure to a drug.

A critical element in moving this field forward has been the active participation of the cardiovascular practice community. This has been important in both identifying and characterizing in detail the phenotypes of probands and family members in kindreds, as well as in defining appropriate phenotypes for analysis in large populations. Thus, paradoxically, the field is emerging into a position where the practitioner is the centerpiece of the phenotyping which must be done to apply genetic information, and yet the practitioner is increasingly detached from the results of the genetic testing. This is especially frustrating since it occurs at a time when new knowledge is rapidly developing, genetic testing is now becoming available for rare and common disease, and individualized therapies hold especially great promise.

A view to the near future

The unraveling of monogenic disease and the advances enabled by the human genome project are but the first steps toward a genome-driven future. Moore's Law tells us that microprocessor power doubles every 18 months. Genome technology is evolving at least as rapidly: extraordinary technology advances will make the 30 minute, $1000 genome—full resequencing of an individual's genome—available by 2010–2012. This data deluge presents astonishing opportunities and challenges. An obvious opportunity is enhanced access to variation in human genomes—faster and earlier diagnosis of potential monogenic disease or variation conferring risk of unusual drug effects. The challenges, however, are enormous: how should millions of variants be interpreted? How can this information be processed and delivered to practitioners and to patients? What are reasonable approaches to the multiple potential ethical issues raised by availability of these data? What economic model might support integration of genetic information into practice? The time has long past when a physician could keep track of his or her own patients' diseases, how these are best treated in populations and in individuals, responses to drugs, and past and family history. Information technology tools are thus a vital component of modern healthcare, and will be absolutely required to exploit advances in genomics.

This monograph represents the commitment of the AHA to practitioner education. I am grateful to the AHA for this commitment, to the authors who devoted their expertise and time to this educational process, and to Wiley-Blackwell for coordinating the editorial process. Major advances in this field are occurring even as this edition is produced. Stay tuned—the future is almost here.

Dan Roden, MD

Foreword

The strategic driving force behind the American Heart Association's mission of reducing disability and death from cardiovascular diseases and stroke is to change practice by providing information and solutions to healthcare professionals. The pillars of this strategy are knowledge discovery, knowledge processing, and knowledge transfer. The books in the AHA Clinical Series, of which *Cardiovascular Genetics and Genomics* is included, focus on high-interest, cutting-edge topics in cardiovascular medicine. This book series is a critical tool that supports the AHA mission of promoting healthy behavior and improved care of patients. Cardiology is a rapidly changing field and practitioners need data to guide their clinical decision-making. The AHA Clinical Series serves this need by providing the latest information on the physiology, diagnosis, and management of a broad spectrum of conditions encountered in daily practice.

Rose Marie Robertson, MD FAHA
Chief Science Officer, American Heart Association

Elliott Antman, MD FAHA
Director, Samuel A. Levine Cardiac Unit,
Brigham and Women's Hospital

PART I

Principles

Chapter 1

Candidate gene and genome-wide association studies

J. Gustav Smith and Christopher Newton-Cheh

Introduction

The recent exciting developments in genomic research have been catalyzed by the generation of a reference sequence of the human genome [1,2] and the identification of millions of sequence variants [3], combinations of which make each human genetically unique. Additionally, correlation patterns among these variants in individuals of diverse continental ancestry have been comprehensively catalogued as part of the International HapMap Project (HapMap, www.hapmap.org) [4,5]. To identify sequence variants in humans that influence disease susceptibility, two general methods have historically been employed by genetic researchers: linkage and association analysis.

Linkage analysis tests for the joint transmission of chromosomal segments and disease within families. Linkage is the method of choice to identify rare variants with a large impact on disease risk that aggregate in families. The diseases caused by such variants show obvious inheritance patterns and are typically called Mendelian diseases, after Gregor Mendel who described the general patterns of inheritance [6]. Mendelian diseases in cardiovascular medicine include the congenital long QT syndrome, hypertrophic cardiomyopathy, and familial hypercholesterolemia.

Association analysis, on the other hand, which simply tests for differences in allele frequencies of variants between cases and controls, is the method of choice to identify functional variants that are common in the general population, termed polymorphisms. These polymorphisms typically have a modest impact on risk for common diseases, such as myocardial infarction, type 2

Cardiovascular Genetics and Genomics. Edited by Dan Roden. © 2009 American Heart Association, ISBN: 978-14051-7540-1.

diabetes, and hypertension. These diseases are called complex diseases because they arise from multiple genetic and environmental causes and, although often aggregating in families, do not show distinct inheritance patterns. Historically, association studies have been able to examine polymorphisms in only those candidate genes known or proposed to play a role in the pathophysiology of disease. More recently, it has become possible to examine large numbers of polymorphisms, in the order of 100 000–1 000 000, throughout the genome using highly parallel genotyping arrays [7]. These genome-wide association (GWA) analyses systematically examine variation throughout the human genome regardless of putative biologic function. Owing to the fact that common polymorphisms are correlated, a smaller number of polymorphisms can be chosen to serve as proxies for the majority of common sequence variations. The GWA study is hypothesis generating in the sense that it can identify polymorphisms near genes without a recognized pathophysiological link to disease. The method has recently been successfully used to identify common variants in previously unsuspected genes associated with diseases including myocardial infarction [8–10], type 2 diabetes [11–14], and atrial fibrillation [15], as well as medication side-effects such as statin-induced myopathy [16] and excessive anticoagulation from warfarin [17].

DNA sequence variants and linkage disequilibrium

Variation in the genetic sequence between any two individuals constitutes approximately 0.1% of the genome and can take different forms, including substitutions, deletions, insertions, duplications, or inversions. Regional and global [18,19] resequencing studies have found smaller sequence variants to be the most common, with single-base substitutions, also termed single nucleotide polymorphisms (SNPs), predominating. Large-scale SNP discovery projects have identified more than 10 million SNPs in human populations, available in such online catalogs as dbSNP (www.ncbi.nlm.nih.gov/projects/SNP) [3–5,20]. Although individually less frequent in the genome, other sequence variants called copy number polymorphisms (CNPs) account for a larger proportion of the total number of bases that differ between individuals. Typically, these variants stretch over just a few nucleotides, but may be long enough that whole genes may be duplicated or absent on a given chromosome. Hundreds of CNPs have recently been identified in large-scale discovery projects [21], and a number of CNPs have been linked to common diseases [22].

Common variants are highly correlated in blocks across stretches of DNA spanning tens of kilobases, a phenomenon termed linkage disequilibrium (LD) [23]. This extensive correlation among neighboring variants results from the few generations since the last common human ancestor relative to the rates of mutation and recombination [24,4] and the restriction of the majority of recombination events to focal hotspots [4,25,26]. In European- and Asian-derived populations these blocks are typically longer than in African-derived populations, in which genetic diversity is somewhat higher owing to the relatively small number of Africans who founded the modern European and Asian populations approximately 50 000 years ago.

Genetic architecture of human traits

Rare Mendelian diseases segregating in families with obvious inheritance patterns have been found to result from rare mutations of strong effect (odds ratios of 100–1000). Variants with such strong effect on disease susceptibility remain rare because of negative selection [27]. Some variants of strong effect may be more common in certain populations owing to founder effects or positive selection in certain environments, as exemplified by sickle cell anemia, caused by variants in the beta-globin gene present at high frequency in regions where malaria is endemic as it confers resistance against malaria [28]. More than 2000 Mendelian diseases have been found to result from rare mutations of strong effect, with population frequencies typically well below 1%. However, the contribution of rare variants to complex human diseases and traits is unknown. These traits have been postulated to result from interactions between multiple genetic variants, both common and rare, and environmental factors, and because of late onset have typically escaped negative selection [27].

In steadily increasing numbers, some genes have been found to harbor both common and rare variants that are associated with human diseases and traits, many of which are described throughout this monograph. For example, rare variants in the low-density lipoprotein (LDL) receptor gene that cause Mendelian familial hypercholesterolemia with very high plasma concentrations of LDL, leading to accelerated atherosclerosis and myocardial infarction if untreated [29]. Common variants in the same gene have also been found in association studies to incrementally increase LDL cholesterol and risk of myocardial infarction in the general population [30]. The effects of common variants are typically smaller, with odds ratios ,2, but can translate into much higher population-attributable risks than mutations underlying Mendelian diseases, owing to the comparatively high population frequency of polymorphisms. The relative contributions of common and rare variants to susceptibility to disease in the general population will become clear only as tests sufficiently sensitive to detect both classes of variants are completed in well-powered samples.

Additionally, the contribution of somatic mutations to common traits is only beginning to be clarified. Some studies have suggested that somatic (as opposed to germline) mutations may play a role in common diseases other than their well-recognized contribution to cancer development. In one such study by Gollob *et al.* [31], the gap junction gene connexin 40 (*GJA5*) was sequenced from cardiomyocytes of patients with atrial fibrillation and compared with DNA from lymphocytes, identifying an apparent excess of somatic mutations and suggesting a potential role in the development of an arrhythmogenic substrate.

Both common and rare germline or somatic variations can affect gene products either in a structural manner, when occurring in sequences encoding amino acids or splice sites and leading to changes in the protein sequence, or in a regulatory manner, when occurring in regulatory regions leading to changes in protein expression. Classic studies showing almost identical protein sequences in primates suggested a central role for regulatory rather than structural variants in species differentiation [32]. Early studies of individual human genomes indicate that regulatory variants are also responsible for the majority of within-species sequence differences [33], whereas variants affecting protein sequences are more rare but more often found in Mendelian disease. Sequencing of additional individual human genomes will increase our understanding of the contribution of regulatory variants, including the relative roles of *cis*-regulatory (located near a gene) and *trans*-regulatory (remote from a gene) sequence variation.

Principles of genetic association studies

Association methods are quite simple in principle: they are used to examine whether a specific version, allele, of a polymorphism is overrepresented in cases compared with controls beyond differences expected by chance. Association studies examine either differences in the frequency of an allele [e.g., copies of adenine (A) or guanine (G) bases for an A/G SNP] or the frequency of a genotype (e.g., AA, AG, or GG). For example, in dichotomous traits (e.g., myocardial infarction or sudden cardiac death) a set of cases and controls are genotyped to determine which alleles each individual has. The null hypothesis of no difference in allele frequency between cases and controls is then examined. An allele overrepresented in cases is considered a risk allele; if underrepresented it is a protective allele.

When linkage analyses were unable to identify polymorphisms underlying complex diseases association studies were suggested to be more powerful [34]. Recognition of the commonality of SNPs and the extensive LD in the human genome sparked the idea of genotyping a number of well-chosen SNPs to scan the genome for disease loci by acting as proxies for most SNPs, whether genotyped or not. To this end, a large-scale SNP discovery project followed the generation of a reference sequence of the human genome, resulting in a map of 1.42 million SNPs [3]. Additional SNPs were then identified through the HapMap project [4,5] and other efforts [20]. The HapMap project defined the frequencies of SNPs and the linkage disequilibrium patterns among them in population samples of European, East Asian, and West African ancestry. These correlation patterns then serve as a reference catalogue for association studies that systematically examine regional (e.g., focused on a candidate gene) or global (genome-wide) genetic variation.

Although correlation among neighboring variants is exploited to detect functional genetic elements without directly genotyping them, once association has been found, great effort is required to identify the causal polymorphism at a locus. Then the hard work of defining the biological action of functional genetic variation in the pathogenesis of disease can begin!

Candidate gene association studies

Historically, limitations in genotyping throughput and cost have restricted association studies to the examination of only a few variants in a narrow genetic region typically focused on a specific gene, termed candidate gene (CG) studies. For example, one of the most extensively studied genetic polymorphisms in cardiovascular disease involves a common 287 base pair sequence in the gene coding for angiotensin I-converting enzyme (ACE) which is either present or absent (insertion or deletion, termed "indel") and determines about 50% of interindividual variability of plasma ACE levels [35]. The *ACE* gene is clearly a strong biological candidate given its well-known role in the activation of vasoactive hormones and the important clinical role of ACE inhibitors in the treatment of hypertension and heart failure. The *ACE* polymorphism has been examined for association with many diseases including myocardial infarction, ventricular hypertrophy, stroke, and hypertension, as well as diabetic nephropathy and Alzheimer's disease. This insertion/deletion polymorphism illustrates several properties of candidate gene association studies.

First, although examined for association with multiple diseases, only findings with diabetic nephropathy and Alzheimer's disease can be considered relatively conclusive with inconsistent findings for other diseases [36], a problem that is well known to have plagued candidate gene association studies [37]. The study of the genetic basis of complex traits was set back by the failure of association findings reported in the 1990s and early 2000s to be replicated, which arose from use of inappropriately permissive *P*-value thresholds and small sample sizes in replication samples [38].

Second, although the association of the *ACE* insertion/deletion polymorphism with changes in circulating ACE concentration is well established, the basic mechanism linking the polymorphism to changes in gene expression is uncertain. Unlike the situation for DNA sequence that encodes amino acid sequence, we have a limited understanding of the determinants of gene expression [39]. The *ACE* indel may be in LD with the underlying causal variant or prove to be causal by an as yet unknown mechanism. Several other polymorphisms have also been identified in the *ACE* gene and examined for association with different diseases, most of them strongly correlated with the insertion/deletion. Long-range LD thus represents both an advantage—association of ungenotyped causal variants is detectable indirectly through genotyping of correlated variants—and a disadvantage—correlation among neighboring variants makes identification of the specific functional variant difficult because of the number of proxies to sort through.

More recently, taking advantage of the catalogue of SNPs and LD patterns in HapMap, candidate gene association studies have moved from the examination of a few variants to systematic studies of all common variations across a gene locus. By genotyping "tagging SNPs" chosen to represent (tag) polymorphisms to which they are correlated, costs are reduced without loss of coverage [40]. Ultimately, discovery of the full spectrum of sequence variants, including variants with minor allele frequency $<5\%$ at a locus, requires resequencing of the gene.

Genome-wide association studies

A genome-wide association study examines the large fraction of common variation throughout the human genome. First proposed in 1996 following the failure of linkage analysis to identify genetic determinants of common diseases, association methods are more powerful to detect the modest effect sizes of common variants which represent a blindspot for linkage approaches [34]. Genome-wide association methods have only recently been made possible by technical and analytic advances as described above.

In a genome-wide association study, between 100 000 and 1 000 000 SNPs are genotyped. Owing to linkage disequilibrium, or correlation among neighboring variants, genome-wide scans have been shown to represent well the 3.1 million SNPs examined in HapMap [41,42]. The SNPs in HapMap in turn capture the majority of common variations in the human genome, as shown by comparison with deep resequencing of randomly chosen genomic regions as part of the ENCODE project [4,5]. Genotyping of larger numbers of variants than those on fixed arrays is likely to result in only a marginal gain in genomic coverage, with the possible exception of populations of African ancestry, in whom linkage disequilibrium extends for shorter distances and the diversity of genetic variants is slightly higher.

In the field of cardiovascular disease and physiology, one of the earliest successes of genome-wide association studies was the finding that common variants at the 59 end of the gene encoding the neuronal nitric oxide synthase adaptor protein (NOS1AP) affect myocardial repolarization as manifest in the electrocardiographic QT interval [43–46]. This gene had not previously been recognized to contribute to myocardial repolarization nor to any process of cardiac physiology. A subsequent study of expression and protein–protein interactions in guinea pig cardiomyocytes has found that NOS1AP interacts with neuronal nitric oxide synthase (NOS1) to accelerate repolarization by inhibition of the L-type calcium channel [47]. The precise causal variant in humans is unknown, but it is clear from early analyses that coding variation does not explain the signal of association, in agreement with findings from other GWA studies suggesting a central role for regulatory variants in complex disease. This highlights the fact that, historically, human genetics has been limited to the identification of recognizable coding mutations within families segregating Mendelian diseases and has been unable to explain the genetic basis of most complex diseases. Other examples of cardiovascular traits and diseases in which previously unsuspected genetic loci have been discovered through GWA studies include blood lipids [30,48], myocardial infarction [8–10], and atrial fibrillation [15]. For the loci on chromosomes 9p and 4q showing strong association with myocardial infarction and atrial fibrillation, respectively, associated SNPs are not only uncorrelated with any known coding variants but also distant from any known gene. These findings could be explained by unrecognized protein coding or regulatory sequence in the region, trans-regulatory regions about which very little is known or long-range LD. The effort to identify causal variants and mechanisms underlying signals of association identified in GWA studies will provide important clues for an improved understanding of genomic structure and function.

GWA studies have identified large numbers of reproducible associations. Additional work will be required to translate these discoveries to clinical utility at the population level as the effect sizes of individual variants are small. Predictive models will need to incorporate multiple genetic variants and, potentially, interactions among variants and environmental factors, a strategy which has shown some promise for cardiovascular disease [49], diabetes [50,51], and age-related macular degeneration [52,53] and which holds some promise for guiding safe treatment with potentially toxic therapies such as warfarin [54].

Utility of candidate gene and genome-wide approaches

Even with the development of global GWA approaches, candidate gene efforts remain an integral tool in the genetics of common traits. GWA studies may be viewed as hypothesis-generating screening tools, whereas candidate gene association studies are useful for more focused examination of genes recognized to have a role in human physiology whether through prior basic investigation or discoveries from GWA approaches.

One disadvantage of genome-wide studies is the higher costs of genotyping (Table 1.1). However, if one considers the costs on a per SNP basis of low-throughput genotyping platforms that can determine 1–50 SNPs per array, genome-wide arrays can produce a genotype for 100- to 1000-fold lower cost. Another disadvantage of GWA studies is the loss of power from the strict significance thresholds required to filter out spurious associations resulting from the large numbers of tests performed. The solution is to maximize the sample size to ensure adequate power to achieve *P*-value thresholds as low as 5×10^{-8}, or similar thresholds proposed in the literature. The 5×10^{-8} threshold has been proposed based on Bonferroni adjustment for the effective 1 000 000 independent tests in the human genome of European and Asian ancestry individuals [4,55]; African ancestry DNA sequence includes a larger number of independent tests owing to its greater diversity as described above. Although the appropriate *P*-value threshold for candidate gene studies remains undetermined and somewhat difficult to estimate, some threshold considering the number of tests performed and the prior probability of any candidate gene to harbor associated variants is required to avoid the false-positive results that hampered the field of complex trait genetics in the late 1990s and early 2000s [56,57]. See further comparisons of global and regional approaches in Table 1.1.

Table 1.1 Comparison of candidate gene versus genome-wide association approaches

	Candidate gene study	**Genome-wide study**
Design	A small number of SNPs across a candidate gene	100 000–1 000 000 SNPs throughout the genome
Sample size	Large	Very large
Cost	Inexpensive per array, but expensive on a per SNP basis	More expensive per array; much less expensive on a per SNP basis
Multiple testing burden	Lower; variants have higher prior probability of association	High; large sample sizes needed to achieve stringent thresholds
False-positive risk	Relatively low owing to low number of tests	Higher; requires careful quality control to avoid technical artifacts and stringent *P*-value thresholds
Detection of/ adjustment for stratification	No; limited number of SNPs and not spread across genome	Yes; very easily handled
Discovers novel loci	No; restricted to known genes	Yes; unbiased by current knowledge
Resequencing	Fully characterize all variation across a gene, identify functional variants	Not feasible on genome-wide scale; methods are evolving

SNP, single nucleotide polymorphism.

Sampling designs

Association studies can be performed in case–control, cohort, and family-based study samples using different analytic methods. A case–control study ascertains cases (e.g., myocardial infarction) after they have occurred and matches on relevant characteristics that might otherwise confound a study. A cohort study prospectively enrolls subjects irrespective of clinical characteristics and examines the distribution of characteristics at a single time point (cross-sectional) or follows for future development of incident cases (longitudinal). Family-based studies can enroll pedigrees (multiple generations) or siblings and can ascertain on an individual case (probands) or sample from the general population.

A case–control or family-based case ascertainment may be better suited for diseases with relatively low population frequency as the number of cases in cohort studies may be insufficient for adequate power to detect the modest effect sizes typically seen in common variants [58]. Even in case–control and family-based designs, however, there are often difficulties in achieving the sample sizes necessary for GWA studies, which typically exceed 1000 cases and 1000 controls as this sample size detects only the few strong variants. This problem is most often solved by investigators forming multicenter consortia. Recently, GWA studies have been performed in several large cohort studies available, including the Framingham Heart Study [59] and Women's Health Study [60], and have primarily focused on quantitative traits (present in every participant) rather than case status (only a minority of individuals for most diseases). The pooling of several studies offers distinct advantages of the cohort design for the possibility to examine, in adequately powered samples, the population predictive value of genetic variants and gene–environment and gene–gene interactions [58]. See further comparisons of different sampling approaches in Table 1.2.

Challenges in association studies

Before the era of GWA studies, only a handful of the thousands of genetic polymorphisms examined in candidate genes showed consistent replication [37,38,61]. As mentioned, this has been attributed to poor study design including small sample sizes, inadequate genotype quality control, population stratification, and permissive thresholds for declaring statistical significance. To address these problems, a working group assembled by the American National Cancer Institute and the National Human Genome Research Institute suggested a set of standards culled from the literature for the performance of genetic association studies targeted to maximizing discovery and minimizing false-positive associations [62]. Through

Table 1.2 Comparison of sampling approaches in association studies

	Case–control	Cohort	Family based
Design	Individuals with disease are matched with individuals without disease from the same population	Individuals are randomly drawn from a population and traits ascertained cross-sectionally or prospectively	An individual with disease (proband) and family members are collected
Cost	Lower	Expensive, especially with longitudinal follow-up, but many traits collected	Lower cost for rare disease; relatively higher for common disease
Time frame	Short	Short, or long if longitudinal	Short
Number of traits that can be examined	Limited to ascertainment and collected clinical characteristics	Typically many	Few
Population stratification susceptibility	High	Intermediate	Low
Technical artifact susceptibility	Higher	Low	Intermediate

the application of these and other careful measures of quality control, GWA studies are currently finding reproducible genetic variant associations with complex traits and have largely avoided the flood of nonreplicable findings that was seen both in candidate gene-based association studies [37] and when genome-wide linkage analysis was first applied to complex diseases [63]. It should be noted that many of the reproducible associations have come at loci containing very strong candidate genes (e.g., identified using linkage and cloning in Mendelian families), thus arguing that methodological problems were the major contributor to poor reproducibility of association studies in the 1990s. Current genetic association studies, whether focused on candidate genes or all genes, benefit from the large samples used, careful study design and quality control, stringent thresholds for statistical significance, and use of independent samples for validation and replication [64].

Genetic epidemiology offers a distinct advantage over nongenetic epidemiology in that a genetic association has an unambiguous causal relationship to an outcome because genetic variation of necessity precedes the development of disease. The association between a clinical factor such as C-reactive protein and coronary heart disease, for example, requires great effort to tease apart the directionality of the association and determine the causal sequence. Aside from technical artifacts, the only potential confounder in a genetic association study is population stratification—differences in ancestry between cases and controls leading to false-positive association of any genetic variants with frequencies that differ by ancestry [65–67]. Population stratification can be efficiently overcome using genome-wide SNP data from which ancestry can be inferred, subgroups with different ancestry identified, and such stratification corrected for using one of several approaches [68–71]. In candidate gene studies, the number of SNPs genotyped is typically too small to infer ancestry. Sampling based on self-reported ancestry is critically important to such studies but does not remove the possibility of stratification, which, for example, has been demonstrated in studies within self-identified Europeans [66]. Optimally, a panel of ancestry-informative markers should be genotyped in all genetic association studies, but the panels developed so far contain more SNPs than most candidate gene studies test [72,73].

Technical artifacts have also been shown to cause false-positive associations [65]. This issue pertains particularly to GWA studies in which large numbers of variants are genotyped and uncommon but extreme chance differences in frequencies between cases and controls are more likely to occur. In particular, technical artifacts may induce spurious associations when cases and controls undergo separate ascertainment, DNA processing, and finally genotyping. In such circumstances, differences in genotyping success (generally biased toward undercalling of heterozygotes) between cases and controls may lead to apparent frequency differences and result in artifactually inflated test statistics (lower P-values). These technical artifacts are best avoided by uniform ascertainment, sample handling and genotyping with cases and controls intermixed in the laboratory process and on plates, and lastly by using careful quality control of genotypes. Use of convenience controls that have undergone different ascertainment, sample processing, or genotyping than cases will generally require more stringent quality control thresholds (more SNPs thrown out) than a study in which these parameters are uniform between cases and controls [74].

Another critical issue in GWA approaches is the problem that arises from the simultaneous testing of association of hundreds of thousands of genetic variants [34]. With the traditional significance threshold of $P = 0.05$ one polymorphism would be expected to show a falsely "significant" association for each 20 SNPs examined. In a genome-wide dataset of 500 000 SNPs the corresponding number would be 25 000 falsely positive SNPs. The problem lies in differentiating this random "noise" from true genetic associations. The solution is to apply much more stringent *P*-value thresholds to association results to filter out the false-positive association. As described above, one threshold applied in several recent studies is the adjustment of the 0.05 threshold for the estimated 1 million effectively independent tests in the genome of European or Asian populations [4,55] using Bonferroni correction, resulting in a significance threshold of 5×10^{-8}. However, to reach these levels of significance very large sample sizes are necessary. Alternative approaches have also been suggested and sporadically utilized [56,75]. Ultimately, differentiation of true from false association signals comes from replication in independent samples.

In summary, most problems with association study designs are generic to whether a regional or global approach is used. The major problems are population stratification, technical artifacts, and multiple testing, which can all be handled with recently developed methods.

Outlook for the future

With the recent wave of discoveries from genome-wide association studies, we have come one step closer to an understanding of the genetic architecture of common diseases and traits, as acknowledged by *Science* as the Breakthrough of the Year 2007 [76]. These studies have confirmed the role of common variants, both SNPs and CNPs assayed on the latest microarrays, in complex diseases and traits. However, the current catalogue of common genomic sequence variants is not complete. In order to be complete, systematic resequencing of large numbers of individuals will have to be performed. To this end, the recently announced sequencing of the full genome from 1000 individuals, the 1000 Genomes Project, will contribute greatly (www.1000genomes.org). Additionally, this project is likely to make whole-genome resequencing more feasible as an approach to identify rare variants associated with common diseases and traits. Until then, the search for rare variants as well as somatic mutations will be restricted to resequencing of candidate genes.

The potential to elucidate the precise genetic architecture of common diseases and traits offers four primary opportunities for the medical sciences: (1) identification of novel markers of disease risk at the population level, (2) identification of novel genes and pathways involved in human pathophysiology, (3) inference of causality to epidemiological observations, and (4) the identification of drug targets for which the in vivo relevance in humans has already been demonstrated. As discussed above, GWA studies have led to identification of several novel pathways in disease pathophysiology and established a causal role for biomarkers which has not been possible with nongenetic epidemiological associations, but the initial incentive for genetic association studies was the prospect of identifying novel risk markers for utilization in prediction of common diseases. However, the polymorphisms that have so far shown significant and replicable association all show at best modest risk estimates with odds ratios of the order of 1.1–1.3, with few exceptions such as polymorphisms near the complement factor H gene for age-dependent macular degeneration [77], FTO for obesity [78], and TCF7L2 for type 2 diabetes [79] with odds ratios in the range of 1.3–1.5. Still, the values of predictive and prognostic models incorporating multiple polymorphisms remain to be examined, with early attempts showing promising results [49–53]. An additional gain in predictive power may come from models incorporating interactions among polymorphisms (epistasis) or between polymorphisms and environmental factors, but to date few such interactions have been demonstrated [80]. Studies testing the population-level relevance of genetic variants in aggregate are still in their earliest stages. Hopefully, with the identification of additional risk variants and creation of models incorporating multiple variants and environmental and clinical risk factors, predictive models can be moved further to clinical trials, some of which are already under way (e.g., warfarin dosing [54]). Finally, sequence variants with known function may inform rational drug therapy design in the same manner that identification of rare variants in the LDL receptor as the cause of familial hyperlipidemia ultimately led to the development of statins [29]. Clearly, the genomic era holds great promise for cardiovascular medicine and genetic association studies represent an important tool for the near term in much the same manner as Mendelian disease gene mapping with linkage was in the 1990s.

References

1 Lander ES, Linton LM, Birren B *et al.* Initial sequencing and analysis of the human genome. *Nature* 2001; **409**: 860–921.
2 Venter JC, Adams MD, Myers EW *et al.* The sequence of the human genome. *Science* 2001; **291**: 1304–51.
3 Sachidanandam R, Weissman D, Schmidt SC *et al.* A map of human genome sequence variation containing 1.42 million single nucleotide polymorphisms. *Nature* 2001; **409**: 928–933.
4 Altshuler D, Brooks LD, Chakravarti A *et al.* A haplotype map of the human genome. *Nature* 2005; **437**: 1299–1320.
5 Frazer KA, Ballinger DG, Cox DR *et al.* A second generation human haplotype map of over 3.1 million SNPs. *Nature* 2007; **449**: 851–861.
6 Mendel G. Experiments in plant hybridization. *Journal of the Brno Natural History Society* 1866; **4**: 3–47.
7 Gresham D, Dunham MJ, Botstein D. Comparing whole genomes using DNA microarrays. *Nature Reviews* 2008; **9**: 291–302.
8 Samani NJ, Erdmann J, Hall AS *et al.* Genomewide association analysis of coronary artery disease. *New England Journal of Medicine* 2007; **357**: 443–453.
9 McPherson R, Pertsemlidis A, Kavaslar N *et al.* A common allele on chromosome 9 associated with coronary heart disease. *Science* 2007; **316**: 1488–1491.
10 Helgadottir A, Thorleifsson G, Manolescu A *et al.* A common variant on chromosome 9p21 affects the risk of myocardial infarction. *Science* 2007; **316**: 1491–1493.

11 Saxena R, Voight BF, Lyssenko V *et al.* Genome-wide association analysis identifies loci for type 2 diabetes and triglyceride levels. *Science* 2007; 3b16: 1331–1336.
12 Scott LJ, Mohlke KL, Bonnycastle LL *et al.* A genome-wide association study of type 2 diabetes in Finns detects multiple susceptibility variants. *Science* 2007; **316**: 1341–1345.
13 Zeggini E, Weedon MN, Lindgren CM *et al.* Replication of genome-wide association signals in UK samples reveals risk loci for type 2 diabetes. *Science* 2007; **316**: 1336–1341.
14 Sladek R, Rocheleau G, Rung J *et al.* A genome-wide association study identifies novel risk loci for type 2 diabetes. *Nature* 2007; **445**: 881–885.
15 Gudbjartsson DF, Arnar DO, Helgadottir A *et al.* Variants conferring risk of atrial fibrillation on chromosome 4q25. *Nature* 2007; **448**: 353–7.
16 Link E, Parish S, Armitage J *et al.* SLCO1B1 variants and statin-induced myopathy: a genomewide study. *New England Journal of Medicine* 2008; **359**: 789–799.
17 Schwarz UI, Ritchie MD, Bradford Y *et al.* Genetic determinants of response to warfarin during initial anticoagulation. *New England Journal of Medicine* 2008; **358**: 999–1008.
18 Levy S, Sutton G, Ng PC *et al.* The diploid genome sequence of an individual human. *PLoS Biology* 2007; **5**: e254.
19 Wheeler DA, Srinivasan M, Egholm M *et al.* The complete genome of an individual by massively parallel DNA sequencing. *Nature* 2008; **452**: 872–876.
20 Hinds DA, Stuve LL, Nilsen GB *et al.* Whole-genome patterns of common DNA variation in three human populations. *Science* 2005; **307**: 1072–1079.
21 Kidd JM, Cooper GM, Donahue WF *et al.* Mapping and sequencing of structural variation from eight human genomes. *Nature* 2008; **453**: 56–64.
22 McCarroll SA, Altshuler DM. *Nature Genetics* 2008; **39**: S37–S42.
23 Slatkin M. Linkage disequilibrium: understanding the evolutionary past and mapping the medical future. *Nature Reviews* 2008; **9**: 477–485.
24 Reich DE, Cargill M, Bolk S *et al.* Linkage disequilibrium in the human genome. *Nature* 2001; **411**: 199–204.
25 McVean GA, Myers SR, Hunt S *et al.* The fine-scale structure of recombination rate variation in the human genome. *Science* 2004; **304**: 581–584.
26 Reich DE, Schaffner SF, Daly MJ *et al.* Human genome sequence variation and the influence of gene history, mutation and recombination. *Nature Genetics* 2002; **32**: 135–142.
27 Reich DE, Lander ES. On the allelic spectrum of human disease. *Trends in Genetics* 2001; **17**: 502–510.
28 Friedman MJ, Trager W. The biochemistry of resistance to malaria. *Scientific American* 1981; **244**: 154–155, 8–64.
29 Goldstein JL, Brown MS. Familial hypercholesterolemia: identification of a defect in the regulation of 3-hydroxy-3-methylglutaryl coenzyme A reductase activity associated with overproduction of cholesterol. *Proceedings of the National Academy of Sciences of the USA* 1973; **70**: 2804–2808.
30 Willer CJ, Sanna S, Jackson AU *et al.* Newly identified loci that influence lipid concentrations and risk of coronary artery disease. *Nature Genetics* 2008; **40**: 161–169.
31 Gollob MH, Jones DL, Krahn AD *et al.* Somatic mutations in the connexin 40 gene (GJA5) in atrial fibrillation. *New England Journal of Medicine* 2006; **354**: 2677–2688.

32 King MC, Wilson AC. Evolution at two levels in humans and chimpanzees. *Science* 1975; **188**: 107–116.
33 Ng PC, Levy S, Huang J *et al*. Genetic variation in an individual human exome. *PLoS Genetics* 2008; **4**: e1000160.
34 Risch N, Merikangas K. The future of genetic studies of complex human diseases. *Science* 1996; **273**: 1516–1517.
35 Rigat B, Hubert C, Alhenc-Gelas F *et al*. An insertion/deletion polymorphism in the angiotensin I-converting enzyme gene accounting for half the variance of serum enzyme levels. *The Journal of Clinical Investigation* 1990; **86**: 1343–1346.
36 Sayed-Tabatabaei FA, Oostra BA, Isaacs A *et al*. ACE polymorphisms. *Circulation Research* 2006; **98**: 1123–1133.
37 Hirschhorn JN, Lohmueller K, Byrne E, Hirschhorn K. A comprehensive review of genetic association studies. *Genetics in Medicine* 2002; **4**: 45–61.
38 Lohmueller KE, Pearce CL, Pike M *et al*. Meta-analysis of genetic association studies supports a contribution of common variants to susceptibility to common disease. *Nature Genetics* 2003; **33**: 177–182.
39 Birney E, Stamatoyannopoulos JA, Dutta A *et al*. Identification and analysis of functional elements in 1% of the human genome by the ENCODE pilot project. *Nature* 2007; **447**: 799–816.
40 de Bakker PI, Yelensky R, Pe'er I *et al*. Efficiency and power in genetic association studies. *Nature Genetics* 2005; **37**: 1217–1223.
41 Pe'er I, de Bakker PI, Maller J, Yelensky R, Altshuler D, Daly MJ. Evaluating and improving power in whole-genome association studies using fixed marker sets. *Nature Genetics* 2006; **38**: 663–7.
42 Barrett JC, Cardon LR. Evaluating coverage of genome-wide association studies. *Nature Genetics* 2006; **38**: 659–662.
43 Post W, Shen H, Damcott C *et al*. Associations between genetic variants in the NOS1AP (CAPON) gene and cardiac repolarization in the old order Amish. *Human Heredity* 2007; **64**: 214–219.
44 Aarnoudse AJ, Newton-Cheh C, de Bakker PI *et al*. Common NOS1AP variants are associated with a prolonged QTc interval in the Rotterdam Study. Circulation. 2007; **116**: 10–6.
45 Lehtinen AB, Newton-Cheh C, Ziegler JT *et al*. Association of NOS1AP genetic variants with QT interval duration in families from the Diabetes Heart Study. *Diabetes* 2008; **57**: 1108–14.
46 Arking DE, Pfeufer A, Post W *et al*. A common genetic variant in the NOS1 regulator NOS1AP modulates cardiac repolarization. *Nature Genetics* 2006; **38**: 644–651.
47 Chang KC, Barth AS, Sasano T *et al*. CAPON modulates cardiac repolarization via neuronal nitric oxide synthase signaling in the heart. *Proceedings of the National Academy of Sciences of the USA* 2008; **105**: 4477–4482.
48 Kathiresan S, Melander O, Guiducci C *et al*. Six new loci associated with blood low-density lipoprotein cholesterol, high-density lipoprotein cholesterol or triglycerides in humans. *Nature Genetics* 2008; **40**: 189–197.
49 Kathiresan S, Melander O, Anevski D *et al*. Polymorphisms associated with cholesterol and risk of cardiovascular events. *New England Journal of Medicine* 2008; **358**: 1240–1249.

50 Lango H, Palmer CN, Morris AD *et al.* Assessing the combined impact of 18 common genetic variants of modest effect sizes on type 2 diabetes risk. *Diabetes* 2008; **57**: 3129–35.
51 Cauchi S, Meyre D, Durand E *et al.* Post genome-wide association studies of novel genes associated with type 2 diabetes show gene–gene interaction and high predictive value. *PLoS ONE* 2008; **3**: e2031.
52 Despriet DD, Klaver CC, Witteman JC *et al.* Complement factor H polymorphism, complement activators, and risk of age-related macular degeneration. *JAMA: The Journal of the American Medical Association* 2006; **296**: 301–309.
53 Maller J, George S, Purcell S *et al.* Common variation in three genes, including a noncoding variant in CFH, strongly influences risk of age-related macular degeneration. *Nature Genetics* 2006; **38**: 1055–1059.
54 Anderson JL, Horne BD, Stevens SM *et al.* Randomized trial of genotype-guided versus standard warfarin dosing in patients initiating oral anticoagulation. *Circulation* 2007; **116**: 2563–2570.
55 Pe'er I, Yelensky R, Altshuler D, Daly MJ. Estimation of the multiple testing burden for genomewide association studies of nearly all common variants. *Genet Epidemiol* 2008; **32**: 381–5.
56 Wacholder S, Chanock S, Garcia-Closas M *et al.* Assessing the probability that a positive report is false: an approach for molecular epidemiology studies. *Journal of the National Cancer Institute* 2004; **96**: 434–442.
57 Newton-Cheh C, Hirschhorn JN. Genetic association studies of complex traits: design and analysis issues. *Mutation Research* 2005; **573**: 54–69.
58 Manolio TA, Bailey-Wilson JE, Collins FS. Genes, environment and the value of prospective cohort studies. *Nature Reviews* 2006; **7**: 812–820.
59 Cupples LA, Arruda HT, Benjamin EJ *et al.* The Framingham Heart Study 100K SNP genome-wide association study resource: overview of 17 phenotype working group reports. *BMC Medical Genetics* 2007; **8** Suppl 1: S1.
60 Ridker PM, Chasman DI, Zee RY *et al.* Rationale, design, and methodology of the Women's Genome Health Study: a genome-wide association study of more than 25,000 initially healthy American women. *Clinical Chemistry* 2008; **54**: 249–255.
61 Ioannidis JP, Ntzani EE, Trikalinos TA, Contopoulos-Ioannidis DG. Replication validity of genetic association studies. *Nature Genetics* 2001; **29**: 306–309.
62 Chanock SJ, Manolio T, Boehnke M *et al.* Replicating genotype–phenotype associations. *Nature* 2007; **447**: 655–660.
63 Altmuller J, Palmer LJ, Fischer G *et al.* Genomewide scans of complex human diseases: true linkage is hard to find. *American Journal of Human Genetics* 2001; **69**: 936–950.
64 Altshuler D, Daly M. Guilt beyond a reasonable doubt. *Nature Genetics* 2007; **39**: 813–815.
65 Clayton DG, Walker NM, Smyth DJ *et al.* Population structure, differential bias and genomic control in a large-scale, case–control association study. *Nature Genetics* 2005; **37**: 1243–1246.
66 Campbell CD, Ogburn EL, Lunetta KL *et al.* Demonstrating stratification in a European American population. *Nature Genetics* 2005; **37**: 868–872.
67 Freedman ML, Reich D, Penney KL *et al.* Assessing the impact of population stratification on genetic association studies. *Nature Genetics* 2004; **36**: 388–393.

68 Devlin B, Roeder K. Genomic control for association studies. *Biometrics* 1999; **55**: 997–1004.
69 Pritchard JK, Stephens M, Rosenberg NA, Donnelly P. Association mapping in structured populations. *American Journal of Human Genetics* 2000; **67**: 170–181.
70 Price AL, Patterson NJ, Plenge RM *et al.* Principal components analysis corrects for stratification in genome-wide association studies. *Nature Genetics* 2006; **38**: 904–909.
71 Purcell S, Neale B, Todd-Brown K *et al.* PLINK: a tool set for whole-genome association and population-based linkage analyses. *American Journal of Human Genetics* 2007; **81**: 559–575.
72 Price AL, Butler J, Patterson N *et al.* Discerning the ancestry of European Americans in genetic association studies. *PLoS Genetics* 2008; **4**: e236.
73 Tian C, Plenge RM, Ransom M *et al.* Analysis and application of European genetic substructure using 300 K SNP information. *PLoS Genetics* 2008; **4**: e4.
74 Wellcome Trust Case Control Consortium. Genome-wide association study of 14,000 cases of seven common diseases and 3,000 shared controls. *Nature* 2007; **447**: 661–678.
75 Benjamini Y, Hochberg Y. Controlling the false discovery rate: a practical and powerful approach to multiple testing. *Journal of the Royal Statistical Society* 1995; **57**: 289–300.
76 Kennedy D. Breakthrough of the year. *Science* 2007; **318**: 1833.
77 Klein RJ, Zeiss C, Chew EY *et al.* Complement factor H polymorphism in age-related macular degeneration. *Science* 2005; **308**: 385–389.
78 Frayling TM, Timpson NJ, Weedon MN *et al.* A common variant in the FTO gene is associated with body mass index and predisposes to childhood and adult obesity. *Science* 2007; **316**: 889–894.
79 Grant SF, Thorleifsson G, Reynisdottir I *et al.* Variant of transcription factor 7-like 2 (TCF7L2) gene confers risk of type 2 diabetes. *Nature Genetics* 2006; **38**: 320–323.
80 Lasky-Su J, Lyon HN, Emilsson V *et al.* On the replication of genetic associations: timing can be everything! *American Journal of Human Genetics* 2008; **82**: 849–858.

Chapter 2

A primer in statistical methods in genetics

Jonathan L. Haines, Dana C. Crawford, and Marylyn D. Ritchie

Introduction

There has been remarkable progress in human genetics over the past 35 years. At the first human gene mapping conference in 1973 there were fewer than 100 genes mapped to any chromosome; the length of the genome and the number of genes were both unknown. There have been innumerable critical advances, including the development of DNA sequencing, polymerase chain reaction (PCR), stunning technological advances in high-throughput methods, and concomitant advances in computational hardware and software. These advances allowed the human genome project to be conceived and delivered, so that we can now interrogate millions of genetic variations in each individual at reasonable cost in a matter of days.

These advances have fostered immense interest in dissecting the genetic architecture of human disease, first through the tools of genetic linkage analysis, and now flourishing through applications in genetic association analysis. This chapter will provide an overview of the current approaches and methods available for understanding the genetic influence on human cardiovascular traits.

Cardiovascular traits are generally complex

The first genetic traits that usually come to mind are rare traits in which mutations in a single gene cause disease, for example Marfan syndrome (*gene symbol*: *FBN*), hypertrophic cardiomyopathy (multiple myofilament genes), atrial

Cardiovascular Genetics and Genomics. Edited by Dan Roden. © 2009 American Heart Association, ISBN: 978-14051-7540-1.

fibrillation (multiple potassium channel genes), and hereditary hemorrhagic telangiectasia (*gene symbol*: *ENG*). While critical and important, these Mendelian diseases are quite rare. The more prevalent cardiovascular diseases, such as myocardial infarction, hypertension, atrial fibrillation (non-Mendelian forms), and atherosclerosis are not caused by rare mutations in one or a few genes. These traits are considered complex for several reasons. First, their clinical expression varies widely, with such aspects as age at onset, length of episodes, response to treatments, and constellation of symptoms all varying widely between individuals. Second, while the evidence for a genetic influence on the trait is strong, it also suggests that multiple genes each with modest or small effect, acting singly or in combination, are necessary for the trait to develop. There may be multiple rare or common variations within each gene that influence the risk or expression of the trait. Third, most if not all of these traits are also influenced by nongenetic (e.g., environmental) factors such as diet. All these factors make each trait unique and complex and we are faced with the difficult challenge of determining the best methods available to tease apart these effects as described in the next sections.

Common study designs

Family based

Table 2.1 outlines the advantages and disadvantages of each study design. The family-based study design consists of related individuals with and without the trait of interest. This design has been the workhorse of gene mapping since the advent of linkage analysis in the mid-twentieth century. As mentioned above, multiple rare cardiovascular traits were localized using family-based study designs and linkage analysis. The same strategy has been less successful for complex human diseases and traits common in the general population such as type 2 diabetes and hypertension. Despite the suggestion that linkage studies are not as powerful in identifying the risk-conferring loci for common disorders [1], the family-based study design continues to be popular because, in addition to linkage analysis, this design is amenable to tests of association, which includes the more contemporary genome-wide approaches powered for complex traits.

The family-based study design is flexible in which family members are targeted for ascertainment, albeit with differing levels of power to detect either linkage or association between the trait of interest and the risk-conferring locus. Ascertainment of study subjects for a family-based study design can be subdivided into three basic categories: (1) nuclear, (2) extended, and (3) pair. The basic unit of ascertainment for the nuclear family pedigree is the mother, the father, and their offspring (who represent independent meiotic events). In traditional linkage analysis, nuclear families of two or more generations are ascertained, and a family is informative for a linkage study if one of the parents

Table 2.1 Common study designs in human genetics and their advantages and disadvantages

Study design	Advantages	Disadvantages
Family based	Flexible study design	Difficult to ascertain large and/ or intact family structures
	Linkage and association	Sensitive to missing or incorrect genotypes
	Robust to population stratification	Not suitable for late-onset diseases or for studies of pharmacogenomics
Case–control	Easier to ascertain compared with family-based studies	Confounding by population stratification
	Suitable for late-onset disorders and studies of pharmacogenetics	Subject to more bias than cohort studies
	Less expensive than cohort studies	
Cohort	Incident cases are collected	Expensive
	Risk estimates can be calculated	Very large sample sizes are needed to ensure a sufficient number of cases for the disorder of interest
	Environmental exposures can be well documented	
	Less bias than case–control studies	

is heterozygous for the loci of interest. This study design is powerful to detect linkage between markers and a trait given that the informative families are large with many offspring. If sufficiently large, a single, multigenerational nuclear family could be used to localize a causative gene without the addition of other, unrelated families—the latter of which can lead to loss of power owing to locus heterogeneity. Another advantage of the nuclear family is that this study design can be used for performing tests of association in addition to linkage, as described below.

A major disadvantage of this study design is that it is often difficult to ascertain large and/or intact nuclear families. Often, parents and/or offspring are unavailable, rendering the family uninformative. For late-onset disorders, the missingness problem is exacerbated: retrospective ascertainment of multiple generations is not possible given that most if not all previous generations are deceased by the time an affected proband is ascertained for study. Missing individuals (or their genotypes) can severely reduce power for testing both linkage and association. Another complicating factor is related to the allele frequency of the disease-causing locus—if the allele is common, large families may not be the optimal approach given that parents are more likely to be homozygous (and uninformative) for the locus of interest.

The extended pedigree is not constrained to ascertaining only parents and offspring and can vary greatly in size. The most extreme extended pedigrees that have been collected for analysis are generally from culturally or geographically isolated populations that have detailed genealogical records (such as the Icelanders and the Anabaptists). The advantage of ascertaining more distant relatives is that it is possible to increase both the number of meiotic events and the determination of marker phase for analysis. This advantage can increase the power to detect linkage; however, depending on the size and complexity of the pedigrees, the ability to analyze the data using available software may be limited. Like the nuclear family, the extended family study design can also be used to test for association.

The final common family-based study design is the relative or sibling pair. The nuclear family ascertained for linkage analysis was a successful study design to identify single locus traits; however, this approach was not successful for traits or disorders that did not follow patterns of Mendelian inheritance that were expected to have arisen from multiple genes each with a small to moderate genetic effect size. The relative pair [2,3] and sibpair methods [4] are considered "model free" because they rely on patterns of allele sharing rather than mode of inheritance to infer linkage. While sibpair methodology was established in the early twentieth century, a renewed interest in the methodology emerged in the mid-1990s as power calculations suggested sibpair approaches [1], such as the extreme discordant sibpair approach [5], would have increased power compared with conventional linkage methods to detect loci relevant to common, complex traits. In practice, though, it has been difficult to ascertain sufficient numbers of affected/unaffected sibpairs for study.

Case–control

The case–control study design is arguably the most popular study design for genetic studies today. Its popularity is owed, in part, to the ease of ascertaining large numbers of unrelated cases with the trait or disorder of interest and unrelated controls. Also, the case–control study design can be used for the study of late-onset disorders and the study of the efficacy of and adverse reactions to medication and vaccines, none of which can be effectively studied using a family-based study design. A major disadvantage of case–control studies is that they can potentially be confounded by population stratification or differing levels of admixture between cases and controls, which can lead to false-positive results (reviewed in [6]). While it is thought that the effects of population stratification on the false-positive rate of published genetic association studies are greatly exaggerated [6], there is still much interest in adjusting or controlling for this possible confounder. The first step in controlling for population stratification is matching the cases with controls drawn from the same population, a basic tenet of epidemiology. Given that even among carefully matched cases and controls there may be some measurable level of population stratification, the most popular method for identifying it is the use of unlinked genetic markers to cluster individuals with similar inferred ancestry [7–9]. If the cases and controls, which were matched to be similar with regard to race or ancestry, do not cluster together, the individuals that fall out of the cluster are typically omitted from the study to make the case–control study more homogeneous. Other methods to control or adjust for population stratification include the genomic control method [10,11], the Eigenstrat method [12], and outlier methods [13].

In the gene discovery process, most case–control studies are designed to exploit the disorder or trait of interest so that cases represent individuals most likely to have developed the disorder or trait owing to genetic susceptibility. Therefore, the high-risk cases are generally not drawn from a general population and thus are biased. Once a genetic variation associated with disease has been identified, population-based cases and controls could be ascertained to better estimate the genetic effect size of the variation associated with the disorder or trait (reviewed in [14]). Population-based cases and controls could also be used to test for gene–environment interactions or modifiers of genetic risk. The main disadvantage of using case–control studies for gene–environment studies is that most case–control studies, whether population based or not, are retrospective, which can lead to biases in collecting exposure information such as recall bias (reviewed in [15]).

Cohort

The prospective cohort is the gold standard study design in epidemiology. In a prospective cohort, a well-defined group of individuals is ascertained before the disorder of interest develops, exposures are defined, and incident cases emerge during follow-up. The prospective cohort has not been used extensively in genetic linkage or association studies mostly because of the substantial time and financial investment they represent [16]. When properly designed, however, the prospective cohort is a rich resource for both gene discovery and gene–environment research [15].

For cardiovascular research, there are several large prospective cohorts with DNA samples available. The most ubiquitous cohort is Framingham, which began in 1948 in Massachusetts for the study of cardiovascular health in men and women [17,18]. More than 9000 DNA samples are available on the Framingham Heart Study, which now represents three generations of

Framingham participants. Other large prospective cohorts available for genetic studies of cardiovascular disease include the Coronary Artery Risk Development in Young Adults (CARDIA) [19], the Cardiovascular Health Study (CHS) [20], the Dallas Heart Study (DHS) [21], the Jackson Heart Study (JHS) [22], and the Women's Health Initiative (WHI) [23], to name a few.

Two complementary approaches to identify genetic variation

Once a dataset has been developed, there are two general approaches toward disease gene discovery. The first, and until recently the more common approach, is to examine a specific set of candidate genes. These genes can be chosen for different reasons, including their proposed biological function that relates to the trait in question, their location in a region of genetic linkage, or the results of gene expression or proteomic studies. This is an example of a direct association analysis. For direct association analysis, preference is given to single nucleotide polymorphisms (SNPs) that are most likely to be functional, such as nonsynonymous SNPs (i.e., SNPs that change protein sequence), or promoter SNPs that may alter gene expression. Investigators may also preferentially include SNPs that are frequent in the population and SNPs at intron/exon boundaries that may affect splicing. The advantage of this approach is that a very detailed (including complete resequencing) examination of each gene (and its variations) is possible at a reasonable cost. In addition, results of direct association analyses tend to be most readily understood and may be testable at the functional level. The disadvantage is that only specific hypotheses, based on prior information of varying quality and relevance, can be tested. Truly novel associations are not likely to be discovered with this approach.

The second approach is to perform a broad genome screen. This has been widely applied in family-based designs for linkage analysis, and is now being extended to all designs for association analysis. In this approach representative variations (typically SNPs) spread across the entire genome are tested for linkage or association to the trait. This strategy is an example of indirect association analysis. Indirect association analyses rely on the fact that, over many human generations, recombination rarely occurs between multiple SNPs that are in close proximity on a chromosome. As a result, SNPs in a relatively small region of a chromosome may exist as a set that is in linkage disequilibrium (LD), which describes the nonrandom association of alleles at multiple genetic loci. Sets of such statistically associated SNPs are often called haplotype blocks (also called LD blocks) [24], although they may not in fact be completely physically contiguous. Since these multiple SNPs are inherited as a unit, knowing the allele at any one SNP in the set may identify all other SNP alleles in that set. Variants that efficiently distinguish among LD sets are called tagging SNPs, since they "tag" other SNPs in the set [25]. The goal of indirect association analysis is to find the LD set (containing the causative polymorphism) that is most strongly associated with the outcome of interest. If an LD set contains the susceptibility SNP, then the tagging SNP for that set will differ in frequency among cases and controls. The advantage of this approach is that it requires no prior assumption about the biology of the trait or the potential influences or interactions of the underlying genes. The disadvantages are that no one gene or region is examined in really fine detail (thus some associations might be missed), an appropriately powered study requires quite large sample sizes (typically in the thousands of samples), and a very substantial analytical effort is required to manage and analyze the resulting large datasets.

The most recent application of genome screening is the genome-wide association (GWA) study, which examines between 500 000 and 1 000 000 SNPs in each individual. This approach has tremendous potential to identify moderate to modest genetic effects in common diseases, and there has been some initial success [26,27]. The power of this approach exploits the concept of indirect association analysis and rests on the assumption that common diseases are influenced, at least in part, by common variation.

Analytical methods

Linkage analysis

Linkage analysis has its roots in Mendelian genetics, which provides a model of heredity and whose second law states that inheritance of one trait does not influence the inheritance of another. Violation of the second law, i.e., coinheritance of a marker and a trait from the affected parent to offspring, implies that the disease-causing locus and the marker are in close physical proximity and are thus "linked." Linkage analysis requires a family-based design in which multiple independent meiotic events can be observed so that cosegregation can be tested. Typically, the statistical measure of linkage (or nonlinkage) is captured in the lod score. Lod (*lo*garithm of the *od*ds) scores >3 are classically regarded as providing strong evidence for linkage, whereas lod scores <-2 provide strong evidence against linkage. Linkage can be performed using one or many markers, with the latter having the advantage of providing greater evidence for the location of the variation linkage to the trait. There are numerous algorithms and programs available to perform linkage analysis under many different situations [28,29].

Association analysis

Association analysis describes the use of families, case–control samples, or cohort data to statistically relate genetic factors to a trait of interest. Because association analysis directly examines the effect of a particular locus, rather than an effect that is diffused across large regions of chromosomes, its greatest applicability is in fine mapping and identification of susceptibility loci. As described above, association analysis can be either direct or indirect.

One of the most important aspects of any association analysis is the careful selection of cases with the phenotype of interest, and appropriate controls lacking the phenotype. Misclassification of cases and controls will decrease power to detect true genetic associations, or can also lead to false associations [30]. Genomic studies can focus on quantitative traits, with similar study designs but different analytical methods. Having classified samples as cases and controls, a strategy to relate phenotypic data to human genomics must be selected.

Detecting main effects

Single locus association tests are a powerful workhorse in statistical genetics. Family-based association methods include the transmission disequilibrium tests (TDT) and all its variations (such as the sib-TDT, the quantitative-TDT (S-TDT), and the pedigree disequilibrium test (PDT) [31–37], the family-based association test (FBAT) [38], and the association in the presence of linkage (APL) test [39]). Population-based association methods include χ^2 [40], Fisher's exact test [40], Armitage trend test [41], and logistic regression [42]. The obvious goal of these methods is to determine which loci are important predictors of clinical outcome. However, most of these methodologies are applied with the hypothesis that a single gene with a major effect will be associated with the disease. Based on the history of human genetic studies, this was an excellent starting hypothesis. Many genetic variations have been elucidated that have strong associations with Mendelian genetic phenotypes. To this end, traditional statistical approaches for discrete dependent variables were used or family-based association methods were developed. However, these methods falter when applied to traits with genes of modest main effects, making results harder to interpret when viewed alone. This is one reason for the movement toward replication of results in an independent dataset as a gold standard.

Detecting epistasis

Most rare Mendelian genetic disorders, such as Marfan syndrome, are influenced by the effects of a single gene. However, common diseases, such as atrial fibrillation, hypertension, and atherosclerosis are influenced by more than one gene, some of which may be associated with disease risk primarily through nonlinear interactions [43]. The possibility of complex interactions makes the detection and characterization of genes associated with common, complex disease difficult. Templeton *et al.* [44] document that gene–gene interactions (or epistasis) are commonly found when properly investigated. Based on recent research, epistasis is not merely a theoretical argument. Epistasis has been identified as a component of complex phenotypes in a number of studies [45]. For example, Mendelian disorders such as retinitis pigmentosa [46], Hirschsprung disease [47], juvenile-onset glaucoma [48], familial amyloid polyneuropathy [49], and cystic fibrosis [50] are documented examples of epistasis in which modifier genes interact with Mendelian inherited main effect genes. More compelling are studies in model organisms where there is both biological and statistical evidence for epistasis. Three arthritis loci have been identified in a quantitative trait locus (QTL) in mice that exhibit epistatic interactions [51,52]. Epistatic effects have also been documented in a number of other phenotypes in mice including obesity [53] and fluctuating asymmetry of tooth size and shape [54]. Similarly, research in other model organisms such as *Saccharomyces cerevisiae* has documented epistasis associated with quantitative variation phenotypes such as metabolism [55]. These model organism studies provide additional evidence that epistasis detected via statistical and computational techniques may be relevant biologically. This is something that is not possible to assess easily in human genetics studies [56].

To deal with the challenge of detecting interactions, much research is under way for improved statistical and computational methodologies. Many researchers are exploring variations and modifications of logistic regression such as logic regression, penalized logistic regression, classification/regression trees (CART) and multivariate adaptive regression splines (MARS), focused interaction testing framework (FITF), and automated detection of informative combined effects (DICE). Additional studies are being conducted in data mining and machine learning research, including data reduction and pattern recognition approaches. Data reduction involves a collapsing or mapping of the data to a lower dimensional space. Examples of data reduction approaches include the combinatorial partitioning method (CPM), restricted partition method (RPM), set association, and multifactor dimensionality reduction (MDR). Pattern recognition, on the other hand, involves extracting patterns from the data to discriminate between groups using the full dimensionality of the data. Examples of pattern recognition methods include cluster analysis [57], cellular automata (CA), support vector machines (SVM), self-organizing maps (SOM), and neural networks (NN). To successfully study complex disease risk factors and analyze GWA data, statistical methods must consider combinations of polymorphisms and environmental factors and must be able to model their interaction effects [58].

The problem of multiple comparisons

With the rapid increase in the number of genetic variations that can be tested, the statistical problem of performing multiple tests, and thus doing multiple comparisons, has become a major issue. The concern arises since increasing the number of tests also increases the number of potential false-positive results unless the *P*-value is adjusted. For example, using a *P*-value of 0.05 and performing a test of association between one SNP in *KCNE2* with atrial fibrillation, one would expect a false-positive result only once out of 20 datasets.

However, if performing an association using 1 000 000 SNPs, one would expect 50 000 false-positive results, hardly encouraging when trying to identify a small number of true effects. The level of correction for multiple comparisons is a point of significant debate, with some arguing that no correction is necessary, and others arguing for an extreme level of correction (most often a Bonferroni correction of 0.05/number of tests; in the above case this would require a *P*-value of 5×10^{-8}). The problem with the former extreme is that almost all results declared significant will be false positives, while the problem with the latter is that a very large dataset is needed or no significant results will be found at all. More moderate levels of correction have been proposed [59,60], but the debate is likely to rage for years.

Future directions

The next few years will see continued advances in genomic technologies and in their application to cardiovascular disease. There is a huge push to improve technologies so that the complete sequence of a person's entire genome can be done at reasonable cost, which will generate a nearly complete compendium of genomic variation for each individual. This wealth of data will carry within it the answers to many questions about the role of genetic variation in cardiovascular disease. However, the analytical and computational challenges of sifting through these data are momentous and will require significant advances in analytical and computational methods. With these in place, we can look toward better diagnostics, interventions, and therapeutics based on our understanding of underlying genetic variation.

References

1 Risch N, Merikangas K. The future of genetic studies of complex human disorders. *Science* 1996; **273**: 1516–1517.
2 Curtis D, Sham PC. Using risk calculation to implement an extended relative pair analysis. *Annals of Human Genetics* 1994; **58** (Part 2): 151–162.
3 Cordell HJ, Wedig GC, Jacobs KB, Elston RC. Multilocus linkage tests based on affected relative pairs. *Annals of Human Genetics* 2000; **66**: 1273–1286.
4 Knapp M, Seuchter S, Bauer M. Linkage analysis in nuclear families. 1. Optimality criteria for affected sib-pair test. *Human Heredity* 1994; **44**: 37–43.
5 Risch N, Zhang H. Extreme discordant sib pairs for mapping quantitative trait loci in humans. *Science* 1995; **268**: 1584–1589.
6 Cardon LR, Palmer LJ. Population stratification and spurious allelic association. *Lancet* 2003; **361**: 598–604.
7 Pritchard JK, Stephens M, Rosenberg NA, Donnelly P. Association mapping in structured populations. *Annals of Human Genetics* 2000; **67**: 170–181.
8 Pritchard JK, Rosenberg NA. Use of unlinked genetic markers to detect population stratification in association studies. *Annals of Human Genetics* 1999; **65**: 220–228.

9 Rosenberg NA, Pritchard JK, Weber JL *et al.* Genetic structure of human populations. *Science* 2002; **298**: 2381–2385.

10 Bacanu SA, Devlin B, Roeder K. The power of genomic control. *Annals of Human Genetics* 2000; **66**: 1933–1944.

11 Marchini J, Cardon LR, Phillips MS, Donnelly P. The effects of human population structure on large genetic association studies. *Nature Genetics* 2004; **36**: 512–517.

12 Price AL, Patterson NJ, Plenge RM *et al.* Principal components analysis corrects for stratification in genome-wide association studies. *Nature Genetics* 2006; **38**: 904–909.

13 Purcell S, Neale B, Todd-Brown K *et al.* PLINK: a tool set for whole-genome association and population-based linkage analyses. *Annals of Human Genetics* 2007; **81**: 559–575.

14 Zondervan KT, Cardon LR, Kennedy SH. What makes a good case–control study? Design issues for complex traits such as endometriosis. *Human Reproduction* 2002; **17**: 1415–1423.

15 Manolio TA, Bailey-Wilson JE, Collins FS. Genes, environment and the value of prospective cohort studies. *Nature Reviews Genetics* 2006; **7**: 812–820.

16 Collins FS. The case for a US prospective cohort study of genes and environment. *Nature* 2004; **429**: 475–477.

17 Dawber TR, Meadors GF, Moore FE, Jr. Epidemiological approaches to heart disease: the Framingham Study. *American Journal of Public Health and the Nation's Health* 1951; **41**: 279–281.

18 Dawber TR, Kannel WB, Lyell LP. An approach to longitudinal studies in a community: the Framingham Study. *Annals of the New York Academy of Sciences* 1963; **107**: 539–556.

19 Hall JG, Friedman JM, Kenna BA *et al.* Clinical, genetic, and epidemiological factors in neural tube defects. *Annals of Human Genetics* 1988; **43**: 827–837.

20 Fried LP, Borhani NO, Enright P *et al.* The Cardiovascular Health Study: design and rationale. *Annals of Epidemiology* 1991; **1**: 263–276.

21 Victor RG, Haley RW, Willett DL *et al.* The Dallas Heart Study: a population-based probability sample for the multidisciplinary study of ethnic differences in cardiovascular health. *American Journal of Cardiology* 2004; **93**: 1473–1480.

22 Wilson JG, Rotimi CN, Ekunwe L *et al.* Study design for genetic analysis in the Jackson Heart Study. *Ethnicity and Disease* 2005; **15** (4 Suppl 6): S6–37.

23 Ridker PM, Chasman DI, Zee RY *et al.* Rationale, design, and methodology of the Women's Genome Health Study: a genome-wide association study of more than 25,000 initially healthy American women. *Clinical Chemistry* 2008; **54**: 249–255.

24 Daly MJ, Rioux JD, Schaffner SF *et al.* High-resolution haplotype structure in the human genome. *Nature Genetics* 2001; **29**: 229–232.

25 Johnson GC, Esposito L, Barratt BJ *et al.* Haplotype tagging for the identification of common disease genes. *Nature Genetics* 2001; **29**: 233–237.

26 International Multiple Sclerosis Genetics Consortium. Risk alleles for multiple sclerosis identified by a genomewide study. *New England Journal of Medicine* 2007; **357**: 851–862.

27 Wellcome Trust Case Control Consortium. Genome-wide association study of 14,000 cases of seven common diseases and 3,000 shared controls. *Nature* 2007; **447**: 661–678.

28 Ott J. *Analysis of Human Genetic Linkage*, 3rd edn. Johns Hopkins University Press, Baltimore, 1999.

29 Haines JL, Korf BR, Morton CC, Seidman CE, Seidman JG, Smith DR. *Current Protocols in Human Genetics*. John Wiley & Sons, New York, 2008.
30 Healy DG. Case–control studies in the genomic era: a clinician's guide. *Lancet Neurology* 2006; **5**: 701–707.
31 Spielman RS, McGinnis RE, Ewens WJ. Transmission test for linkage disequilibrium: the insulin gene region and insulin-dependent diabetes mellitus (IDDM). *Annals of Human Genetics* 1993; **52**: 506–516.
32 Martin ER, Monks SA, Warren LL, Kaplan NL. A test for linkage and association in general pedigrees: the pedigree disequilibrium test. *Annals of Human Genetics* 2000; **67**: 146–154.
33 Martin ER, Bass MP, Gilbert JR *et al*. Genotype-based association test for general pedigrees: the genotype-PDT. *Genetic Epidemiology* 2003; **25**: 203–213.
34 Spielman RS, Ewens WJ. The TDT and other family-based tests for linkage disequilibrium and association. *Annals of Human Genetics* 1996; **59**: 983–989.
35 Spielman RS, Ewens WJ. A sibship test for linkage in the presence of association: the sib transmission/disequilibrium test. *Annals of Human Genetics* 1998; **61**: 450–458.
36 Horvath S, Laird NM. A discordant-sibship test for disequilibrium and linkage: no need for parental data. *Annals of Human Genetics* 1998; **63**: 1886–1897.
37 Boehnke M, Langefeld CD. Genetic association mapping based on discordant sib pairs: the discordant alleles test (DAT). *Annals of Human Genetics* 1998; **62**: 950–961.
38 Horvath S, Xu X, Laird NM. The family based association test method: strategies for studying general genotype: phenotype associations. *European Journal of Human Genetics* 2001; **9**: 301–306.
39 Martin ER, Bass MP, Hauser ER, Kaplan NL. Accounting for linkage in family-based tests of association with missing parental genotypes. *Annals of Human Genetics* 2003; **73**: 1016–1026.
40 Agresti A. *Categorical Data Analysis*. John Wiley & Sons, New York, 1990.
41 Slager SL, Schaid DJ. Case–control studies of genetic markers: power and sample size approximations for Armitage's test for trend. *Human Heredity* 2001; **52**: 149–153.
42 Hosmer D, Lemeshow S. *Applied Logistic Regression*. John Wiley & Sons Inc., New York, 2000.
43 Moore JH, Williams SM. New strategies for identifying gene–gene interactions in hypertension. *Annals of Medicine* 2002; **34**: 88–95.
44 Templeton AR. Epistasis and complex traits. In: Wolf J, Brodie III ED, Wade MJ, eds. *Epistasis and the Evolutionary Process*. Oxford University Press, Inc., New York, 2000: 41–57.
45 Ming JE, Muenke M. Multiple hits during early embryonic development: digenic diseases and holoprosencephaly. *Annals of Human Genetics* 2002; **71**: 1017–1032.
46 Kajiwara K, Berson EL, Dryja TP. Digenic retinitis pigmentosa due to mutations at the unlinked peripherin/RDS and ROM1 loci. *Science* 1994; **264**: 1604–1608.
47 Auricchio A, Griseri P, Carpentieri ML *et al*. Double heterozygosity for a RET substitution interfering with splicing and an EDNRB missense mutation in Hirschsprung disease. *Annals of Human Genetics* 1999; **64**: 1216–1221.
48 Vincent AL, Billingsley G, Buys Y *et al*. Digenic inheritance of early-onset glaucoma: CYP1B1, a potential modifier gene. *Annals of Human Genetics* 2002; **70**: 448–460.

49 Soares ML, Coelho T, Sousa A *et al.* Susceptibility and modifier genes in Portuguese transthyretin V30M amyloid polyneuropathy: complexity in a single-gene disease. *Human Molecular Genetics* 2005; **14**: 543–553.
50 Dipple K, McCabe E. Modifier genes convert "simple" Mendelian disorders to complex traits. *Molecular Genetics and Metabolism* 2000; **71**: 43–50.
51 Johannesson M, Karlsson J, Wernhoff P *et al.* Identification of epistasis through a partial advanced intercross reveals three arthritis loci within the Cia5 QTL in mice. *Genes and Immunity* 2005; **6**: 175–185.
52 Johannesson M, Olsson LM, Lindqvist AK *et al.* Gene expression profiling of arthritis using a QTL chip reveals a complex gene regulation of the Cia5 region in mice. *Genes and Immunity* 2005; **6**: 575–583.
53 Warden CH, Yi N, Fisler J. Epistasis among genes is a universal phenomenon in obesity: evidence from rodent models. *Nutrition* 2004; **20**: 74–77.
54 Leamy LJ, Workman MS, Routman EJ, Cheverud JM. An epistatic genetic basis for fluctuating asymmetry of tooth size and shape in mice. *Heredity* 2005; **94**: 316–325.
55 Duggal P, Klein AP, Lee KE *et al.* A genetic contribution to intraocular pressure: the beaver dam eye study. *Investigative Ophthalmology and Visual Science* 2005; **46**: 555–560.
56 Moore JH, Boczko EM, Summar ML. Connecting the dots between genes, biochemistry, and disease susceptibility: systems biology modeling in human genetics. *Molecular Genetics and Metabolism* 2005; **84**: 104–111.
57 Weeks DE, Lehner T, Squires-Wheeler E *et al.* Measuring the inflation of the lod score due to its maximization over model parameter values in human linkage analysis. *Genetic Epidemiology* 1990; **7**: 237–243.
58 Motsinger AA, Ritchie MD, Reif DM. Novel methods for detecting epistasis in pharmacogenomics studies. *Pharmacogenomics* 2007; **8**: 1229–1241.
59 Nyholt DR. A simple correction for multiple testing for single-nucleotide polymorphisms in linkage disequilibrium with each other. *Annals of Human Genetics* 2004; **74**: 765–769.
60 Benjamini Y, Hochberg Y. Controlling the false discovery rate: a practical and powerful approach to multiple testing. *Journal of the Royal Statistical Society B* 1995; **57**: 289–300.

Chapter 3

The role of ethnicity in managing cardiovascular patients

Raymond Hreiche, Veronique Michaud, and Jacques Turgeon

Introduction

Historically, the North American population was formed by episodic migration flows. While the majority of these flows initiated from Europe—mainly England, Spain, and France—North America's current demographic makeup is much more diversified. In 2005, the US Census Bureau (www.census.gov/popest/estimates.php) estimated the national population to be 296410404. Of this total, 14.4% self-identified as being of Hispanic or Latino origin, 12.8% as Black, 4.3% as Asian, and 1% as American Indian and Alaskan Native among other less numerous groups. This heterogeneity can be easily found in the majority of the world's metropolitan areas, and therefore raises major issues related to disparities, ranging from health risk factors to disease prevalence, life expectancy, and adequate healthcare delivery. All these issues are inevitably related to genetic and environmental factors.

The term *ethnicity* stems from the Greek *ethnos* [1,2], meaning *people* or *nation*. It is "a multi-faced quality that refers to the group to which people belong, and/or are perceived to belong, as a result of certain shared characteristics, including geographical and ancestral origins, but particularly cultural traditions and languages" [1]. However, the concept of ethnicity in healthcare and public health remains a controversial variable, with many ethical and definition issues. In clinical studies, it is still difficult to have a good grasp of terms such as *Asians*, *Blacks*, or *Hispanic* because of their inconsistent usage, intragroup heterogeneity (many studies do not mention the subgroups), and an absence of internationally recognized definitions. In this chapter, the "Asian" term in one clinical study, for example, may not be as representative of a subpopulation as the same term used in another study.

Cardiovascular Genetics and Genomics. Edited by Dan Roden. © 2009 American Association, ISBN: 978-14051-7540-1.

According to the World Heart Federation, heart disease is the world's number one killer and is responsible for one in every three deaths. This prevalence is even more pronounced in the Western industrialized world. In the USA, heart disease has been the leading cause of death for the past 80 years [3]. Moreover, it is worth noting that rapid economic development, urbanization, and lifestyle changes in developing countries are heavily responsible for an impressive increase in cardiovascular disease (CVD) [4]. Owing to many genetic and environmental factors, not all individuals are equal with regard to prevalence of CVD or in treatment responses, which inevitably leads to inequalities in their health management. In addition, the majority of clinical studies have been conducted using white men, and their results have been generalized to all patients irrespective of their ethnic group. This has led to the rise of "ethnopharmacology," which Munoz and Hilgenberg [5] define as "the study of the effect of ethnicity on responses to prescribed medication."

Environmental and cultural factors in treatment response

Environmental factors, such as climate, pollution, smoking, alcohol, drug intake, diet, and so on, can be responsible for an important variation in drug response within the same individual [6]. Furthermore, these factors can cause disparities among groups of individuals, which could be related ethnicity.

For example, in addition to its proven direct effect on the prevalence of CVD [7], tobacco use has been implicated in drug interactions with the widely prescribed anticoagulant warfarin. It is well known that tobacco smoke is a potent inducer of the cytochrome P450 (CYP) 1A2, which is partially responsible for the metabolism of warfarin in humans. Therefore, many clinical cases of increase in warfarin efficacy have been described in people who have recently stopped smoking [8]. In addition, possible warfarin treatment failure has been associated with smokeless tobacco. This failure was explained by an increased dietary source of vitamin K from tobacco [9]. These interactions can be of significant importance owing to variations of prevalence of cigarette smoking within each population. According to the 2005 National Health Interview Survey, American Indians and Alaskan Natives had the highest prevalence of cigarette smoking (32.0%), followed by non-Hispanic whites (21.9%), non-Hispanic blacks (21.5%), Hispanics (16.2%), and Asians (13.3%) [10].

On the other hand, chronic and acute ethanol consumption can modulate the response and toxicity of many cardiovascular treatments. For example, ethanol can cause additive vasodilatation with such agents as nitroglycerin, methyldopa, and hydralazine [11]. Moreover, ethanol can decrease plasma clearance of propranolol, leading to a decrease in the latter's efficacy [12]. Because of historical, religious, and cultural factors, alcohol consumption varies among ethnic groups, which leads to a disparity in the toxicity observed with these drugs among these groups [13].

Treatment adherence is a key factor among cultural factors that could also modulate drug response, For example, many studies have correlated mediocre blood pressure control to poor treatment adherence, equally correlated to ethnicity [14].

Role of genetic factors in treatment efficacy and toxicity

Polymorphisms are naturally occurring variations in the sequence of genetic information on a segment of DNA in more than 1% of the population. These variations lead to a modulation in the gene products—mostly proteins—which interact directly or indirectly with drugs. This could result in absence of the gene product (e.g., absence of a specific enzyme), presence of an inactive gene product (e.g., presence of an inactive enzyme), or increased gene product activity (e.g., presence of higher copies of this enzyme).

According to Burroughs *et al.* [6], three processes or mechanisms are involved in the polymorphisms–drug response interaction, namely drug metabolism, drug targets, and disease pathway. However, polymorphisms in drug metabolism are usually considered the most relevant because of their recurrence in many important therapeutic classes. This is especially true in comparison with the other two mechanisms, which may affect only one drug or one class of drugs [6].

Polymorphisms of drug metabolism can influence individual response to drug therapy as a result of highly variable plasma concentrations of the parent compound or its metabolites [15]. Oxidation, acetylation, and/or methylation are the main processes of biotransformation. The CYP family is the major oxidative system and is implicated in the oxidation—and elimination—of more than 50% of all marketed drugs [16]. More importantly, many polymorphisms in CYP activity have been described.

Drug targets are extremely numerous and consist of enzymes, cell surface receptors, nuclear hormone receptors, ion channels, and transporters [17]. Many polymorphisms are observed within the genes encoding for these drug targets and can cause an alteration in sensitivity to several therapies.

Many of the above-mentioned polymorphisms are not uniformly distributed among ethnic groups [18]. This ethnicity-related discrepancy results in significant variation of drug response and takes one of the following forms: (1) alteration in treatment efficacy and responsiveness or (2) alteration in treatment toxicity and adverse reactions (Fig. 3.1).

Alteration in treatment responsiveness and efficacy

One of the best illustrations of the polymorphism of drug metabolism and its relation to ethnicity and treatment responsiveness may be the polymorphisms observed in *CYP2D6* (as discussed in Chapter 14). Indeed, *CYP2D6* polymorphisms are clinically very important owing to the fact that around 20–25%

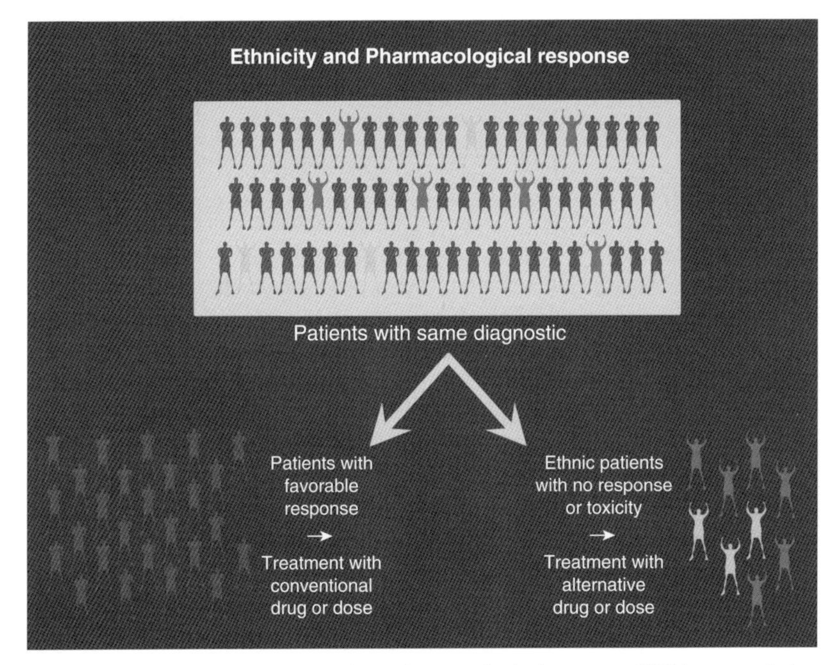

Fig. 3.1 Ethnicity can play a major role in pharmacological response. Within a population, patients with the same diagnosis can be divided into two groups: (1) patients with favorable response and (2) ethnic patients with no response or toxicity. The latter group requires a treatment adjustment with an alternative drug or dose. (Adapted and reprinted with permission from the *Annual Review of Genomics and Human Genetics*, Volume 2 © 2001 by Annual Reviews www.annualreviews.org [51].)

of all drugs are metabolized by this enzyme. Mutations in the *CYP2D6* locus result in a non-encoded enzyme, a deficient enzyme, or an enzyme with increased activity [19]. This leads to four activity levels (or phenotypes): poor metabolizers (PMs); intermediate metabolizers (IMs); extensive metabolizers (EMs); and ultrarapid metabolizers (UMs) [20,21]. Presently, more than 46 different major polymorphic *CYP2D6* alleles are known [22]. However, few are clinically and quantitatively relevant, namely *CYP2D6*2*, *CYP2D6*4*, *CYP2D6*5*, *CYP2D6*10*, *CYP2D6*17*, and *CYP2D6*41* (Table 3.1). In particular, the *2 allele variant, resulting from a gene multiduplication, increases enzyme activity, which leads to an extensive CYP2D6-mediated metabolism and a decrease in the efficacy of CYP2D6 substrates (many cardiovascular drugs). An excellent review by Bernard *et al.* [23] provides a list of numerous studies conducted in many countries that demonstrated significant interethnic differences in *CYP2D6* allele frequencies (Table 3.2). These interethnic differences lead to significant variations in treatment efficacy among ethnic groups.

Table 3.1 Major human polymorphic variant *CYP2D6* alleles and their global distribution

			Allele frequencies (%)			
Major variant alleles	**Mutation**	**Consequence**	**Caucasians**	**Asians**	**Black Africans**	**Ethiopians and Saudi Arabians**
*CYP2D6*2xn*	Gene duplication/ multiduplication	Increased enzyme activity	1–5	0–2	2	10–16
*CYP2D6*4*	Defective splicing	Inactive enzyme	12–21	1	2	1–4
*CYP2D6*5*	Gene deletion	No enzyme	2–7	6	4	1–3
*CYP2D6*10*	P34S, S486T	Unstable enzyme	1–2	51	6	3–9
*CYP2D6*17*	T107I, R296C, S486T	Altered affinity for substrates	0	0	20–35	3–9

Reproduced from Ingelman-Sundberg *et al.* [22] with permission from *The Pharmacogenomics Journal.*

Table 3.2 Incidence of CYP2D6 enzyme phenotypes among different ethnic populations

Population	PM phenotype (%)	Diminished activity of IMs (%)	UM phenotype (%)	Reference
White		1–2		[1]
American	7.7		4.3	[20,40]
British	8.9			[26]
Polish	8.3			
Swiss	10			[25]
Danish			0.8	[22]
German	7.7		0.8	[49]
Swedish			1	[50]
Spanish			10	[23]
Turkish	1.5		8.7	
Croatian	3.0		4.0	
African				
African American	1.9–7.3		4.9	[20,39–42]
Nigerian	0–8.1			[35,36]
Ghanaian	6.0			[37]
Ethiopian	1.8		29	[21]
South African	19			[38]
Asian		51		[1]
Japanese	0			[29]
Chinese	<1.0		0.9	[28]
Thai	1.2			[27]
Indian	1.8–4.8			[30–33]
Saudi Arabian	1–2	3–9	21.0	[1,52]
Hispanic				
Colombian	6.6		1.7	[47]
Mexican	3.2			[46]
Panamanian (Amerindian)	2.2–4.4			[45]
Nicaraguan	3.6			[48]

IM, intermediate metabolizer; PM, poor metabolizer, UM, ultrarapid metabolizer.

Reproduced from Bernard *et al.* [23] with permission from *Oncologist*.

To cite some examples, many beta-blockers such as bufuralol, bupranolol, carvedilol, labetalol, metoprolol, propranolol, and timolol [22] are partially or entirely cleared via a CYP2D6-mediated metabolism. An increase in their metabolic clearance decreases their plasmatic concentrations and efficacy. In Ethiopian and Saudi Arabian descendants, for example, special attention—and probably higher doses—should be given to management of their hypertension with many beta-blockers [22,23], since 29% of Ethiopians and 21% of Saudi Arabians are UMs for CYP2D6 compared with whites (4%).

Other polymorphisms could diminish the efficacy and response of beta-blockers. In fact, many polymorphisms have been observed in β_1-adrenergic receptors, showing altered functions or regulations [24]. These receptors are the drug targets of beta-blockers and could therefore reduce their responsiveness. However, many clinical studies still need to be conducted in order to gain a better understanding of these polymorphisms and the way to use them in managing cardiovascular patients from different ethnic groups.

As is the case with beta-blockers, several antiarrhythmics are also metabolized by CYP2D6. Indeed, propafenone and flecainide can be less effective in UMs for CYP2D6 and higher doses may be required [25]. Special attention should be given to these drugs.

Angiotensin-converting enzyme (ACE) inhibitors are currently the cornerstone of managing patients with cardiovascular and renal disease [26]. However, responsiveness to equivalent doses of ACE inhibitors fluctuates significantly between individuals within the same group or from different ethnic groups [27] (Fig. 3.2). Rigat *et al.* [28] were among the first to explain interindividual variability in the response to ACE inhibitor treatment. They found that the ACE insertion/deletion (I/D) polymorphism—corresponding to an insertion or a deletion of a 287bp Alu repeat polymorphism in intron 16—explained around 50% of the variance in serum ACE levels. While many studies have been conducted since then in order to elucidate the impact of this polymorphism, the results have been inconclusive [29]. Still, a trend has been observed towards a better response to ACE inhibitors in white DD carriers than in II carriers [30]. Moreover, some studies have found that ACE inhibitors do not normalize hypertension in African Americans as effectively as in whites, and therefore the addition of a second antihypertensive agent, such as a diuretic, would be an excellent strategy [31–33].

Alteration in treatment toxicity and adverse reactions

Anticoagulant therapy is an excellent example for describing the variation of adverse reactions and its correlation with ethnicity. Indeed, warfarin—an oral anticoagulant from the coumarin family—is one of the most widely prescribed anticoagulant drugs for prophylaxis and treatment of pulmonary embolism and venous and arterial thrombosis [34]. However, its use requires very close patient monitoring [international normalized ratio (INR) should fluctuate

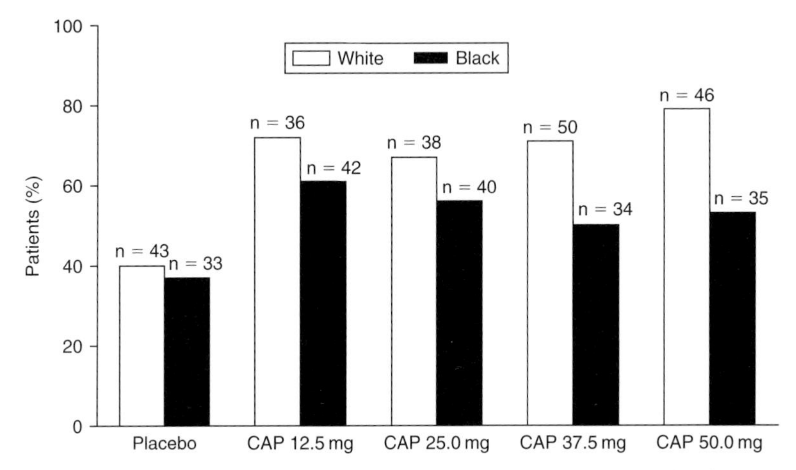

Fig. 3.2 Percentage of patients by race/ethnicity who achieved goal blood pressure with the ACE inhibitor captopril (CAP). (Reproduced from Materson *et al.* [52] with permission.)

between 2 and 3] because of the clinical importance of observed adverse reactions. More precisely, bleeding is observed in up to 16% of patients per year and serious hemorrhages are observed at a rate of 1.3–4.2 per 100 patients per year of exposure [35,36]. These adverse reactions and the variability in warfarin dosage requirements have been related, *inter alia*, to genetic polymorphisms in *CYP2C9* (polymorphism of drug metabolism) and *VKORC1* (polymorphism of drug target).

First, CYP2C9 is the main metabolic enzyme responsible for the metabolism of S-warfarin, the isomer with the most pharmacological activity [37]. In addition, numerous allele variants have been identified for *CYP2C9*. Two of these allele variants (**3* and **6*) are associated with a loss of activity, whereas **2*, **4*, **5*, and **11* are associated with weaker enzyme activities [38–41]. However, a decrease in the metabolic capability of warfarin has been described only in carriers of *2 and *3 variants [42]. Diminution of the metabolic clearance of warfarin in PMs leads inevitably to an increase in plasma concentrations of S-warfarin and an increase in the drug's activity compared with an equivalent dose in EMs. A risk of severe adverse reactions is very frequent in PMs, making a dose adjustment necessary. Health management in warfarin-treated patients is complicated by the fact that these polymorphisms are not uniformly distributed in all ethnic groups. A review by Lee *et al.* [43] describes the heterogenic distribution of CYP2C9 polymorphisms among ethnic groups (Table 3.3). For example, although one-third of whites express either the *2 or *3 genotypes, no individuals of Japanese, Chinese, Korean, or Taiwanese origin express the *2 variant, and few express the *3 variant.

Table 3.3 Population distribution of *CYP2C9* genotype among ethnicity

Ethnic group	Reference	*1*1 (%)	*1*2 (%)	*1*3 (%)	*2*2 (%)	*2*3 (%)	*3*3 (%)	*n*
White	Scordo *et al.*	102 (65.0)	24 (16.8)	22 (14.0)	4 (2.5)	3 (1.9)	2 (1.3)	157
	Taube *et al.*	392 (70.0)	107 (19.0)	53 (9.5)	3 (0.5)	6 (1.0)	0 (0)	561
	Margaglione *et al.*	88 (48.9)	62 (34.4)	28 (15.6)	0 (0)	2 (1.1)	0 (0)	180
	Yasar *et al.*	287 (66.7)	80 (18.6)	50 (11.6)	2 (0.5)	8 (1.9)	3 (0.7)	430
	Lee *et al.*	34 (61.8)	9 (16.4)	8 (14.5)	3 (5.5)	1 (1.8)	0 (0)	55
	Total (%)	903 (65.3)	282 (20.4)	161 (11.6)	12 (0.9)	20 (1.4)	5 (0.4)	1383
African American	Sullivan-Klose *et al.*	97 (97.0)	2 (2.0)	1 (1.0)	0 (0)	0 (0)	0 (0)	100
African	Scordo *et al.*	130 (87.0)	13 (8.7)	7 (4.3)	0 (0)	0 (0)	0 (0)	150
Turkish	Aynacioglu *et al.*	308 (61.7)	90 (18.0)	86 (17.2)	5 (1.0)	6 (1.1)	4 (0.8)	499
Spanish	Garcia-Martin *et al.*	78 (49.7)	25 (15.9)	37 (23.5)	3 (1.9)	14 (8.9)	0 (0)	157
Japanese	Nasu *et al.*	209 (95.9)	0 (0)	9 (4.1)	0 (0)	0 (0)	0 (0)	218
Chinese	Wang *et al.*	111 (96.5)	0 (0)	4 (3.5)	0 (0)	0 (0)	0 (0)	115
Taiwanese	Sullivan-Klose *et al.*	93 (91.8)	0 (0)	5 (8.2)	0 (0)	0 (0)	0 (0)	98
Korean	Yoon *et al.*	561 (97.7)	0 (0)	13 (2.3)	0 (0)	0 (0)	0 (0)	574

Reproduced from Lee *et al.* [43] with permission from *Pharmacogenetics*.

Another factor that can explain the variability in warfarin treatment is the polymorphisms expressed in the warfarin pharmacodynamical target, namely the vitamin K epoxide reductase (VKOR). These polymorphisms may lead to warfarin resistance and to a decrease in its activity. Many variants in the VKOR complex subunit 1 (*VKORC1*) gene have recently been described, including many haplotypes—based on single nucleotide polymorphisms. Moreover, it would appear that individuals carrying the H1 and H2 haplotypes require significantly lower doses of warfarin than those carrying the H7, H8, and H9 haplotypes [44,45]. This is more pronounced in Asian subpopulations where, contrary to *CYP2C9* polymorphisms, *VKORC1* haplotypes account for the difference in warfarin requirements between Chinese, Malays, and Indians [46]. Indeed, the *VKORC1* H1 haplotype is common among Chinese (87%) and Malays (65%) and less so among Indians (12%), while H7, H8, and H9 haplotypes were inversely distributed among these groups [46]. In short, according to ethnic group, *CYP2C9* and *VKORC1* account for 5–22% and 6–37% of warfarin variability respectively [47]. In light of this, new studies are needed to elucidate all the mechanisms and parameters that account for genetic-related variability of warfarin treatment [48].

ACE inhibitors have also been associated with an increase in treatment toxicity according to the ethnic background of the patient. Indeed, many studies have concluded that black patients treated with ACE inhibitors had a threefold increase in relative risk of angioedema episodes compared with non-blacks [49]. It has also been suggested that American Asian patients have a high risk (50%) of cough with ACE inhibitors, making this therapeutic class less tolerable in this ethnic population [50]. On the other hand, some small clinical trials have reported more depression incidence with hydrochlorothiazide in black patients than in white patients [49].

Towards an individualized therapy for better management of cardiovascular patients from ethnic minorities?

As shown above, many examples of ethnicity-related pharmacogenetics can be listed to illustrate variability of drug efficacy and toxicity and, therefore, the difficulty of health management in these cases.

The genomic revolution, with the Human Genome Project as its center piece, has made many strides in providing a better understanding of the relationship between drug therapy and ethnicity. However, we are still at the very beginning of this knowledge development process. Indeed, many studies confirm that the impact of genetic ethnicity-related polymorphisms is still very controversial. This uncertainty can be explained by the fact that there have been only a few large clinical trials that have closely studied the impact of ethnicity on drug response. Moreover, even many published comparative trials between ethnic groups remain controversial because of the small number of black, Asian, or Hispanic subjects included compared with white subjects. This imbalance can create many biases and could lead to false conclusions.

In addition, we still lack an understanding of the clinical impact of every polymorphism discovered and of their impact on observed interethnic variability. For example, polymorphisms in *VKOR1* and *CYP2C9* can explain only some of the variability in warfarin therapy. Many other yet-to-be-discovered genetic polymorphisms and environmental factors remain to be elucidated.

The dilemma that every physician faces remains the same: what is the optimal approach to, say, a self-described black patient. Will he or she respond less with an ACE inhibitor? It is well established that even though blacks in general respond less to ACE inhibitors, this therapeutic family should not be avoided for all black patients. Even though physicians can ask—at a relatively high cost with many pharmacoeconomic doubts—for the genetic "fingerprints" of their patients, there is still a problem with the predictability of this information. Although genetic fingerprints are undoubtedly very useful in predicting plasmatic concentrations of a drug and its clearance, they do not necessarily predict its pharmacological response.

The pharmacogenetic gaps we are currently facing in our understanding and prediction of drug response and toxicity can be overcome by continuing research in pharmacogenomics at the basic and clinical levels. The direction this research should take should be based on discovering new genetic markers followed by their validation in large clinical trials in different ethnic groups. Subsequently, this research could be used as a tool for physicians in everyday clinical practice. In addition, pharmaceutical companies should be pressed to include more individuals from ethnic groups in their clinical studies before drug launching.

Good health is our birthright, with no discrimination according to ethnic background. As such, healthcare should seek to eliminate disparities in cardiovascular health and healthcare delivery. All socioeconomic and environmental parameters indicate that population migrations will constantly increase over the next decades. As such, many societies that had genetically homogenous populations are being transformed into a mix of various ethnic backgrounds. Physicians will face new challenges in healthcare management because of greater variability in drug response.

The goal of rational drug treatment is to maximize benefits and to minimize harm. Despite the fact that we are not yet adequately able to predict drug effect and determine which treatment to use based on the patient's genetic characteristics, physicians should base their treatment plan on their clinical judgment, keeping in mind that a particular individual interacts with his or her environment and can have phenotypic characteristics that might be different from genotype-based predictions.

In conclusion, the pharmacogenomic tools currently at our disposition (i.e., genetics chips, etc.) are—and even more so in the future—very useful for developing better individualized therapies, especially for ethnic groups.

References

1 Bhopal R. Glossary of terms relating to ethnicity and race: for reflection and debate. *Journal of Epidemiology and Community Health* 2004; **58**: 441–445.

2 McKenzie K, Crowcroft NS. Describing race, ethnicity, and culture in medical research. *BMJ* 1996; **31**: 1054.

3 Prevalence of heart disease: United States, 2005. *Morbidity and Mortality Weekly Report* 2007; **56**: 113–118.

4 Cappuccio FP. Commentary: epidemiological transition, migration, and cardiovascular disease. *International Journal of Epidemiology* 2004; **33**: 387–388.

5 Munoz C, Hilgenberg C. Ethnopharmacology: understanding how ethnicity can affect drug response is essential to providing culturally competent care. *Holistic Nursing Practice* 2006; **20**: 227–234.

6 Burroughs VJ, Maxey RW, Levy RA. Racial and ethnic differences in response to medicines: towards individualized pharmaceutical treatment. *Journal of the National Medical Association* 2002; **94** (10 Suppl): 1–26.

7 Chen Z, Boreham J. Smoking and cardiovascular disease. *Seminars in Vascular Medicine* 2002; **2**: 243–252.

8 Evans M, Lewis GM. Increase in international normalized ratio after smoking cessation in a patient receiving warfarin. *Pharmacotherapy* 2005; **25**: 1656–1659.

9 Kuykendall JR, Houle MD, Rhodes RS. Possible warfarin failure due to interaction with smokeless tobacco. *The Annals of Pharmacotherapy* 2004; **38**: 595–597.

10 Tobacco use among adults: United States, 2005. *Morbidity and Mortality Weekly Report* 2006; **55**: 1145–1148.

11 DiPiro JT. *Pharmacotherapy : a Pathophysiologic Approach*, 6th edn. McGraw-Hill, New York, 2005.

12 Sotaniemi EA, Anttila M, Rautio A *et al.* Propranolol and sotalol metabolism after a drinking party. *Clinical Pharmacology and Therapeutics* 1981; **29**: 705–710.

13 Caetano R, Clark CL, Tam T. Alcohol consumption among racial/ethnic minorities: theory and research. *Alcohol Health and Research World* 1998; **22**: 233–241.

14 Bosworth HB, Dudley T, Olsen MK *et al.* Racial differences in blood pressure control: potential explanatory factors. *The American Journal of Medicine* 2006; **119**: e9–15.

15 Labbe L, Turgeon J. Clinical pharmacokinetics of mexiletine. *Clinical Pharmacokinetics* 1999; **37**: 361–384.

16 Rendic S, Di Carlo FJ. Human cytochrome P450 enzymes: a status report summarizing their reactions, substrates, inducers, and inhibitors. *Drug Metabolism Reviews* 1997; **29**: 413–580.

17 Robertson JG. Mechanistic basis of enzyme-targeted drugs. *Biochemistry* 2005; **44**: 5561–5571.

18 Engen RM, Marsh S, Van Booven DJ, McLeod HL. Ethnic differences in pharmacogenetically relevant genes. *Current Drug Targets* 2006; **7**: 1641–1648.

19 Bertilsson L. Geographical/interracial differences in polymorphic drug oxidation. Current state of knowledge of cytochromes P450 (CYP) 2D6 and 2C19. *Clinical Pharmacokinetics* 1995; **29**: 192–209.

20 Jann MW, Cohen LJ. The influence of ethnicity and antidepressant pharmacogenetics in the treatment of depression. *Drug Metabolism and Drug Interactions* 2000; **16**: 39–67.

21 Meyer UA. Pharmacogenetics: the slow, the rapid, and the ultrarapid. *Proceedings of the National Academy of Sciences of the USA* 1994; **91**: 1983–1984.

22 Ingelman-Sundberg M. Genetic polymorphisms of cytochrome P450 2D6 (CYP2D6): clinical consequences, evolutionary aspects and functional diversity. *Pharmacogenomics Journal* 2005; **5**: 6–13.

23 Bernard S, Neville KA, Nguyen AT, Flockhart DA. Interethnic differences in genetic polymorphisms of CYP2D6 in the U.S. population: clinical implications. *Oncologist* 2006; **11**: 126–135.

24 Mialet-Perez J, Liggett SB. Pharmacogenetics of beta1-adrenergic receptors in heart failure and hypertension. *Archives des Maladies du Coeur et des Vaisseaux* 2006; **99**: 616–620.

25 Poolsup N, Li Wan Po A, Knight TL. Pharmacogenetics and psychopharmacotherapy. *Journal of Clinical Pharmacy and Therapeutics* 2000; **25**: 197–220.

26 Masoudi FA, Rathore SS, Wang Y *et al.* National patterns of use and effectiveness of angiotensin-converting enzyme inhibitors in older patients with heart failure and left ventricular systolic dysfunction. *Circulation* 2004; **110**: 724–731.

27 Haas M, Yilmaz N, Schmidt A *et al.* Angiotensin-converting enzyme gene polymorphism determines the antiproteinuric and systemic hemodynamic effect of enalapril in patients with proteinuric renal disease. Austrian Study Group of the Effects of Enalapril Treatment in Proteinuric Renal Disease. *Kidney and Blood Pressure Research* 1998; **21**: 66–69.

28 Rigat B, Hubert C, Alhenc-Gelas F *et al.* An insertion/deletion polymorphism in the angiotensin I-converting enzyme gene accounting for half the variance of serum enzyme levels. *The Journal of Clinical Investigation* 1990; **86**: 1343–1346.

29 Costa-Scharplatz M, van Asselt AD, Bachmann LM *et al.* Cost-effectiveness of pharmacogenetic testing to predict treatment response to angiotensin-converting enzyme inhibitor. *Pharmacogenetics and Genomics* 2007; **17**: 359–368.

30 Scharplatz M, Puhan MA, Steurer J *et al.* Does the angiotensin-converting enzyme (ACE) gene insertion/deletion polymorphism modify the response to ACE inhibitor therapy? A systematic review. *Current Controlled Trials in Cardiovascular Medicine* 2005; **6**: 16.

31 Saunders E, Weir MR, Kong BW *et al.* A comparison of the efficacy and safety of a beta-blocker, a calcium channel blocker, and a converting enzyme inhibitor in hypertensive blacks. *Archives of Internal Medicine* 1990; **150**: 1707–1713.

32 Cushman WC, Reda DJ, Perry HM *et al.* Regional and racial differences in response to antihypertensive medication use in a randomized controlled trial of men with hypertension in the United States. Department of Veterans Affairs Cooperative Study Group on Antihypertensive Agents. *Archives of Internal Medicine* 2000; **160**: 825–831.

33 Richardson AD, Piepho RW. Effect of race on hypertension and antihypertensive therapy. *International Journal of Clinical Pharmacology and Therapeutics* 2000; **38**: 75–79.

34 Abdelhafiz AH. A review of anticoagulation with warfarin in patients with nonvalvular atrial fibrillation. *Clinical Therapeutics* 2001; **23**: 1628–1636.

35 Aithal GP, Day CP, Kesteven PJ, Daly AK. Association of polymorphisms in the cytochrome P450 CYP2C9 with warfarin dose requirement and risk of bleeding complications. *Lancet* 1999; **353**: 717–719.

36 Taube J, Halsall D, Baglin T. Influence of cytochrome P-450 CYP2C9 polymorphisms on warfarin sensitivity and risk of over-anticoagulation in patients on long-term treatment. *Blood* 2000; **96**: 1816–1819.

37 Wingard LB, Jr, O'Reilly RA, Levy G. Pharmacokinetics of warfarin enantiomers: a search for intrasubject correlations. *Clinical Pharmacology and Therapeutics* 1978; **23**: 212–217.

38 Sullivan-Klose TH, Ghanayem BI, Bell DA *et al.* The role of the CYP2C9-Leu359 allelic variant in the tolbutamide polymorphism. *Pharmacogenetics* 1996; **6**: 341–349.
39 Dickmann LJ, Rettie AE, Kneller MB *et al.* Identification and functional characterization of a new CYP2C9 variant (CYP2C9*5) expressed among African Americans. *Molecular Pharmacology* 2001; **60**: 382–387.
40 Kidd RS, Curry TB, Gallagher S *et al.* Identification of a null allele of CYP2C9 in an African-American exhibiting toxicity to phenytoin. *Pharmacogenetics* 2001; **11**: 803–808.
41 Tai G, Farin F, Rieder MJ *et al.* In-vitro and in-vivo effects of the CYP2C9*11 polymorphism on warfarin metabolism and dose. *Pharmacogenetics and Genomics* 2005; **15**: 475–481.
42 Linder MW, Looney S, Adams JE, 3rd *et al.* Warfarin dose adjustments based on CYP2C9 genetic polymorphisms. *Journal of Thrombosis and Thrombolysis* 2002; **14**: 227–232.
43 Lee CR, Goldstein JA, Pieper JA. Cytochrome P450 2C9 polymorphisms: a comprehensive review of the in-vitro and human data. *Pharmacogenetics* 2002; **12**: 251–263.
44 Rieder MJ, Reiner AP, Gage BF *et al.* Effect of VKORC1 haplotypes on transcriptional regulation and warfarin dose. *The New England Journal of Medicine* 2005; **352**: 2285–2293.
45 Takahashi H, Wilkinson GR, Nutescu EA *et al.* Different contributions of polymorphisms in VKORC1 and CYP2C9 to intra- and inter-population differences in maintenance dose of warfarin in Japanese, Caucasians and African-Americans. *Pharmacogenetics and Genomics* 2006; **16**: 101–110.
46 Lee SC, Ng SS, Oldenburg J *et al.* Interethnic variability of warfarin maintenance requirement is explained by VKORC1 genotype in an Asian population. *Clinical Pharmacology and Therapeutics* 2006; **79**: 197–205.
47 Yin T, Miyata T. Warfarin dose and the pharmacogenomics of CYP2C9 and VKORC1: rationale and perspectives. *Thrombosis Research* 2007; **120**: 1–10.
48 Sconce EA, Khan TI, Wynne HA *et al.* The impact of CYP2C9 and VKORC1 genetic polymorphism and patient characteristics upon warfarin dose requirements: proposal for a new dosing regimen. *Blood* 2005; **106**: 2329–2333.
49 McDowell SE, Coleman JJ, Ferner RE. Systematic review and meta-analysis of ethnic differences in risks of adverse reactions to drugs used in cardiovascular medicine. *BMJ* 2006; **332**: 1177–1181.
50 Hunt SA, Baker DW, Chin MH *et al.* ACC/AHA Guidelines for the Evaluation and Management of Chronic Heart Failure in the Adult: Executive Summary. A Report of the American College of Cardiology/American Heart Association Task Force on Practice Guidelines (Committee to Revise the 1995 Guidelines for the Evaluation and Management of Heart Failure): Developed in Collaboration with the International Society for Heart and Lung Transplantation; Endorsed by the Heart Failure Society of America. *Circulation* 2001; **104**: 2996–30007.
51 Evans W, Johnson J. PHARMOCOGENOMICS: The Inherited Basis for Interindividual Differences in Drug Response. *Annual Review of Genomics and Human Genetics* 2001; **2**: 9–39.
52 Materson BJ. Variability in response to antihypertensive drugs. *The American Journal of Medicine* 2007; **120** (4 Suppl 1): S10–20.

Chapter 4

Genetic testing: moving to the bedside—when and how?

Jacqueline S. Danik and Paul M. Ridker

Introduction

An ideal genetic test for clinical purposes would have 100% sensitivity and specificity, identify a genetic disorder that is highly penetrable but easily treated, and provide information that could not otherwise have been obtained in usual practice. Unfortunately, few genetic tests have these characteristics. Much more commonly, the presence of a particular genetic polymorphism or haplotype pattern is associated with only a modest increase in risk of developing a given disease, having a specific biochemical abnormality, or a differential response to a therapeutic agent. This is particularly true for complex cardiovascular disorders where large gene–environment interactions are known to exist and where behavioral interventions have proven highly effective at lowering patient risk and in secondary prevention.

Nonetheless, genetic tests are having an increasingly important clinical role for cardiovascular practice and questions from patients and their families regarding genetic predisposition are common. Both commercial and academic medical centers now provide an array of genetic tests that have a potential role in cardiovascular management, some of which are commonly ordered (such as factor V Leiden among those with a history of recurrent or idiopathic venous thrombosis) as well as those more selectively used in certain high-risk settings (such as screening for long QT syndrome). Other uses of genetic testing have been advocated, but their utility in clinical practice remains controversial (such as screening for several polymorphisms known to be associated with warfarin metabolism). To demonstrate the complexity and speed with which

Cardiovascular Genetics and Genomics. Edited by Dan Roden. © 2009 American Heart Association, ISBN: 978-14051-7540-1.

choices for genetic testing have become available, a representative listing of genetic tests related to cardiovascular diseases that are available to physicians at the Brigham and Women's Hospital in Boston, MA, is provided in Table 4.1.

In other chapters of this text, core ethical, legal, and social issues surrounding clinical genetic testing are described, as is the need for genetic counseling both before and after test results are available. By contrast, the goal of this chapter is to begin addressing how and when genetic testing should be considered for individual cardiovascular patients, and to touch on the minimum criteria needed for a genetic test to move to the bedside.

To accomplish this, genetic tests for four cardiovascular conditions – venous thromboembolism, long QT syndrome (LQTS), hypertrophic cardiomyopathy (HCM), and warfarin initiation—will be used to illustrate several questions that should be asked before considering genetic testing for individual patients: What is the prevalence of the genetic risk factor in the population being screened? What is the magnitude of risk associated with the genetic test? How reliable is the genetic test itself, and have putative associations been confirmed in diverse patient groups? And, most importantly, how might my behavior as a physician or the behavior of my patient change based on the knowledge of a given genotype?

Using these four conditions, we hope to illustrate both the benefits and potential hazards that can come from genetic testing. At the same time we hope to illustrate the potential for a future where we believe better understanding will lead to second-generation genetic tests that not only will be useful for diagnosis but also will allow us to avoid toxicities and greatly improve therapeutic benefits for our patients.

Venous thromboembolism and the genetics of hypercoagulable states

After myocardial infarction, stroke, and heart failure, venous thrombosis and pulmonary embolism are the most common causes of cardiovascular hospitalization in the USA. As early as 1856, Rudolf Virchow recognized that venous thrombosis had a heritable component as his triad of risk factors for thromboembolism included not only local trauma and stasis but also hypercoagulability [1]. The translation of this work to genetics initially focused on rare disorders such as deficiencies of antithrombin III, protein C, or protein S. However, with the descriptions of factor V Leiden [2–5] as well as a G20210A [6] single point mutation in the prothrombin gene, genetic testing for hypercoagulability now involves consideration of two common polymorphisms.

Factor V Leiden (FVL) has a prevalence of between 5 % and 7% among whites in the USA, but is much less prevalent in African Americans and Asian Americans [7,8], groups that also have lower relative risks of developing venous thromboembolism. Heterozygous carriers of factor V Leiden have a condition characterized by activated protein C resistance, a blunted partial thromboplastin time (PTT) prolongation, and a marked hereditary predisposition to idiopathic venous thrombosis. In general, the risk of venous thrombosis increases three- to fivefold among carriers [3,4,9–12], and by eightfold among women who are also taking oral contraceptives [13]. These latter data demonstrate the importance of gene–environment interactions for this disorder.

In general, FVL has been found in 20–50% of patients with documented venous thrombosis [3,14], and estimates of the annual incidence of venous thrombosis among heterozygous carriers for FVL range from 0.19% to 0.58%, suggesting a lifetime risk of 12–30% [15–17]. Not surprisingly, risks are even higher for those rare individuals who are homozygous carriers of the FVL mutation. By contrast, the G20210A prothrombin mutation has a prevalence between 1% and 3% in the USA and confers an approximate doubling of risk [18–22]. Although both of these polymorphisms increase risk of venous thrombosis, neither appears to substantially affect arterial thrombosis.

The fact that a gene is prevalent, penetrant, and highly associated with a disease state does not, however, imply that broad screening is necessarily a clinically effective approach. For example, with regard to FVL, broad screening is not recommended as the absolute risk of venous thromboembolism in the general population is low [23]. Even in analyses limited to young women in whom one might wish to avoid oral contraception among known FVL carriers, it has been suggested that the number of thrombotic events caused by proactively withholding oral contraception and thus leading to unwanted pregnancy might well be greater than the number of venous thromboses avoided. Thus, for the general population, a careful family history remains the most cost-effective method for identifying those at heightened thromboembolic risk.

On the other hand, screening for FVL and the G20210A prothrombin mutation are often done among those with a personal or family history of venous thromboembolism. In this setting, efficiency is greatly increased, particularly when the index event is idiopathic (i.e., not associated with surgery or trauma) [23]. Among those found to carry either of these mutations, recommendations to avoid prolonged immobility and consider long-term prophylaxis are often made. In practice, it is generally more efficient to screen for FVL than to evaluate plasma for activated protein C resistance, especially since the latter cannot be done in patients taking anticoagulation.

Despite the consistency of data regarding hypercoagulable risk on a genetic basis, there remains substantial controversy about whether or not screening has a net clinical utility [15,24,25]. A cogent argument can be made that all patients with a history of idiopathic venous thromboembolism should avoid periods of prolonged stasis, and that all women with a personal history of venous thrombosis should elect an alternative method of birth control, whether or not they carry FVL or the G20210A prothrombin mutation. There is also little evidence that either of these genetic polymorphisms substantially increases the risk of recurrence when the initial event was secondary to surgery or trauma.

Last, it remains highly controversial as to whether those with FVL or the G20210A prothrombin mutation require more prolonged anticoagulation to prevent recurrent disease [24]. In the National Institutes of Health-funded Prevention of Recurrent Thromboembolism (PREVENT) trial [26], long-term low-intensity warfarin [international normalized ratio (INR) 1.5–2.0] was highly effective at preventing recurrent events, regardless of genetic status. Specifically, among genetically affected individuals, low-intensity warfarin reduced the rate of recurrent venous thromboembolism by 75%, a reduction that was not statistically different from that observed among noncarriers (58%) or for the study population as a whole (64%).

Thus, while evaluation of FVL and the G20210A prothrombin mutation are often done in clinical practice—and while these defects are both common and clearly associated with increased risk—the impact on clinical decision-making is typically modest in most situations.

Long QT syndrome

LQTS is an inherited disorder associated with life-threatening ventricular arrhythmias. Although rare in the general population, those with documented syncope or fainting who are found to have LQTS represent a group with significantly high lifetime risk for sudden death. There are two major forms of LQTS, one transmitted as an autosomal dominant trait (Romano–Ward syndrome) and one transmitted as an autosomal recessive disease that is also associated with deafness (Jervell and Lange-Nielsen syndrome).

Clinical diagnosis of LQTS can be complex and typically includes the finding of prolonged corrected QT interval on electrocardiograms in asymptomatic individuals or in individuals after an event such as syncope. Clinical criteria for diagnosis include the Schwartz score [27], which uses factors such as family history of long QT syndrome, corrected QTc interval on ECG, and clinical history of syncope for diagnosis. The severity of the clinical manifestations of LQTS vary widely; at one end of the spectrum are patients with borderline QT prolongation and no history of syncope or arrhythmia, whereas others come from families with a clear history of sudden death in multiple generations. Thus, LQTS represents a diffuse group of disorders in which risk stratification is a crucial step for management, and one in which genetics can play a major role.

LQTS can arise as a result of mutations in multiple genes that encode structural units of ion channels. Mutations in the potassium channel and sodium channel genes are the most common causes of LQTS [28,29]. In Romano–Ward LQTS, for example, screening of five LQTS genes—*KCNQ1*, *KCNE1*, *KCNE2*, *KCNH2*, and *SCN5A*—allows identification of the genetic defect in 50–70%

of affected individuals [30]. The recessive form of LQTS (Jervell and Lange-Nielsen disease) associates with homozygous or compound heterozygous mutations in two genes, *KCNQ1* and *KCNE1*, that characterize at least 80% of cases [30]. Private, uncommon mutations may also appear and be causal within specific families. When potentially causal genes are relatively few and of normal size, sequencing is feasible. Sequencing is performed of exons and splice sites believed to constitute the coding regions of implicated genes rather than assays for single point mutations, because different mutations within the same gene can lead to the same disease (alleleic heterogeneity). If a causal mutation is found, then "cascade" screening of other family members for that mutation is relatively easy. The implication of a sequencing approach is the need for common polymorphisms within the genes to be known, to avoid falsely positive diagnoses.

For patients suspected of having LQTS, genetic testing serves multiple roles. First, genetic testing often can clarify a heterogeneous or misdiagnosed phenotype. A high proportion of patients (up to 40%) may be misdiagnosed with the LQTS phenotype by cardiologists based on clinical criteria alone [31], resulting in significant morbidity such as unnecessary automatic defibrillator implantation, profound lifestyle changes, and high anxiety for patients and families [32].

Second, clinical studies have shown that the addition of genetic testing for the most common LQTS genes can greatly help to confirm clinical diagnoses. In one study of patients considered to have "definite" LQTS by clinicians, a LQTS-causing mutation was identified in 78% of the patients with LQTS who underwent genetic testing, with LQT1 and LQT2 genotypes being the most common [31]. By contrast, LQTS-causing genes were identified among 34% of those considered to have "probable" LQTS, and in none of those classified as "unlikely" LQTS. Clinical diagnosis, not surprisingly, significantly increases pretest probability for disease and the positive predictive value of a test. Thus, it has been suggested that genetic diagnosis can address prognosis [33], impact on risk stratification [29], and selection of therapy [34], and can be useful for the prevention of factors that precipitate arrhythmias [35].

Genetic testing has also led to a better understanding of the triggers for arrhythmic events. As specific examples, those with LQT1 tend to have an increased risk of lethal arrhythmia during physical or emotional stress, whereas those with LQT3 have most of their events while asleep [35]. Interestingly, clinical work suggests that almost all cardiac events that occur while swimming in LQTS patients do so among those with LQT1 [36], whereas auditory stimuli are typically involved for those with LQT2 [37]. However, there can be incomplete penetrance and highly variable clinical presentations, even among individuals carrying the same mutations [38].

Therapy for LQTS typically includes beta-blockade and, in patients with documented lethal arrhythmias, implantation of a defibrillator device. Over the past several years there has been discussion about the concept of "gene-specific" therapy for patients with LQTS, in part owing to small studies suggesting that, in contrast to those with LQT1 and LQT2, those with LQT3 may have less benefit from this approach [29]. Such data, however, are not conclusive because of the small number of families affected. Because different forms of LQTS are due to different ion channel effects, it is also possible that different therapeutic approaches are needed. Among those with LQT2, it has been proposed that increasing potassium concentration might have greater benefit [39]. Ongoing clinical trials are being conducted to address whether or not genetic differences in etiology merit different therapeutic choices.

While genotyping for LQTS has a clear clinical role in cardiovascular practice, an important issue to remember is that genotyping of the best-known causal genes is not comprehensive. It has been estimated that about 30% of genes or location of gene mutations have not yet been identified for LQTS. Thus, it is appropriate to consider the genetic basis of even this most studied of Mendelian diseases to be in its infancy.

Hypertrophic cardiomyopathy

HCM is a condition typically characterized by inappropriate myocardial hypertrophy, often but not always involving the interventricular septum, that appears in the absence of other causes such as systemic hypertension or aortic stenosis. Classically, the distinctive feature of patients with HCM has been considered the presence of a dynamic outflow tract obstruction leading to an intracavitary pressure gradient. However, as is now well understood, the phenotypic expression of HCM varies greatly and less than one-fourth of all affected individuals share these classic hemodynamic findings [40–42].

Histologic changes in HCM are more consistent and usually include marked myocyte cellular disarray. While the majority of patients with HCM are asymptomatic, the first clinical expression of disease is often sudden death, which can occur at young age. Thus, a high index of suspicion is needed in clinical practice when there is a personal or family history of pre-syncope, frank syncope, or sudden death, or when abnormalities are found on echocardiogram suggestive of unexplained left ventricular hypertrophy, whether segmental or not. While the pathologic abnormalities of HCM can lead to hemodynamic collapse or ischemic complications, the most common problems stem from ventricular tachycardia and fibrillation.

From a genetic perspective, familial HCM is an excellent example of an autosomal dominant disease with substantial genetic and phenotypic heterogeneity. The same genotypes can have varied features such as the age of presentation, the extent of septal hypertrophy, outflow obstruction, and propensity towards arrhythmias or sudden death.

The first report of a genetic basis for HCM came from Seidman, Seidman and colleagues [43], who first mapped a gene for familial hypertrophic cardiomyopathy to chromosome 14q1, then to chromosome 14q11–12 [44], and subsequently reported a beta-cardiac myosin heavy chain gene missense mutation [44]. Since that initial description, several hundred mutations within 19 genes that encode components of the sarcomere, including the cardiac beta- and alpha-myosin heavy chains, cardiac troponins T, I, and C, cardiac myosin binding protein C, and α-tropomyosin have been identified among affected individuals [43,45]. Thus, as was the case for LQTS, initial hopes that a small set of common polymorphisms could be used to screen for most cases of HCM is unlikely. Rather, a diverse set of genic pathways that commonly involve sarcomere structure and function seem to result in similar clinical phenotypes.

Some have suggested that sequencing of the reading frames of the most commonly implicated HCM genes such as *MYH7, MYBPC3, TNN13, TNNT2, MYL2, MYL3, TPM1, ACTC,* and *TNNC1*, may identify genetic variants in over 60% of patients with HCM. In particular, more than 80% may carry mutations in the *MYH7* and *MYBPC3* genes [46–48]. However, sequencing such a number of genes is not trivial, even with the current advances in technology. Thus, as with LQTS, high clinical suspicion in conjunction with genetic data contribute to diagnosis. Increased pretest probability of disease in family members with high-risk clinical features helps to improve testing. Alternatively, if broad population screening were performed, there would be a low negative predictive value of the genetic tests.

Given this situation, questions have arisen as to whether or not evaluation for specific HCM mutations provides clinically important information for management. Carriers of troponin T mutations, for example, may have an increased risk of sudden cardiac death, even in the absence of significant left ventricular hypertrophy [45]. Carriers of specific mutations in *MYBPC3* mutations may have higher incidence of sudden cardiac death and later onset of disease than noncarriers [49]. Different mutations within the same gene, furthermore, may confer more adverse prognosis (R403Q, R719W, and R453C mutations within *MHY7*) than others (V1606M, L908V, G256Q, and P513C in *MHY7*) [50–52].

Thus, while it is possible that genetics in addition to high-risk clinical features such as syncope and profound septal hypertrophy may guide clinical decisions [53–55], consistent clinical studies are needed to address this hypothesis and to evaluate impact on clinical care. Genetic studies of patients with HCM may in the future become useful for determining whether or not to perform echocardiography in asymptomatic children found to be mutation positive, whether to prophylactically place implantable defibrillators or whether there are differential gene-specific responses to therapy. At this time, however, there remain substantial technical challenges as well as expense associated with HCM genetic screening that are likely to keep this approach from becoming routine. As with factor V Leiden and with LQTS, a careful history and physical examination remain of great importance for both the diagnosis and screening of those at risk for HCM. Almost half of those with idiopathic HCM observable on echocardiograms within the left ventricle have affected first-degree relatives, and thus, despite phenotypic heterogeneity, echocardiography has been widely applied for familial screening.

Warfarin initiation

A fourth clinical arena in which genetic screening has been proposed is the management and initiation of patients taking warfarin therapy. Since its introduction over 50 years ago, more than 20 million prescriptions have been written for warfarin in the USA [56] and this form of anticoagulation is standard care for those with atrial fibrillation or mechanical heart valves, and for prophylaxis and treatment of venous thromboembolism. However, warfarin has a relatively narrow toxic-to-therapeutic ratio and both hemorrhagic and thrombotic complications remain a substantial problem.

Several clinical factors are involved in selecting the appropriate warfarin dose including age, liver function, ethnicity, and obesity. However, most clinicians follow a standard dosing monogram for warfarin initiation, an approach that has not shown great efficacy. For this reason, there has been considerable discussion about using genetic polymorphisms that are known to affect warfarin metabolism as a novel method to select warfarin dose.

Broadly, two sets of genes appear to have potential efficacy for this purpose. The first are those involved in the cytochrome P450 system that partly controls warfarin metabolism. While the human cytochrome P450 (CYP) system comprises more than 50 separate genes, *CYP2C9* is largely responsible for metabolism of the *S*-warfarin enantiomer and within that gene two variants (*CYP2C9*2* and *CYP2C9*3*) differ from the wild-type *CYP2C9*1* by a single amino acid substitution that results in impaired hydoxylation of warfarin. To date, multiple clinical studies have shown that these polymorphisms are associated with increased risk during anticoagulation and that they may have utility in predicting warfarin dosing [57–59].

The second gene set understood to be involved in warfarin metabolism are those of the vitamin K epoxide reductase complex (*VKORC1*) [60,61]. In the general population, five haplotypes have been constructed within this gene set and it has been shown that two of these haplotypes (A and B) can also be used to determine warfarin dosing [62]. For example, AA individuals appear to require less daily warfarin on average (3 mg) than do AB individuals (4 mg) or BB individuals (6 mg). Clinical studies suggest that these polymorphisms are responsible for approximately 20–25% of the variance in warfarin dosing.

Not surprisingly, clinical genetic tests for both *CYP2C9*1/2/3* and for *VCOKC1* have rapidly become available and are being promoted for clinical use. It is unclear, however, how such information would truly change practice. Much of the alleleic variance in these genes is on an ethnic basis, so clinical algorithms that simply take into account ethnicity may also improve selection of warfarin dose. Further, since measurement of the INR is unlikely to be replaced in clinical practice because there remains wide variation in response that goes well beyond these genes, it is not clear that such an approach would reduce warfarin monitoring nor necessarily lead to more rapid achievement of steady-state dosing. Perhaps of greatest importance, a major clinical problem of warfarin therapy is the risk of bleeding long after stable therapy has been initiated, and it is uncertain how knowledge of genotype would impact upon this risk. For this reason, clinical studies are being designed that seek to address whether or not clinical outcomes will be improved with knowledge of this genetic information [63]. The best designed of these studies will compare genetic-based warfarin dosing with dosing based on clinical factors already known to influence warfarin, including ethnicity.

Other diseases in which genotyping can be considered

As these four examples demonstrate, how and when to consider using genetic tests is uncertain even when there are clear links between the genetic information and risk of disease or complications of therapy. It is not surprising then that these decisions are even more complex in other cardiovascular settings such as those selected below.

Dilated cardiomyopathy

Dilated cardiomyopathy (DCM) is the final result of multiple pathways, but some idiopathic cardiomyopathies appear to have a genetic basis. Understanding the genetics of DCM began when DCM was found to be a feature of Duchenne and Becker muscular dystrophies. Most genes implicated since then have been associated with cardiomyopathy in the context of skeletal myopathies. Only a small proportion of idiopathic DCM is due to known genes thus far [64]. Mutations in the dystrophic muscle-promoter region [65], the lamin A/C gene [66], and six sarcomeric genes previously known to cause HCM have been implicated in different types of DCM. Clinically recognized syndromes of skeletal myopathies and conduction defects may prompt genotyping.

However, there is as yet insufficient replication of these data in large cohorts to have wide impact on treatment or clinical decision-making. Overestimation of penetrance can be anticipated in initial studies that emerge from referral centers because patients with the most severe phenotypic expressions will self-refer for further testing and specialized care. Nonetheless, genotyping can be performed on the most commonly implicated genes which typically include a panel for genes *MYBPC3*, *MYH7*, *TNNT2*, *TNNI3*, and *TPM1* and a panel for genes *ACTC*, *LDB3*, *PLN*, *LMNA*, and *TAZ* (Table 4.1).

Table 4.1 Genetic tests related to cardiovascular diseases available to physicians at the Brigham and Women's Hospital

Disease	Genes tested*
Hypertrophic cardiomyopathy	Panel A (*MYBPC3, MYH7, TNNT2, TNNI3, TPM1* sequencing[†])
	Panel B (*ACTC, MYL2, MYL3* sequencing)
Unexplained cardiac hypertrophy	*PRKAG2* and *LAMP2* sequencing
Dilated cardiomyopathy	Panel A (*MYBPC3, MYH7, TNNT2, TNNI3, TPM1* sequencing)
	Panel B (*ACTC, LDB3, PLN, LMNA* and *TAZ* sequencing)
Arrhythmogenic right ventricular dysplasia	*DSP, DSG2, DSC2* and *PKP2* sequencing
Fabry disease	*GLA* sequencing
Familial amyloidosis	*TTR* sequencing
Marfan and Loeys–Dietz syndromes	*FBN1, TGFBR1, TGFBR2* sequencing
Noonan syndrome	*PTPN11, SOS1, KRAS* sequencing
LEOPARD syndrome	*PTPN11* sequencing
Cardio-facio-cutaneous syndrome	*BRAF* and *KRAS* sequencing
Costello syndrome	*HRAS* sequencing
Warfarin metabolism	*VKORC1* at 16p11.2[‡]
	CYP2C9 at 10q24
Venous thromboembolism	Factor V G1691A Leiden mutation[‡]
	Prothrombin gene G20210A mutation
Long QT syndrome	
Romano–Ward Syndrome	*KCNQ1, KCNE1, KCNE2, KCNH2, SCN5A* sequencing
Jervell and Lange-Nielsen syndrome	*KCNQ1, KCNE1* sequencing

*Laboratories that offer specific tests can be found at www.genetests.com.

[†]Sequencing of exons and splice sites believed to comprise the coding regions of the gene is usually performed.

[‡]Allele states at specific point locations are assessed rather than sequencing within genes. For warfarin metabolism, Third Wave Invader reagents are used to identify the allele state for *CYP2C9* (*1, *2, *3) and *VKORC1* (haplotype A or haplotype B). With the Factor V Leiden and the Prothrombin G20210A gene mutations, hybridization-based assays are often used (Third Wave Invader assay, Madison, WI, USA).

Arrhythmogenic right ventricular dysplasia/cardiomyopathy

Arrhythmogenic right ventricular dysplasia/cardiomyopathy (ARVD/C) is an autosomal dominant condition with variable expression, in which the right, and sometimes the left, ventricle is involved with thinning and replacement of the myocardium by fat and fibrosis. At least five genes have been implicated in ARVD, including plakoglobin (*JUP*), desmoplakin (*DSP*), plakophilin-2 (*PKP2*), desmoglein-2 (*DSG2*), and desmocollin-2 (*DSC2*). These are different components of the desmosome junction complex involved in the tensile strength and resilience of the epithelium. Functional mutations within this complex may result in myocyte detachment and death, and subsequent replacement with fiber and fat [67]. While *PKP2* mutations may account for 25% of patients with disease [68,69], multiple replication and clinical studies have yet to be done. Tests that will soon be available at BWH include *DSP*, *DSG2*, *DSC2*, and *PKP2*.

Other arrhythmogenic disorders

Other diseases relevant to cardiovascular disease include catecholaminergic polymorphic ventricular tachycardia, in which screening of two genes, *RYR2* and *CASQ2*, may be able to identify mutations in many patients with the disease. The exact percentage of variance explained remains to be investigated. Furthermore, *RYR2*, because of its large size, is difficult to assay.

Another disease is the Brugada syndrome, which is characterized by right bundle branch block and ST segment elevation in leads V1–V3, and potentially sudden death. The only gene associated with this phenotype so far has been the gene encoding for the cardiac sodium channel (*SCN5A*) [70].

Caution in genetic screening for complex cardiovascular diseases: the problem of atherothrombosis

Thus far we have considered disorders that largely follow a Mendelian pattern of inheritance and have shown that, even in these cases, clinical decision-making is complex and that clinical application is at best in the earliest stages. Most cardiovascular conditions, however, are not the result of single or polygenic disorders, but are highly complex involving many genes across multiple pathways, each intimately interacting with environmental factors. Such is the case for atherothrombosis, the underlying cause of most cases of myocardial infarction, stroke, and congestive heart failure.

From a research perspective, it is clear that family history of premature atherothrombosis is an important risk factor for coronary disease and stroke. In both the Framingham Heart Study [71] and in the recently presented Reynolds Risk Score [72], the presence of a parental history of myocardial infarction before age 60 has been shown to approximately double the relative risk of atherothrombotic disease in offspring. It is widely recognized, however, that families share environments as well as genes, and that common patterns of diet, exercise, and smoking are also often passed from one generation to the next.

Despite these concerns, the past few years have seen success in the initiation of large-scale genome-wide association studies seeking evidence of common allelic risk variants for myocardial infarction and stroke. Recent advances include identification of a locus on chromosome 17 for coronary artery disease [73] and genetic variants in chromosome 9p21 for myocardial infarction [74] and coronary heart disease [75]. Genetic variants in 5-lipoxygenase-activating protein (*ALOX5AP*) [76], complement factor H (*CFH*), toll-like receptor 4 (*TLR4*) [77], lipopolysaccharide receptor CD14 (*CD14*) [78], cyclooxygenase 2 (*COX-2*) [79], and galectin-2, a member of the galactose-binding lectin family (*LGALS2*) [80], are but a few polymorphisms that have been linked to myocardial infarction. In a similar manner, genetic variants in *CDKN2A*, *CDKN2B* [81], *IGF2BP2*, and *CDKAL1* have been linked to type 2 diabetes [81,82], while genes such as *CRP* have been implicated in the degree of inflammation both during the chronic stage of atherosclerosis [83–87] and during acute myocardial infarction [88].

Although exciting at a population level, caution must be exercised when considering any of these observations for individual patients. The contribution of any single common gene variant to complex disease risk is generally small, usually in the range $<1\%$ per single nucleotide polymorphism, much less than the genetic contribution of diseases that follow Mendelian inheritance. Although several commercial entities offer screening for atherothrombotic risk, clinicians should be aware that no unique set of genetic polymorphisms has to date demonstrated any improvement in risk stratification. Equally important, there is little evidence that many of the genes being screened in commercial applications replicate across (or even within) different population samples. At this time, results from both candidate gene studies and genome-wide studies targeting atherothrombosis should be considered hypothesis-generating only and are not ready for clinical application.

That being said, several large-scale studies have been undertaken with the hopes of moving forward a better biologic understanding of complex vascular disease on the basis of genomic findings. These include, among others, the Wellcome Trust Case Control Consortium [89], the Icelandic DeCode projects [74], the Women's Genome Health Study [90–92], and several federally funded cardiovascular studies being done as part of the SHARE and GAIN program which includes genetic data from the Framingham Heart Study. Each of these programs aims to use genome-wide technologies to survey for genetic differences among tens of thousands of individuals, and to use population-based epidemiology to evaluate for crucial gene–gene and gene–environment interactions. Some, such as the Women's Genome Health Study, also have full phenotypic data on plasma-based intermediate phenotypes, whereas others such as the Framingham cohort have imaging-based data on atherosclerotic burden. In an initial report from the Wellcome Trust group [89], several promising gene targets emerged but were not always in gene-coding regions, a finding also found in recent data from the Ottowa Heart and Dallas Heart Studies [75]. Careful coordination between these and other major studies will be required to fully exploit the power of genome-wide analyses.

How, then, do we answer the question of when and how genetic tests can be used for the detection of cardiovascular risk in the general population? We believe the most reasonable approach is to remain conservative for immediate clinical care, but remain open-minded about the future given the speed with which genetic work is advancing in the cardiovascular arena. As genetic tests become increasingly available, multiple questions with regard to direct-to-consumer marketing, costs, ethics, and clinical application will need to be simultaneously addressed. How will appropriate counseling and interpretation of test information occur? Will insurance reimburse the cost of genetic testing? Could tests performed and documented in patients' medical records result in potential genetic discrimination? And, ultimately, how will genetic data affect our ability as physicians to make earlier and better diagnoses, avoid misdiagnoses, and hopefully improve our ability to target therapies toward those at greatest need and away from those with the greatest likelihood of adverse outcomes?

References

1 Virchow R. *Phlogose und Thrombose im GefaBsystem; Gesammelte Abhandlungen zur Wissenschaftlichen Medizin*. Staatsdruckerei, Frankfurt, 1856.

2 Dahlback B, Carlsson M, Svensson PJ. Familial thrombophilia due to a previously unrecognized mechanism characterized by poor anticoagulant response to activated protein C: prediction of a cofactor to activated protein C. *Proceedings of the National Academy of Sciences of the USA* 1993; **90**: 1004–1008.

3 Svensson PJ, Dahlback B. Resistance to activated protein C as a basis for venous thrombosis. *New England Journal of Medicine* 1994; **330**: 517–522.

4 Voorberg J, Roelse J, Koopman R *et al*. Association of idiopathic venous thromboembolism with single point-mutation at Arg506 of factor V. *Lancet* 1994; **343**: 1535–1536.

5 Bertina RM, Koeleman BP, Koster T *et al*. Mutation in blood coagulation factor V associated with resistance to activated protein C. *Nature* 1994; **369**: 64–67.

6 Poort SR, Rosendaal FR, Reitsma PH, Bertina RM. A common genetic variation in the 3′-untranslated region of the prothrombin gene is associated with elevated plasma prothrombin levels and an increase in venous thrombosis. *Blood* 1996; **88**: 3698–3703.

7 Ridker PM, Miletich JP, Hennekens CH, Buring JE. Ethnic distribution of factor V Leiden in 4047 men and women. Implications for venous thromboembolism screening. *JAMA: The Journal of the American Medical Association* 1997; **277**: 1305–1307.

8 Rees DC, Cox M, Clegg JB. World distribution of factor V Leiden. *Lancet* 1995; **346**: 1133–1134.

9 Rosendaal FR. Venous thrombosis: a multicausal disease. *Lancet* 1999; 353: 1167–73.

10 Meyer G, Emmerich J, Helley D *et al*. Factors V leiden and II 20210A in patients with symptomatic pulmonary embolism and deep vein thrombosis. *American Journal of Medicine* 2001; **110**: 12–15.

11 Ridker PM, Hennekens CH, Lindpaintner K *et al.* Mutation in the gene coding for coagulation factor V and the risk of myocardial infarction, stroke, and venous thrombosis in apparently healthy men. *New England Journal of Medicine* 1995; **332**: 912–917.
12 Desmarais S, de Moerloose P, Reber G *et al.* Resistance to activated protein C in an unselected population of patients with pulmonary embolism. *Lancet* 1996; **347**: 1374–1375.
13 Vandenbroucke JP, Koster T, Briet E *et al.* Increased risk of venous thrombosis in oral-contraceptive users who are carriers of factor V Leiden mutation. *Lancet* 1994; **344**: 1453–1457.
14 Koster T, Rosendaal FR, de Ronde H *et al.* Venous thrombosis due to poor anticoagulant response to activated protein C: Leiden Thrombophilia Study. *Lancet* 1993; **342**: 1503–1506.
15 Middeldorp S, Meinardi JR, Koopman MM *et al.* A prospective study of asymptomatic carriers of the factor V Leiden mutation to determine the incidence of venous thromboembolism. *Annals of Internal Medicine* 2001; **135**: 322–327.
16 Simioni P, Sanson BJ, Prandoni P *et al.* Incidence of venous thromboembolism in families with inherited thrombophilia. *Thrombosis and Haemostasis* 1999; **81**: 198–202.
17 Martinelli I, Bucciarelli P, Margaglione M *et al.* The risk of venous thromboembolism in family members with mutations in the genes of factor V or prothrombin or both. *British Journal of Haematology* 2000; **111**: 1223–1229.
18 Ridker PM, Hennekens CH, Miletich JP. G20210A mutation in prothrombin gene and risk of myocardial infarction, stroke, and venous thrombosis in a large cohort of US men. *Circulation* 1999; **99**: 999–1004.
19 Makris M, Preston FE, Beauchamp NJ *et al.* Co-inheritance of the 20210A allele of the prothrombin gene increases the risk of thrombosis in subjects with familial thrombophilia. *Thrombosis and Haemostasis* 1997; **78**: 1426–1429.
20 Arruda VR, Annichino-Bizzacchi JM, Goncalves MS, Costa FF. Prevalence of the prothrombin gene variant (nt20210A) in venous thrombosis and arterial disease. *Thrombosis and Haemostasis* 1997; **78**: 1430–1433.
21 Hillarp A, Zoller B, Svensson PJ, Dahlback B. The 20210 A allele of the prothrombin gene is a common risk factor among Swedish outpatients with verified deep venous thrombosis. *Thrombosis and Haemostasis* 1997; **78**: 990–992.
22 Cumming AM, Keeney S, Salden A *et al.* The prothrombin gene G20210A variant: prevalence in a U.K. anticoagulant clinic population. *British Journal of Haematology* 1997; **98**: 353–355.
23 Grody WW, Griffin JH, Taylor AK *et al.* American College of Medical Genetics consensus statement on factor V Leiden mutation testing. *Genetic Medicine* 2001; **3**: 139–148.
24 Vossen CY, Conard J, Fontcuberta J *et al.* Risk of a first venous thrombotic event in carriers of a familial thrombophilic defect. The European Prospective Cohort on Thrombophilia (EPCOT). *Journal of Thrombosis and Haemostasis* 2005; **3**: 459–464.
25 Simioni P, Tormene D, Prandoni P *et al.* Incidence of venous thromboembolism in asymptomatic family members who are carriers of factor V Leiden: a prospective cohort study. *Blood* 2002; **99**: 1938–1942.
26 Ridker PM, Goldhaber SZ, Danielson E *et al.* Long-term, low-intensity warfarin therapy for the prevention of recurrent venous thromboembolism. *New England Journal of Medicine* 2003; **348**: 1425–1434.

27 Schwartz PJ, Moss AJ, Vincent GM, Crampton RS. Diagnostic criteria for the long QT syndrome. An update. *Circulation* 1993; **88**: 782–784.

28 Splawski I, Shen J, Timothy KW *et al.* Spectrum of mutations in long-QT syndrome genes. KVLQT1, HERG, SCN5A, KCNE1, and KCNE2. *Circulation* 2000; **102**: 1178–1185.

29 Priori SG, Schwartz PJ, Napolitano C *et al.* Risk stratification in the long-QT syndrome. *New England Journal of Medicine* 2003; **348**: 1866–1874.

30 Priori SG, Napolitano C. Role of genetic analyses in cardiology: part I: mendelian diseases: cardiac channelopathies. *Circulation* 2006; **113**: 1130–1135.

31 Taggart NW, Haglund CM, Tester DJ, Ackerman MJ. Diagnostic miscues in congenital long-QT syndrome. *Circulation* 2007; **115**: 2613–2620.

32 Hendriks KS, Grosfeld FJ, van Tintelen JP *et al.* Can parents adjust to the idea that their child is at risk for a sudden death? Psychological impact of risk for long QT syndrome. *American Journal of Medical Genetics A* 2005; **138**: 107–112.

33 Zareba W, Moss AJ, Schwartz PJ *et al.* Influence of genotype on the clinical course of the long-QT syndrome. International Long-QT Syndrome Registry Research Group. *New England Journal of Medicine* 1998; **339**: 960–965.

34 Priori SG, Napolitano C, Schwartz PJ *et al.* Association of long QT syndrome loci and cardiac events among patients treated with beta-blockers. *JAMA: The Journal of the American Medical Association* 2004; **292**: 1341–1344.

35 Schwartz PJ, Priori SG, Spazzolini C *et al.* Genotype-phenotype correlation in the long-QT syndrome: gene-specific triggers for life-threatening arrhythmias. *Circulation* 2001; **103**: 89–95.

36 Ackerman MJ, Tester DJ, Porter CJ. Swimming, a gene-specific arrhythmogenic trigger for inherited long QT syndrome. *Mayo Clinic Proceedings* 1999; **74**: 1088–1094.

37 Wilde AA, Jongbloed RJ, Doevendans PA *et al.* Auditory stimuli as a trigger for arrhythmic events differentiate HERG-related (LQTS2) patients from KVLQT1-related patients (LQTS1). *Journal of the American College of Cardiology* 1999; **33**: 327–332.

38 Roden DM, Spooner PM. Inherited long QT syndromes: a paradigm for understanding arrhythmogenesis. *Journal of Cardiovascular Electrophysiology* 1999; **10**: 1664–1683.

39 Etheridge SP, Compton SJ, Tristani-Firouzi M, Mason JW. A new oral therapy for long QT syndrome: long-term oral potassium improves repolarization in patients with HERG mutations. *Journal of the American College of Cardiology* 2003; **42**: 1777–1182.

40 Maron BJ, Seidman JG, Seidman CE. Proposal for contemporary screening strategies in families with hypertrophic cardiomyopathy. *Journal of the American College of Cardiology* 2004; **44**: 2125–2132.

41 Niimura H, Patton KK, McKenna WJ *et al.* Sarcomere protein gene mutations in hypertrophic cardiomyopathy of the elderly. *Circulation* 2002; **105**: 446–451.

42 Rosenzweig A, Watkins H, Hwang DS *et al.* Preclinical diagnosis of familial hypertrophic cardiomyopathy by genetic analysis of blood lymphocytes. *New England Journal of Medicine* 1991; **325**: 1753–1760.

43 Jarcho JA, McKenna W, Pare JA *et al.* Mapping a gene for familial hypertrophic cardiomyopathy to chromosome 14q1. *New England Journal of Medicine* 1989; **321**: 1372–1378.

44 Solomon SD, Geisterfer-Lowrance AA, Vosberg HP *et al.* A locus for familial hypertrophic cardiomyopathy is closely linked to the cardiac myosin heavy chain genes, CRI-L436, and CRI-L329 on chromosome 14 at q11-q12. *American Journal of Human Genetics* 1990; **47**: 389–394.

45 Watkins H, McKenna WJ, Thierfelder L *et al.* Mutations in the genes for cardiac troponin T and alpha-tropomyosin in hypertrophic cardiomyopathy. *New England Journal of Medicine* 1995; **332**: 1058–1064.

46 Richard P, Charron P, Carrier L *et al.* Hypertrophic cardiomyopathy: distribution of disease genes, spectrum of mutations, and implications for a molecular diagnosis strategy. *Circulation* 2003; **107**: 2227–2232.

47 Fokstuen S, Blouin JL, Lyle R *et al.* [The contribution of molecular genetics to clinical cardiology: the example of hypertrophic cardiomyopathy]. *Revue Médicale Suisse* 2005; **1**: 1448, 1450, 1452–1453.

48 Alders M, Jongbloed R, Deelen W *et al.* The 2373insG mutation in the MYBPC3 gene is a founder mutation, which accounts for nearly one-fourth of the HCM cases in the Netherlands. *European Heart Journal* 2003; **24**: 1848–1853.

49 Niimura H, Bachinski LL, Sangwatanaroj S *et al.* Mutations in the gene for cardiac myosin-binding protein C and late-onset familial hypertrophic cardiomyopathy. *New England Journal of Medicine* 1998; **338**: 1248–1257.

50 Anan R, Greve G, Thierfelder L *et al.* Prognostic implications of novel beta cardiac myosin heavy chain gene mutations that cause familial hypertrophic cardiomyopathy. *Journal of Clinical Investigation* 1994; **93**: 280–285.

51 Watkins H, Rosenzweig A, Hwang DS *et al.* Characteristics and prognostic implications of myosin missense mutations in familial hypertrophic cardiomyopathy. *New England Journal of Medicine* 1992; **326**: 1108–1114.

52 Epstein ND, Cohn GM, Cyran F, Fananapazir L. Differences in clinical expression of hypertrophic cardiomyopathy associated with two distinct mutations in the beta-myosin heavy chain gene. A 908Leu–Val mutation and a 403Arg–Gln mutation. *Circulation* 1992; **86**: 345–352.

53 Maron BJ, Shen WK, Link MS *et al.* Efficacy of implantable cardioverter-defibrillators for the prevention of sudden death in patients with hypertrophic cardiomyopathy. *New England Journal of Medicine* 2000; **342**: 365–373.

54 Havndrup O, Bundgaard H, Andersen PS *et al.* Outcome of clinical versus genetic family screening in hypertrophic cardiomyopathy with focus on cardiac beta-myosin gene mutations. *Cardiovascular Research* 2003; **57**: 347–357.

55 MacRae CA, Ellinor PT. Genetic screening and risk assessment in hypertrophic cardiomyopathy. *Journal of the American College of Cardiology* 2004; **44**: 2326–2328.

56 Marketos M. The top 200 generic drugs in 2003 (by units). *Drug Topics* 2004; **148**: 76.

57 Higashi MK, Veenstra DL, Kondo LM *et al.* Association between CYP2C9 genetic variants and anticoagulation-related outcomes during warfarin therapy. *JAMA: The Journal of the American Medical Association* 2002; **287**: 1690–1698.

58 Rettie AE, Korzekwa KR, Kunze KL *et al.* Hydroxylation of warfarin by human cDNA-expressed cytochrome P-450: a role for P-4502C9 in the etiology of (S)-warfarin-drug interactions. *Chemical Research in Toxicology* 1992; **5**: 54–59.

59 Voora D, Eby C, Linder MW *et al.* Prospective dosing of warfarin based on cytochrome P-450 2C9 genotype. *Thrombosis and Haemostasis* 2005; **93**: 700–705.

60 Rost S, Fregin A, Ivaskevicius V *et al.* Mutations in VKORC1 cause warfarin resistance and multiple coagulation factor deficiency type 2. *Nature* 2004; **427**: 537–541.

61 Li T, Chang CY, Jin DY *et al.* Identification of the gene for vitamin K epoxide reductase. *Nature* 2004; **427**: 541–544.

62 Rieder MJ, Reiner AP, Gage BF *et al.* Effect of VKORC1 haplotypes on transcriptional regulation and warfarin dose. *New England Journal of Medicine* 2005; **352**: 2285–2293.

63 Goldhaber SZ. Creating an optimal warfarin nomogram (CROWN) trial. Available from: Clinicaltrials.gov identifier NCT00401414 (accessed June 18, 2007).

64 Fatkin D, Graham RM. Molecular mechanisms of inherited cardiomyopathies. *Physiology Reviews* 2002; **82**: 945–980.

65 Muntoni F, Cau M, Ganau A *et al.* Brief report: deletion of the dystrophin muscle-promoter region associated with X-linked dilated cardiomyopathy. *New England Journal of Medicine* 1993; **329**: 921–925.

66 Bonne G, Di Barletta MR, Varnous S *et al.* Mutations in the gene encoding lamin A/C cause autosomal dominant Emery-Dreifuss muscular dystrophy. *Nature Genetics* 1999; **21**: 285–288.

67 MacRae CA, Birchmeier W, Thierfelder L. Arrhythmogenic right ventricular cardiomyopathy: moving toward mechanism. *Journal of Clinical Investigations* 2006; **116**: 1825–1828.

68 Gerull B, Heuser A, Wichter T *et al.* Mutations in the desmosomal protein plakophilin-2 are common in arrhythmogenic right ventricular cardiomyopathy. *Nature Genetics* 2004; **36**: 1162–1164.

69 van Tintelen JP, Entius MM, Bhuiyan ZA *et al.* Plakophilin-2 mutations are the major determinant of familial arrhythmogenic right ventricular dysplasia/cardiomyopathy. *Circulation* 2006; **113**: 1650–1658.

70 Priori SG, Napolitano C, Gasparini M *et al.* Clinical and genetic heterogeneity of right bundle branch block and ST-segment elevation syndrome: a prospective evaluation of 52 families. *Circulation* 2000; **102**: 2509–2515.

71 Lloyd-Jones DM, Nam BH, D'Agostino RB, Sr.,*et al.* Parental cardiovascular disease as a risk factor for cardiovascular disease in middle-aged adults: a prospective study of parents and offspring. *JAMA: The Journal of the American Medical Association* 2004; **291**: 2204–2211.

72 Ridker PM, Buring JE, Rifai N, Cook NR. Development and validation of improved algorithms for the assessment of global cardiovascular risk in women: the Reynolds Risk Score. *JAMA: The Journal of the American Medical Association* 2007; **297**: 611–619.

73 Farrall M, Green FR, Peden JF *et al.* Genome-wide mapping of susceptibility to coronary artery disease identifies a novel replicated locus on chromosome 17. *PLoS Genetics* 2006; **2**: e72.

74 Helgadottir A, Thorleifsson G, Manolescu A *et al.* A common variant on chromosome 9p21 affects the risk of myocardial infarction. *Science* 2007; **316**: 1491–1493

75 McPherson R, Pertsemlidis A, Kavaslar N *et al.* A common allele on chromosome 9 associated with coronary heart disease. *Science* 2007; **316**: 1488–1491.

76 Helgadottir A, Manolescu A, Thorleifsson G *et al.* The gene encoding 5-lipoxygenase activating protein confers risk of myocardial infarction and stroke. *Nature Genetics* 2004; **36**: 233–239.

77 Kiechl S, Lorenz E, Reindl M *et al.* Toll-like receptor 4 polymorphisms and atherogenesis. *New England Journal of Medicine* 2002; **347**: 185–192.

78 Unkelbach K, Gardemann A, Kostrzewa M *et al.* A new promoter polymorphism in the gene of lipopolysaccharide receptor CD14 is associated with expired myocardial infarction in patients with low atherosclerotic risk profile. *Arteriosclerosis Thrombosis and Vascular Biology* 1999; **19**: 932–938.

79 Cipollone F, Toniato E, Martinotti S *et al.* A polymorphism in the cyclooxygenase 2 gene as an inherited protective factor against myocardial infarction and stroke. *JAMA: The Journal of the American Medical Association* 2004; **291**: 2221–2228.

80 Ozaki K, Inoue K, Sato H *et al.* Functional variation in LGALS2 confers risk of myocardial infarction and regulates lymphotoxin-alpha secretion in vitro. *Nature* 2004; **429**: 72–75.

81 Scott LJ, Mohlke KL, Bonnycastle LL *et al.* A genome-wide association study of type 2 diabetes in Finns detects multiple susceptibility variants. *Science* 2007; **316**: 1341–1345.

82 Saxena R, Voight BF, Lyssenko V *et al.* Genome-wide association analysis identifies loci for type 2 diabetes and triglyceride levels. *Science* 2007; **316**: 1331–1336.

83 Suk HJ, Ridker PM, Cook NR, Zee RY. Relation of polymorphism within the CRP gene and plasma CRP levels. *Atherosclerosis* 2005; **178**: 139–145.

84 Zee RY, Ridker PM. Polymorphism in the human C-reactive protein (CRP) gene, plasma concentrations of CRP, and the risk of future arterial thrombosis. *Atherosclerosis* 2002; **162**: 217–219.

85 Brull DJ, Serrano N, Zito F *et al.* Human CRP gene polymorphism influences CRP levels: implications for the prediction and pathogenesis of coronary heart disease. *Arteriosclerosis Thrombosis and Vascular Biology* 2003; **23**: 2063–2069.

86 Miller DT, Zee RY, Suk Danik J *et al.* Association of common CRP gene variants with CRP levels and cardiovascular events. *Annals of Human Genetics* 2005; **69**: 623–638.

87 Carlson CS, Aldred SF, Lee PK *et al.* Polymorphisms within the C-reactive protein (CRP) promoter region are associated with plasma CRP levels. *American Journal of Human Genetics* 2005; **77**: 64–77.

88 Suk Danik J, Chasman DI, Cannon CP *et al.* Influence of genetic variation in the C-reactive protein gene on the inflammatory response during and after acute coronary ischemia. *Annals of Human Genetics* 2006; **70**: 705–716.

89 Wellcome Trust Case Control Consortium. Genome-wide association study of 14,000 cases of seven common diseases and 3,000 shared controls. *Nature* 2007; **447**: 661–678.

90 Danik JS, Pare G, Chasman DI, *et al.* Multiple novel loci, including those related to Crohn's disease, psoriasis and inflammation, identified in a genome-wide association study of fibrinogen in 17,686 women: the Women's Genome Health Study. Circulation: *Cardiovascular Genetics* 2009: *in press.*

91 Ridker PM, Chasman DI, Zee RY, *et al.* Rationale, design, and methodology of the Women's Genome Health Study: a genome-wide association study of more than 25,000 initially healthy american women. *Clin Chem* 2008; **54**: 249–55.

92 Ridker PM, Pare G, Parker A, *et al.* Loci related to metabolic-syndrome pathways including LEPR,HNF1A, IL6R, and GCKR associate with plasma C-reactive protein: the Women's Genome Health Study. *Am J Hum Genet* 2008; **82**: 1185–92.

PART II

Specific Cardiovascular Disease

Chapter 5

Genomics and atrial arrhythmias

Dawood Darbar and Calum A. MacRae

Introduction

The most far-reaching consequences of genetics and genomics in many ways have been on the sheer scale of biologic investigation, not only in genotyping but also in phenotyping [1]. Genome-derived technologies such as array-based expression profiling enable the study not just of individual genes or pathways but rather the investigation of all known genes in parallel. This in turn has stimulated less biased approaches to phenotyping, redefining our understanding of syndromes first defined over 100 years ago. Ultimately, the true benefit of genomic and "postgenomic" technologies may be the resolution of etiologic heterogeneity in both heritable and acquired conditions. The potential of such technologies is already being realized in the study of atrial arrhythmias.

Atrial fibrillation

Atrial fibrillation (AF), the most common cardiac arrhythmia in clinical practice, affects approximately 2% of the US population and results in substantial morbidity and mortality [2]. The increasing prevalence of AF parallels the increasing age of the general population [3]. AF is also the most common arrhythmia requiring drug therapy, but the limited success of current interventions for AF is in part due to our poor understanding of its molecular pathophysiology [4]. Although some of the risk factors associated with the development of AF have been identified, relatively little is known about the underlying molecular events leading to the arrhythmia [5]. One approach to unraveling the molecular pathogenesis of AF is through the identification of genes responsible for familial forms of the disease. Evidence for the

Cardiovascular Genetics and Genomics. Edited by Dan Roden. © 2009 American Heart Association, ISBN: 978-14051-7540-1.

heritability of AF has come from several sources, including the study of AF kindreds who exhibit the arrhythmia as a primary disease, the analysis of AF presenting in the setting of another familial cardiac disease, and the analysis of common population genetic variants, i.e., DNA polymorphisms, that may predispose to AF.

Monogenic forms of lone atrial fibrillation

Monogenic familial AF was first reported in 1943 [6], and, while it may be uncommon, there has been no attempt to determine the overall prevalence of familial AF. Heritability of AF is further suggested by two recent population-based studies demonstrating that the presence of AF in first-degree relatives was associated with an increased risk of developing AF [7,8]. We and others have shown that 5% of patients with AF and up to 15% of individuals with lone AF may have a familial form of the disease [9,10]. A gene locus for AF was first reported in 1997, based on genetic mapping in three Spanish families [11]. However, the gene responsible for AF in these kindreds has not yet been identified, but resides within a relatively large chromosomal region spanning 14 centi-Morgans (cM). In addition, three other loci on chromosomes 6q14–16 [12], 5p13 [13], and 10p11–q21 [14] have been reported, with no defective genes yet identified. Recently, a novel AF locus on chromosome 5p15 was identified by genome-wide linkage analysis of a four-generation kindred. Importantly, this study established an abnormally prolonged P wave (>155 ms) determined by signal-averaged ECG analysis as an "endophenotype" that improved statistical power of the linkage study in this family [15]. Taken together, these reports support the idea that familial AF is a genetically heterogeneous disease much like many other inherited arrhythmia syndromes [9].

Recently, the first genes for AF have been identified, providing a tentative link between ion channelopathies and the arrhythmia. In a four-generation Chinese family in which long QT syndrome (LQTS) and early-onset AF cosegregate, a mutation (S140G) in the *KCNQ1* gene on chromosome 11p15.5 has been reported [16]. Functional analysis of the S140G mutant revealed a gain-of-function effect in KCNQ1/KCNE1 and KCNQ1/KCNE2 currents, which contrasts with the dominant negative or loss-of-function effects of *KCNQ1* mutations previously associated with LQTS. More recently, the same group established a link between *KCNE2* and AF by identification of a mutation in two families with AF [17]. The mutation, R27C, also caused a gain-of-function when coexpressed with *KCNQ1* but had no effect when expressed with *KCNH2* (HERG). Most recently, a truncating mutation in *KCNA5* encoding a voltage-gated potassium channel ($K_V1.5$) underlying the ultrarapid delayed rectifier current (I_{Kur}) was associated with familial AF [18]. These studies firmly establish the role of potassium channels in the pathogenesis of some forms of familial AF, but resequencing studies in large cohorts suggest that mutations in these channels are a rare cause of the arrhythmia [19].

Atrial fibrillation associated with other monogenic diseases

Studies of other cardiac monogenic disorders have also provided evidence for the genetic contribution to the etiology of AF. These include diseases such as hypertrophic cardiomyopathy, skeletal myopathies, familial amyloidosis, and atrial myopathies. It is likely that AF in these cases is related at least in part to nonspecific structural changes in the atria caused by the underlying cardiac pathology, but AF is undoubtedly uniquely prominent in some kindreds with each of these conditions [20]. AF can also present in other ion channelopathies, such as LQTS type 4 [21], Brugada syndrome [22], and short QT syndrome [23]. The high incidence of atrial arrhythmias in patients with the short QT syndrome and the gain-of-function mutations in I_{Ks} [24] point to an important role for shortening of the action potential in the development of AF. Sodium channel gene (*SCN5A*) defects have also been associated with a syndrome of early-onset dilated cardiomyopathy (DCM) and AF [25]. Moreover, mutations in the gene for the nuclear membrane protein lamin A/C (LMNA) have pleiotropic noncardiac and cardiac manifestations including DCM, AF, and conduction system disease [26]. Collectively, these studies attest to the heterogeneous nature of AF and strongly suggest that defects in many more genes remain to be identified.

Association studies

Most patients with AF have one or more identifiable risk factors, but many or even most patients with these same risk factors do not develop AF. Thus, it is likely that genetic determinants favor AF in some individuals with identifiable risk factors. Studies comparing cases of nonfamilial AF with age-related and gender-matched controls (association studies) have provided some insight into the genetic basis of "acquired" AF. One study evaluated a polymorphism in *KCNE1* and AF and identified an association with the 38G allele. While the 38G allele appears to reduce I_{Ks} [27], mice lacking *KCNE1* are prone to AF owing to an unexpected increase in I_{Ks} [28], suggesting that the consequences of ion channel protein mutations are not always straightforward. In addition, common DNA polymorphisms in *GNB3* [29],*KCNE5* [30], and *SCN5A* have all been associated with AF [31]. Over the last several years there is increasing evidence that activation of the renin–angiotensin–aldosterone (RAAS) activation may be an important risk factor for the development of AF. Retrospective analyses suggest that angiotensin-converting-enzyme (ACE) inhibitor therapy is associated with a lower incidence of AF and a placebo-controlled trial found a similar beneficial effect of adding the angiotensin receptor blocker (ARB) irbesartan to amiodarone [32]. Additionally, a case–control study of 250 Taiwanese subjects with AF and 250 controls identified polymorphisms in this pathway as risk factors for AF [33]. Added support for the increasingly important role of RAAS activation in the pathophysiology of AF comes from a recent study which demonstrated a pharmacogenetic interaction between the ACE I/D polymorphism and efficacy of antiarrhythmic drug therapy in patients with lone AF [34].

The above studies in aging patients with nonfamilial AF in the presence of underlying heart disease suggest some form of heritable contribution to the pathogenesis of the more common forms of AF. Obviously, these data are promising and may help clarify why some people develop AF under specific circumstances while others may not.

Resequencing

The positional cloning strategy identifies a disease gene in the absence of any *a priori* assumptions regarding mechanism, but rather based solely on its chromosomal location. The first gene linked to familial AF (*KCNQ1*) was identified by such a strategy after linkage analysis refined the locus to a critical region on chromosome 11p15.5. *KCNQ1* was an obvious candidate gene in the critical region. Sequence analysis of the *KCNQ1* coding region revealed a missense mutation, S140G, in all of the affected family members with AF [16]. However, most of the other AF genes (Table 5.1) have been identified through a true candidate gene approach. Nonetheless, resequencing of potential candidate genes has successfully identified variants which cosegregate with familial AF in isolated kindreds. Another gene that has recently been identified as a candidate gene

Table 5.1 Loci and genes associated with atrial arrhythmias

	Mode	Locus	Protein	Gene
AF	AD	10q22–24	I_{Ks}	–
	AR	11p15	I_{Kr}	*KCNQ1, KvLQT1*
		6q14–16	I_{K1}	–
		21q22	K_{Kur}	*KCNE2, MiRP1*
		17q23		*KCNJ2, Kir2.1*
		5p13		*KCNA5*
		5p15		
		10p11		
SND, AF	AD	3q21	I_{Na}	*SCN5A*
SND, AF	AD	–		–
AVRT	AD	–		*PRKAG2*
AVB	AD	19q13	I_{Na}	*SCN5A*
		3q21		

AF, atrial fibrillation; AD, autosomal dominat; AR, auto somal recessive; SND, Sinus node dysfunction; AVRT, atrioventricular reentrant. tachycardia; AVB, atrioventricular block.

for AF is the human cardiac sodium channel gene (*SCN5A*) with recent studies demonstrating a link between a syndrome of DCM and AF [25,35]. Although variants in *SCN5A* have been reported to occur in disorders that are sometimes associated with AF, there have been no studies that have systematically evaluated the prevalence of *SCN5A* variants in a cohort of patients with AF. Taken together, these studies provide a strong rationale for *SCN5A* as a candidate gene for AF. Recently, we have resequenced *SCN5A* in 375 patients with AF including a large subgroup with lone AF. We observed novel as well as rare variants in nearly 6% of the population including alleles that segregate with AF in other family members, indicating that *SCN5A* is an important AF susceptibility gene. The relatively high prevalence of such sequence variants and the rather variable functional consequences of these variants in simple model systems reflect the need for innovative tools, especially integrative functional assays, to allow discrimination between genetic signal and genetic noise in candidate gene resequencing studies.

Uncovering common genes for atrial fibrillation

The genetic basis for the majority of patients with AF remains unknown. Although Mendelian forms of lone AF are not rare, large kindreds such as those used to identify disease genes in other inherited arrhythmia syndromes, for example congenital LQTS [36], are unusual. One possible explanation for such complexity may be a smaller genetic contribution to the ultimate clinical phenotype, and thus reduced penetrance with less apparent heritability. Another possible mechanism is that the phenotype may be the result of interaction of several genes, i.e., polygenic, each with a small overall contribution. Finally, AF may require additional perturbations, for example hypertension, to reduce the "AF threshold" sufficiently to trigger an episode of arrhythmia [37].

The paroxysmal nature and variable symptoms in AF, a high prevalence in the general population, and a late age of onset in many individuals all make assignment of the clinical phenotype challenging. A number of strategies can be used to minimize misphenotyping, including "affecteds only" analysis and "diagnosis by offspring," all of which unfortunately reduce the power and maximum potential LOD [logarithm of the odds] score. This complexity has compelled a search for new more effective methods for investigating the genetics of complex diseases, such as AF [38]. One approach is to use the families of affected individuals as an enriched target population for the definition and evaluation of novel phenotypes. The psychiatric field has pioneered systematic approaches to phenotyping in an attempt to discover intermediate or endophenotypes, i.e., subtle or novel phenotypes which are causally related to the poorly penetrant classical clinical syndromes [39]. This strategy, which is only now beginning to bear fruit in genetic studies, has already established, for example, the mechanistic links between conditions such as obsessive–compulsive disorder and depression. In the case of AF, examples of potential endophenotypes include signal-averaged P-wave duration [15], pulmonary venous anatomy as assessed by computed tomography or magnetic resonance imaging, and profiles of biomarkers such as atrial natriuretic peptide [40,41]. If such markers of a reduced threshold for AF can be defined, then not only will they be useful clinically (i.e., to subset patients with AF) but they will also accelerate the identification of causal AF genes.

Alternative approaches

Because of these limitations, researchers have begun to use other strategies to identify genes that are involved in complex diseases such as AF. Genetic association studies using a candidate gene approach are likely to be more effective tools than linkage studies for studying complex traits because they have greater statistical power to detect several genes of small effect [42]. Rather than rely on markers that are evenly spaced throughout the genome without regard to their function or context in a specific gene, candidate gene studies focus on genes that are selected because of *a priori* hypotheses about their etiological role in disease. Furthermore, a candidate gene study is usually conducted in a population-based sample of affected and unaffected individuals (a case–control study). A candidate gene study therefore takes advantage of both the increased statistical efficiency of association analysis of complex diseases and the biological understanding of the phenotype, tissues, genes, and proteins that are likely to be involved in the disease. However, in spite of their promise, candidate gene studies do have two important limitations. First, the significant findings of association in many candidate gene studies have not been replicated when followed up in subsequent association studies. Second, because candidate gene studies are based on the ability to predict functional candidate genes and variants, current knowledge may be insufficient to make these predictions.

A logical consequence of the availability of comprehensive genomic maps is the advent of high-density genome-wide searches for modest gene effects using large-scale testing of single nucleotide polymorphisms (SNPs). Such an approach has been suggested to tackle complex human diseases such as AF. Early proponents suggested the study of coding or promoter variants with potential functional significance [43]. Collins *et al.* [44] subsequently proposed that noncoding or evenly spaced SNPs with high density could be used to track disease loci through linkage disequilibrium. The availability of high-density mapping of marker SNPs and assessment of genomic structure, together with emerging information on functional pathways, have begun to provide powerful means of identifying genetic susceptibilities to AF. In the first genome-wide association study of AF, a novel locus on chromosome 4q25 has recently been identified which confers a 1.6- to 2.0-fold (95% confidence intervals) increased risk of the arrhythmia across multiple different populations [45].

One of the most vexing problems with non-Mendelian genetic approaches is the differentiation of signal from noise. Association studies may be confounded by etiologic heterogeneity, population stratification, or false positives, while the bias toward small effects may miss major genetic contributions relevant only in a subset of study subjects. It may also prove difficult to define the fundamental mechanisms of any true associations, as the responsible gene may be remotely linked to the locus identified. The development of more efficient models for the rapid validation of genome-wide association study results and improved understanding of the underlying biology will facilitate the interpretation of such studies [42].

Novel genetic mechanisms

Advances in genomic technologies and in our understanding of novel genetic mechanisms have also begun to affect our study of these emerging pathways in disease. Somatic mutation is a major cause of neoplastic disease, especially in rapidly dividing cell types, with "second hits" thought to inactivate the wild-type allele in the context of germline inactivation of one copy of the gene. It is not clear how such mechanisms would operate in the heart where postmitotic cell division is thought to occur at an extremely low rate, if at all. Nevertheless, apparently myocardially restricted somatic mutations in the connexin 40 gene, encoding the major component of the cardiac gap junctions, were recently described in a small series of subjects with lone AF [46]. Another form of tissue-specific mutation has also been described. Mitochondrial mutations have been reported in multiple small series of subjects with AF, as for many other conditions associated with aging [47]. The issues surrounding the validation of somatic mutation in nonclonal tissues are complex, but it should be possible to prove this disease mechanism through *in vivo* modeling.

Other forms of inheritance have already been indirectly implicated in AF. The disparate atrial and ventricular phenotypes seen in the context of mutations in the *KCNQ1* gene may reflect the regional expression of individual alleles of this gene or longer range effects on neighboring genes as this locus is heavily imprinted [48]. Finally, as genomic advances uncover novel gene classes, including micro-RNAs that affect the mRNA stability or translation efficiency of many different genes, these will each be explored in a broad range of human diseases [49].

Atrial flutter

Although there is significant overlap among the risk factors for AF and atrial flutter, in general these arrhythmias exhibit quite distinct biology and electrophysiology [50]. Atrial flutter is commonly associated with the later stages of a broad range of congenital heart disease (CHD). There is extensive heterogeneity particularly in the most profound structural disorders, but increasing evidence is accumulating of a substantial heritable component to many forms of

CHD. The association of CHD with atrial flutter has been attributed to abnormal atrial patterning, which may range from the extreme to the subtle, often with no other obvious manifestations. Interestingly, atrial flutter was found to be more strongly associated with the locus on chromosome 4q25 than AF, at least suggesting that there may be common factors underlying the clinical presentation of some forms of these two arrhythmias [45]. Given the intrinsic biases of genome-wide association studies, these links might be far downstream of the primary causation, but nevertheless may have substantial effects on a population basis.

Sinus nodal failure

Classic Mendelian genetics have revealed several distinctive mechanisms for sinus nodal disease. Mutations in the cardiac transcription factors Nkx 2.5 and Tbx 2.5 both cause defects in the differentiation and maintenance of specialized conduction tissues [particularly those of the atrioventricular (AV) node], and each causes subtle abnormalities of sinus impulse generation [51–54]. Similarly, several primary arrhythmic syndromes including some forms of the LQTS also result in perturbations of sinus rhythm [36]. While in many instances potential mechanisms have been framed in terms of effects on transmembrane ionic currents, data from genetic models of SCN5A and AnkB disease suggest that subtle trophic effects on myocardial structures may also play a role [21,55]. Genetic models may also inform human studies at an earlier stage. Murine null alleles of the pacemaker channels HCN2 and HCN4 first directly implicated these channels in normal sinus rhythm, and subsequent human genetic studies have identified mutations in the HCN4 gene in sinoatrial disease [56–58]. Model organisms may also help to parse out potential discrete effects of such mutations on the autonomic innervation of the heart.

The broad number of influences on resting heart rate may confound genome-wide association studies of this trait, but the precise quantitation feasible allows this to be treated as a true quantitative trait. Such traits are perhaps the best suited to genome-wide association studies, and usually exhibit substantially greater power than dichotomous phenotypes, but to date no studies using this approach to identify genes underlying variation in heart rate have been published [42].

Other atrial arrhythmias

Virtually every known myocardial disease has been associated with some form of atrial arrhythmia. However, there are some rare associations which appear to be considerably more specific. A number of metabolic disorders, including mitochondrial diseases and glycogen or other storage disorders, are strongly associated with prominent evidence of AV conduction disease, often with overt ventricular preexcitation as well as frequent macro-reentrant and other atrial arrhythmias. For example, dominant mutations in the adenosine monophosphate (AMP)-activated protein kinase gamma subunit (PRKAG2) have recently been shown to result in massive myocardial thickening, AV conduction system disease, and ventricular preexcitation [59]. These families had previously been included under the rubric of hypertrophic cardiomyopathy on the basis of their inheritance patterns, adult onset, and echocardiographic features. AF and atrial flutter are common, but high-grade AV block is the dominant clinical arrhythmia in these kindreds. Clinical studies suggest that in many cases asymptomatic individuals are maximally preexcited at rest, and therefore probably dependent on accessory AV connections from an early age [60]. These data defined a novel subset of "hypertrophic cardiomyopathy" illustrating the potential utility of molecular nosology for cardiac disease, and also offering some unique insights into the mechanisms of normal AV electrical development [61].

Pharmacogenomics

One of the first ways in which genetics may affect the clinical care of atrial arrhythmias is through the prediction of variable individual drug responses [62]. Understanding relevant differences in drug absorption and metabolism, as well as the extent of on-target effects, will allow drugs to be deployed in those who will gain the most benefit with the fewest adverse events. Clinical use of pharmacogenetic data has already begun to impact on anticoagulation with coumadin in which the incorporation of genotypes at the vitamin K epoxide reductase complex 1 (VKORC1) and cytochrome P450 isoform CYP2C9 loci with clinical and demographic data allow robust prediction of the therapeutic dose [63]. Real world clinical trials are currently under way, and similar genetic data may also have a future role in the choice of antiarrhythmic agents in AF [64].

Future directions

Paradoxically, genetics and genomics have had the greatest impact to date at the phenotypic level, highlighting the need for much finer resolution in our clinical diagnostic repertoire. Atrial arrhythmias are an archetype for many other complex traits, in which dilution of genetic effects by etiologic heterogeneity and substantial environmental influences make systematic dissection difficult [43]. Phenotyping issues are further complicated by the paroxysmal and often asymptomatic nature of the arrhythmias, and consistent stable endophenotypes directly related to the underlying myocardial disorder will be required for a comprehensive understanding of the genetic architecture of many conditions. Ultimately, such endophenotypes are likely to incorporate functional genomic and physiologic data [1,65].

Systematic approaches to gene expression, directly resulting from the availability of comprehensive sequence, have stimulated related efforts designed to allow genome-scale or global profiling of proteins, distinct post-translation modifications such as phosphorylation states, metabolites, and other biological molecules. Inroads are now being made into unraveling the information contained in genome modifications such as methylation, mapping transcription factor binding sites, and histones [66]. The combination of novel biology with *in silico* mining of genomic sequence has uncovered several new classes of genes that do not encode proteins, but rather regulatory RNAs [49,66]. Large genomic regions may be transcriptionally regulated by intronic RNAs, while tiny micro-RNAs may switch off multiple genes to initiate major phenotypic switches. The difficulties intrinsic to understanding the functions of the noncoding sequences that represent over 95% of the human genome are exemplified by the amazing conservation of regulatory functions across species in the absence of any evidence of homology at the level of the primary structure. Many human diseases are highly complex and heterogeneous in their etiology, displaying evidence of interactions between multiple genes (polygenic) and between these genes and environmental exposures. Ultimately, these interactions will require to be integrated in assays that can be performed at a clinical level. Recent efforts to begin cellular profiling using chemical libraries may be the harbinger of the diversity and scale of future phenotyping.

The challenges for translational science in the next decade will include developing technologies for *in vitro* and *in vivo* modeling on a scale capable of integrating vast datasets in a quantitative fashion as algorithms are defined for deriving truly predictive individual profiles to enable molecular diagnosis, risk prediction, and therapeutic tailoring.

References

1 Freimer N, Sabatti C. The human phenome project. *Nature Genetics* 2003; **34**: 15–21.
2 Feinberg WM, Blackshear JL, Laupacis A *et al.* Prevalence, age distribution, and gender of patients with atrial fibrillation. Analysis and implications. *Archives of Internal Medicine* 1995; **155**: 469–473.
3 Lloyd-Jones DM, Wang TJ, Leip EP *et al.* Lifetime risk for development of atrial fibrillation: the Framingham Heart Study. *Circulation* 2004; **110**: 1042–1046.
4 Waldo AL. A perspective on antiarrhythmic drug therapy to treat atrial fibrillation: there remains an unmet need. *American Heart Journal* 2006; **151**: 771–778.
5 Waldo AL. Mechanisms of atrial fibrillation. *Journal of Cardiovascular Electrophysiology* 2003; 14 (12 Suppl): S267–274.
6 Wolff L. Familial auricular fibrillation. *New England Journal of Medicine* 1943; **229**: 396–398.
7 Fox CS, Parise H, D'Agostino RB, Sr.,*et al.* Parental atrial fibrillation as a risk factor for atrial fibrillation in offspring. *JAMA: The Journal of the American Medical Association* 2004; **291**: 2851–2855.
8 Arnar DO, Thorvaldsson S, Manolio TA *et al.* Familial aggregation of atrial fibrillation in Iceland. *European Heart Journal* 2006; **27**: 708–712.

9 Darbar D, Herron KJ, Ballew JD *et al.* Familial atrial fibrillation is a genetically heterogeneous disorder. *Journal of the American College of Cardiologists* 2003; **41**: 2185–2192.
10 Ellinor PT, Yoerger DM, Ruskin JN, MacRae CA. Familial aggregation in lone atrial fibrillation. *Human Genetics* 2005; **118**: 179–184.
11 Brugada R, Tapscott T, Czernuszewicz GZ *et al.* Identification of a genetic locus for familial atrial fibrillation. *New England Journal of Medicine* 1997; **336**: 905–911.
12 Ellinor PT, Shin JT, Moore RK *et al.* Locus for atrial fibrillation maps to chromosome 6q14–16. *Circulation* 2003; **107**: 2880–2883.
13 Oberti C, Wang L, Li L *et al.* Genome-wide linkage scan identifies a novel genetic locus on chromosome 5p13 for neonatal atrial fibrillation associated with sudden death and variable cardiomyopathy. *Circulation* 2004; **110**: 3753–3759.
14 Volders PG, Zhu Q, Timmermans C *et al.* Mapping a novel locus for familial atrial fibrillation on chromosome 10p11–q21. *Heart Rhythm* 2007; **4**: 469–475.
15 Darbar D, Jahangir A, Hammill SC, Gersh BJ. P wave signal-averaged electrocardiography to identify risk for atrial fibrillation. *Pacing and Clinical Electrophysiology* 2002; **25**: 1447–1453.
16 Chen YH, Xu SJ, Bendahhou S *et al.* KCNQ1 gain-of-function mutation in familial atrial fibrillation. *Science* 2003; **299**: 251–254.
17 Yang Y, Xia M, Jin Q *et al.* Identification of a KCNE2 gain-of-function mutation in patients with familial atrial fibrillation. *American Journal of Human Genetics* 2004; **75**: 899–905.
18 Olson TM, Alekseev AE, Liu XK *et al.* Kv1.5 channelopathy due to KCNA5 loss-of-function mutation causes human atrial fibrillation. *Human Molecular Genetics* 2006; **15**: 2185–2191.
19 Ellinor PT, Petrov-Kondratov VI, Zakharova E *et al.* Potassium channel gene mutations rarely cause atrial fibrillation. *BMC Medical Genetics* 2006; **7**: 70.
20 Gruver EJ, Fatkin D, Dodds GA *et al.* Familial hypertrophic cardiomyopathy and atrial fibrillation caused by Arg663His beta-cardiac myosin heavy chain mutation. *American Journal of Cardiology* 1999; **83** (12A): 13H–8H.
21 Mohler PJ, Schott JJ, Gramolini AO *et al.* Ankyrin-B mutation causes type 4 long-QT cardiac arrhythmia and sudden cardiac death. *Nature* 2003; **421**: 634–639.
22 Morita H, Kusano-Fukushima K, Nagase S *et al.* Atrial fibrillation and atrial vulnerability in patients with Brugada syndrome. *Journal of the American College of Cardiologists* 2002; **40**: 1437–1444.
23 Priori SG, Pandit SV, Rivolta I *et al.* A novel form of short QT syndrome (SQT3) is caused by a mutation in the KCNJ2 gene. *Circulation Research* 2005; **96**: 800–807.
24 Gaita F, Giustetto C, Bianchi F *et al.* Short QT Syndrome: a familial cause of sudden death. *Circulation* 2003; **108**: 965–970.
25 Olson TM, Michels VV, Ballew JD *et al.* Sodium channel mutations and susceptibility to heart failure and atrial fibrillation. *JAMA: The Journal of the American Medical Association* 2005; **293**: 447–454.
26 Fatkin D, MacRae C, Sasaki T *et al.* Missense mutations in the rod domain of the lamin A/C gene as causes of dilated cardiomyopathy and conduction-system disease. *New England Journal of Medicine* 1999; **341**: 1715–1724.
27 Ehrlich JR, Zicha S, Coutu P *et al.* Atrial fibrillation-associated minK38G/S polymorphism modulates delayed rectifier current and membrane localization. *Cardiovascular Research.* 2005; **67**: 520–528.
28 Temple J, Frias P, Rottman J *et al.* Atrial fibrillation in KCNE1-null mice. *Circulation Research* 2005; **97**: 62–69.

29 Schreieck J, Dostal S, von Beckerath N *et al.* C825T polymorphism of the G-protein beta3 subunit gene and atrial fibrillation: association of the TT genotype with a reduced risk for atrial fibrillation. *American Heart Journal* 2004; **148**: 545–550.
30 Ravn LS, Hofman-Bang J, Dixen U *et al.* Relation of 97T polymorphism in KCNE5 to risk of atrial fibrillation. *American Journal of Cardiology* 2005; **96**: 405–407.
31 Chen LY, Ballew JD, Herron KJ *et al.* A common polymorphism in SCN5A is associated with lone atrial fibrillation. *Clinical Pharmacology and Therapeutics* 2007; **81**: 35–41.
32 Madrid AH, Bueno MG, Rebollo JM *et al.* Use of irbesartan to maintain sinus rhythm in patients with long-lasting persistent atrial fibrillation: a prospective and randomized study. *Circulation* 2002; **106**: 331–336.
33 Tsai CT, Lai LP, Lin JL *et al.* Renin-angiotensin system gene polymorphisms and atrial fibrillation. *Circulation* 2004; **109**: 1640–1646.
34 Darbar D. Polymorphism modulates symptomatic response to antiarrhythmic drug therapy in patients with atrial fibrillation. *Heart Rhythm* 2007; **4**: 743–749.
35 McNair WP, Ku L, Taylor MR *et al.* SCN5A mutation associated with dilated cardiomyopathy, conduction disorder, and arrhythmia. *Circulation* 2004; **110**: 2163–2167.
36 Keating MT, Sanguinetti MC. Molecular and cellular mechanisms of cardiac arrhythmias. *Cell* 2001; **104**: 569–580.
37 Otway R, Vandenberg JI, Guo G *et al.* Stretch-sensitive KCNQ1 mutation A link between genetic and environmental factors in the pathogenesis of atrial fibrillation? *Journal of the American College of Cardiologists* 2007; **49**: 578–586.
38 Ellinor PT, Macrae CA. The genetics of atrial fibrillation. *Journal of Cardiovascular Electrophysiology* 2003; **14**: 1007–1009.
39 Garver DL, Holcomb JA, Christensen JD. Heterogeneity of response to antipsychotics from multiple disorders in the schizophrenia spectrum. *Journal of Clinical Psychiatry* 2000; **61**: 964–972; quiz 73.
40 Ellinor PT, Low AF, Macrae CA. Reduced apelin levels in lone atrial fibrillation. *European Heart Journal* 2006; **27**: 222–226.
41 Ellinor PT, Low AF, Patton KK *et al.* Discordant atrial natriuretic peptide and brain natriuretic peptide levels in lone atrial fibrillation. *Journal of the American College of Cardiologists* 2005; **45**: 82–86.
42 Cardon LR, Bell JI. Association study designs for complex diseases. *Nature Reviews Genetics* 2001; **2**: 91–99.
43 Risch NJ. Searching for genetic determinants in the new millennium. *Nature* 2000; **405**: 847–856.
44 Collins A, Ennis S, Taillon-Miller P *et al.* Allelic association with SNPs: metrics, populations, and the linkage disequilibrium map. *Human Mutation* 2001; **17**: 255–262.
45 Gudbjartsson DF, Arnar DO, Helgadottir A *et al.* Variants conferring risk of atrial fibrillation on chromosome 4q25. *Nature* 2007; **448**: 353–357.
46 Gollob MH, Jones DL, Krahn AD *et al.* Somatic mutations in the connexin 40 gene (GJA5) in atrial fibrillation. *New England Journal of Medicine* 2006; **354**: 2677–2688.
47 Lai LP, Tsai CC, Su MJ *et al.* Atrial fibrillation is associated with accumulation of aging-related common type mitochondrial DNA deletion mutation in human atrial tissue. Chest 2003; **123**: 539–544.
48 Cerrato F, Vernucci M, Pedone PV *et al.* The 5′ end of the KCNQ1OT1 gene is hypomethylated in the Beckwith-Wiedemann syndrome. *Human Genetics* 2002; **111**: 105–107.

49 Ambros V, Chen X. The regulation of genes and genomes by small RNAs. *Development* 2007; **134**: 1635–1641.
50 Waldo AL. Inter-relationships between atrial flutter and atrial fibrillation. *Pacing and Clinical Electrophysiology* 2003; **26** (7 Pt 2): 1583–1596.
51 Schott JJ, Benson DW, Basson CT *et al.* Congenital heart disease caused by mutations in the transcription factor NKX2–5. *Science* 1998; **281**: 108–111.
52 Basson CT, Huang T, Lin RC *et al.* Different TBX5 interactions in heart and limb defined by Holt-Oram syndrome mutations. *Proceedings of the National Academy of Sciences of the USA* 1999; **96**: 2919–2924.
53 Moskowitz IP, Pizard A, Patel VV *et al.* The T-Box transcription factor Tbx5 is required for the patterning and maturation of the murine cardiac conduction system. *Development* 2004; **131**: 4107–4116.
54 Kasahara H, Wakimoto H, Liu M *et al.* Progressive atrioventricular conduction defects and heart failure in mice expressing a mutant Csx/Nkx2.5 homeoprotein. *Journal of Clinical Investigation* 2001; **108**: 189–201.
55 Papadatos GA, Wallerstein PM, Head CE *et al.* Slowed conduction and ventricular tachycardia after targeted disruption of the cardiac sodium channel gene Scn5a. *Proceedings of the National Academy of Sciences of the USA* 2002; **99**: 6210–6215.
56 Ludwig A, Budde T, Stieber J *et al.* Absence epilepsy and sinus dysrhythmia in mice lacking the pacemaker channel HCN2. *Embo Journal* 2003; **22**: 216–224.
57 Stieber J, Herrmann S, Feil S *et al.* The hyperpolarization-activated channel HCN4 is required for the generation of pacemaker action potentials in the embryonic heart. *Proceedings of the National Academy of Sciences of the USA* 2003; **100**: 15235–15240.
58 Milanesi R, Baruscotti M, Gnecchi-Ruscone T, DiFrancesco D. Familial sinus bradycardia associated with a mutation in the cardiac pacemaker channel. *New England Journal of Medicine* 2006; **354**: 151–157.
59 Arad M, Benson DW, Perez-Atayde AR *et al.* Constitutively active AMP kinase mutations cause glycogen storage disease mimicking hypertrophic cardiomyopathy. *Journal of Clinical Investigation* 2002; **109**: 357–362.
60 Mehdirad AA, Fatkin D, DiMarco JP *et al.* Electrophysiologic characteristics of accessory atrioventricular connections in an inherited form of Wolff-Parkinson-White syndrome. *Journal of Cardiovascular Electrophysiology* 1999; **10**: 629–635.
61 Arad M, Seidman JG, Seidman CE. Phenotypic diversity in hypertrophic cardiomyopathy. *Human Molecular Genetics* 2002; **11**: 2499–2506.
62 Roden DM, Altman RB, Benowitz NL *et al.* Pharmacogenomics: challenges and opportunities. *Annals of Internal Medicine* 2006; **145**: 749–757.
63 Sconce EA, Khan TI, Wynne HA *et al.* The impact of CYP2C9 and VKORC1 genetic polymorphism and patient characteristics upon warfarin dose requirements: proposal for a new dosing regimen. *Blood* 2005; **106**: 2329–2333.
64 Roden DM, George AL, Jr. The genetic basis of variability in drug responses. *Nature Reviews Drug Discovery* 2002: 37–44.
65 Schadt EE, Lamb J, Yang X *et al.* An integrative genomics approach to infer causal associations between gene expression and disease. *Nature Genetics* 2005; **37**: 710–717.
66 ENCODE Project Consortium, Birney E, Stamatoyannopoulos JA *et al.* Identification and analysis of functional elements in 1% of the human genome by the ENCODE pilot project. *Nature* 2007; **447**: 799–816.

Chapter 6

Ventricular arrhythmias and sudden death

Jonas S.S.G. de Jong, Lukas R.C. Dekker and Arthur A.M. Wilde

Introduction

Sudden cardiac death (SCD) in the young has a tremendous impact on the families in which it occurs. SCD in this age group is often caused by hereditary primary arrhythmia syndromes and research into these syndromes has led to a huge advancement in our understanding of the different pathophysiologic mechanisms that can lead to life-threatening arrhythmias. However, the absolute number of SCDs in the young is small.

The majority of the 200,000–450,000 SCDs that occur each year in the USA are caused by coronary artery disease [1]. Patients with acute myocardial infarction have up to 30% risk of dying suddenly in the acute phase. Postinfarction patients with a reduced left ventricular ejection fraction also have an increased risk for SCD. It is thought that the number of sudden deaths will rise in the current aging population. In some regions, the rate of SCD is reported to be declining, which is probably the result of improvement in resuscitation techniques as well as medical treatment [2–4]. Nevertheless, SCD is still a major health concern and if we want to prevent SCD in the future we will have to understand its etiology. Unraveling the pathophysiological mechanisms involved in the primary arrhythmia syndromes is a first step in this process.

Primary arrhythmia syndromes

The cardiac action potential is directed by the precisely timed opening and closing of various ion channels (Fig. 6.1a). Small changes in timing, amount, or

Cardiovascular Genetics and Genomics. Edited by Dan Roden. © 2009 American Heart Association, ISBN: 978-14051-7540-1.

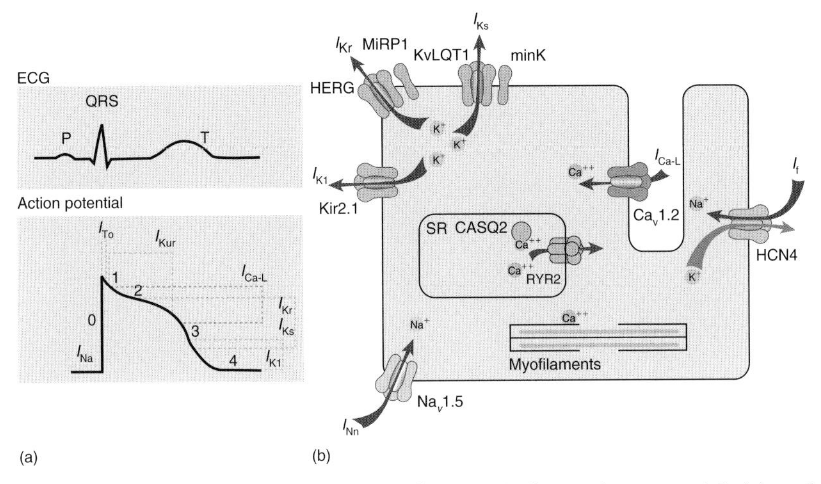

Fig. 6.1 Ionic currents contributing to the ventricular action potential (a) and representation of a cardiomyocyte displaying (only) those proteins involved in the pathogenesis of primary arrhythmia syndromes (b). In (a), the action potential is aligned with its approximate time of action during the ECG. (Reproduced with permission from the BMJ publishing group [39].)

kinetics of ion channels can lead to ECG changes and arrhythmias. Such changes can be brought about by changes in genes that encode for ion channels, their subunits, or transport. In recent decades, many of such genes have been found to underlie heritable arrhythmias and sudden cardiac death. Here, we will briefly review these primary arrhythmia syndromes, also known as "channelopathies."

Long QT syndromes

The long QT syndrome (LQTS) is a repolarization disorder and can be identified on the ECG. It has an estimated prevalence of 1:2000 to 1:5000 [5,6]. Patients with LQTS carry an increased risk of polymorphic ventricular tachycardia (torsades de pointes), leading to syncope if reverted, or sudden death if not. The association between a prolonged QTc interval on the ECG and familial sudden death has long been established in the autosomal recessive Jervell and Lange-Nielsen syndrome and the autosomal dominant Romano–Ward syndrome. Ten congenital long QT subtypes have since been recognized, LQTS1, -2, and -3 are clinically most relevant (Table 6.1).

In LQTS1 the *KCNQ1* gene coding for the KvLQT1 potassium channel is dysfunctional, leading to a reduced (slow) potassium efflux (I_{Ks}, Fig. 6.1b). LQTS1 is present in about 40–50% of patients with LQTS. More than 70 different *KCNQ1* mutations have been described in LQTS1 and genotype–phenotype studies have shown a correlation between the degree of ion channel dysfunction and the clinical course [7]. Arrhythmias are often triggered by exercise,

Table 6.1 An overview of primary arrhythmias syndromes

Phenotype	Gene	Protein	Chromosomal locus	Inheritance	Ion current	References	OMIM
BrS1	*SCN5A*	Na_v1.5	3p21	Dominant	$I_{Na}\downarrow$	[40]	601144
BrS2	*GPD1L*	GPD1L	3p22.3	Dominant	$I_{Na}\downarrow$	[14]	611777
BrS3	*CACNA1C*	Ca_v1.2	12p13.3	Dominant	$I_{Ca\text{-}L}\downarrow$	[41]	611875
BrS4	*CACNB2b*	Ca_v β2	10p12	Dominant	$I_{Ca\text{-}L}\downarrow$	[41]	611876
CPVT1	*RYR2*	RYR2	1q42.1–q43	Dominant	$\uparrow[Ca^{2+}]$	[21]	180902
CPVT2	*CASQ2*	CASQ2	1p13.3–p11	Recessive	$\uparrow[Ca^{2+}]$	[22]	114251
JLN1	*KCNQ1*	K_v7.1 α	11p15.5	Recessive	$I_{Ks}\downarrow$	[42]	220400
JLN2	*KCNE1*	minK β	21q22.1–q22.2	Recessive	$I_{Ks}\downarrow$	[43]	220400
LQT1	*KCNQ1*	K_v7.1 α	11p15.5	Dominant	$I_{Ks}\downarrow$	[44]	192500
LQT2	*KCNH2*	K_v11.1 α	7q35–q36	Dominant	$I_{Kr}\downarrow$	[45]	152427
LQT3	*SCN5A*	Na_v1.5	3p21	Dominant	$I_{Na}\uparrow$	[34]	603830
LQT4	*ANK2*	Ankyrin-B	4q25–q27	Dominant	$I_{Na,K}\downarrow$	[46]	600919
LQT5	*KCNE1*	minK β	21q22.1–q22.2	Dominant	$I_{Ks}\downarrow$	[47]	176261
LQT6	*KCNE2*	MiRP1 β	21q22.1	Dominant	$I_{Kr}\downarrow$	[48]	603796
LQT7 = ATS1	*KCNJ2*	kir2.1	17q23.1–q24.2	Dominant	$I_{K1}\downarrow$	[49]	170390

LQT8 = TS1	*CACNA1C*	Ca_v1.2	12p13.3	Dominant	$I_{Ca\text{-}L}\uparrow$	[50]	601005
LQT9	CAV3	Caveolin3	3p25	Dominant	$I_{Na}\uparrow$	[51]	601253
LQT10	SCN4B	Na_v1.5 β4	11q23.3	Dominant	$I_{Na}\uparrow$	[52]	608256
LQT11	Akap9	AKAP	7q21–q22		$I_{Ks}\downarrow$	[53]	611820
SQT1	*KCNH2*	HERG	7q35–q36	Dominant	$I_{Kr}\uparrow$	[54]	152427
SQT2	*KCNQ1*	KvLQT1	11p15.5	Dominant	$I_{Ks}\uparrow$	[55]	192500
SQT3	*KCNJ2*	Kir2.1, IRK1	17q23.1–q24.2	Dominant	$I_{K1}\uparrow$	[56]	170390

ATS, Andersen–Tawil syndrome; BrS, Brugada syndrome; CASQ2, calsequestrin 2; CPVT, catecholaminergic polymorphic VT; $I_{ca\text{-}L}$, voltage dependent Calcium channel L-type; I_{k1}, inward rectifying K+ current; I_{Kr}, rapid potassium efflux; I_{Ks}, slow potassium efflux; I_{Na}, sodium influx; LQT, long QT syndrome; OMIM, Online Mendelian Inheritance of Man (www.ncbi.nlm.nih.gov/omim); RYR2, ryanodine receptor 2; SQT, short QT syndrome; TS1, Timothy syndrome. Dark shading, involvement of potassium ion currents; white, involvement of sodium ion currents; light shading, involvement of calcium ion currents.

especially swimming [8]. Yearly SCD incidence is about 0.30% per year [9] and patients often present at young age (<5 years old) [10].

In LQTS2 the *KCNH2* gene coding for the HERG potassium channel is affected, leading to a reduced (rapid) potassium efflux (I_{Kr}). LQTS2 is present in about 40–45% of LQTS patients. Emotion or auditory stimuli during sleep are typical triggers for arrhythmias [8].

In LQTS3 the *SCN5A* gene is affected that encodes for the $Na_v1.5$ protein of the sodium channel, leading to a slowed closing of the channel and a prolonged cardiac sodium influx (I_{Na}). LQTS3 is present in about 5–10% of patients with LQTS. Arrhythmias often occur at rest or during sleep without arousal [8].

LQTS4–11 are rare and each represent less than 1% of patients with LQTS.

Treatment recommendations for all patients with LQTS include lifestyle changes (avoiding triggers) and beta-blockers. Implantable cardioverter-defibrillator (ICD) implantation is indicated in those with a previous cardiac arrest or syncope/ventricular tachycardia (VT) during -locker therapy [1].

Short QT syndromes

It is only recently that the short QT syndrome (SQTS) has been described. In this entity the QT interval is typically ≤300 ms [11]. It should be considered in patients with a QT interval <350 ms. In the first 5 years after its discovery only 30 new cases were described. So far, three different causal genes have been identified (Fig. 6.1a), all involving gain of function of potassium channels [12]. SCD risk seems high in patients with SQTS, but treatment is still poorly defined. Quinidine may be useful in patients with a mutation in the *KCNH2* gene. In others, ICD implantation may be necessary [13].

Brugada syndrome

Patients with Brugada syndrome (BrS) have arrhythmic events that mostly occur during the night at an average age of 40 years. BrS has a prevalence of about 5 per 10 000 and is endemic in East and southeast Asia. Of affected individuals, 80% are male. In only 10–30% of patients a gene defect can be identified. In these patients the cause is most often a defect in the *SCN5A* gene that leads to a loss of function of the sodium channel. Recently, three new genes that can cause BrS have been identified. Van Norstrand *et al.* [14] described GDP1L as an ion channel modulator that causes a decrease in inward cardiac sodium current Antezelevich *et al.* [15] found that mutations in *CACNA1C* and *CACNB2*, genes that encode for the α_1- and β_{2b}-subunits of the calcium channel, respectively, can cause BrS by loss of function of the cardiac L-type calcium channel. Diagnosis of BrS is based on typical electrocardiographic characteristics; however, these typically vary within the same patient. Based on morphology, three ECG subtypes can be distinguished. Elevated body temperature and sodium channel blockers such as flecainide, procainamide, and ajmaline can provoke or worsen the typical ECG changes. Only a documented spontaneous or drug-induced type 1 ECG qualifies for a definite diagnosis [16]. Patients with a spontaneous Brugada pattern have a worse prognosis than those with a drug-induced type 1 Brugada ECG [17]. The role of electrophysiologic studies in risk stratification is controversial [18]. Treatment by ICD is indicated in high-risk patients with previous cardiac arrest or documented VT/ventricular fibrillation (VF) or patients with spontaneous type 1 ECG and syncope [1,19,20].

Catecholaminergic polymorphic ventricular tachycardia

Typically, patients with catecholaminergic polymorphic VT (CPVT) experience bidirectional and polymorphic ventricular arrhythmias as the heart rate reaches a threshold of 120–130 beats per minute. An autosomal dominant form is seen in the majority of cases, in 50% of whom the *RYR2* gene is involved [21]. This gene encodes for the ryanodine receptor channel, which regulates Ca^{2+} release from the sarcoplasmic reticulum in response to Ca^{2+} entry through the sarcolemma L-type Ca^{2+} channels during the plateau phase of the action potential. Also, an autosomal recessive form exists in which the *CASQ2* gene is mutated which encodes for calsequestrin, a Ca^{2+}-buffering enzyme within the sarcoplasmic reticulum [22]. This form is associated with more severe symptoms and often occurs at younger age. The genetic defects in both forms lead to a Ca^{2+} overload in the sarcoplasmic reticulum, which worsens during higher heart rates and can result in triggered activity due to delayed afterdepolarizations. Patients in both forms often present in early childhood. Treatment is by beta-blockers in clinically diagnosed patients with CPVT. An ICD is indicated in patients with CPVT who survived cardiac arrest or who have syncope or documented sustained VT while receiving beta-blocker therapy [1].

Screening

The cause of death in young SCD victims has been the subject of several studies (Table 6.2). No structural cardiac abnormalities could be found in 20.9% of sudden death cases (<40 years old) in pathology studies and a primary arrhythmia could be presumed. The question arises whether screening of surviving relatives of these sudden unexplained death victims is warranted. Two studies have addressed this question. Behr *et al.* [23] studied 184 members of 57 families with one or more sudden unexplained death (SUD) between 4 and 64 years with normal autopsy findings. In all evaluated family members a normal and stress ECG, echocardiography, and Holter analysis were performed. Stepwise, other investigations were added which included signal-averaged ECG, ajmaline testing, cardiac magnetic resonance imaging, and mutation analysis. These authors could find a diagnosis in 30 families (57%). A study by our group that examined the same question found that a rigorous and extensive cardiological evaluation, encompassing normal and stress ECG, flecainide

Table 6.2 Cause of death in pathologic examination of sudden death cases <40 years.

Reference	Year	Age (years)	*N*	*N* NC	*N* SCD	Unresolved (%)	CAD (%)	HCM (%)	DCM (%)	ARVD (%)	LVH (%)	Myocarditis (%)	Vascular (%)	Valvular (%)	Conduction (%)	Other (%)
Burke *et al.* [57]	1990	14–40	690		690	15.9	45.8	4.1	0.0	0.1	11.0	4.8	4.2	3.3		10.7
Drory *et al.* [58]	1991	<40	162	25	118	13.9	50.8	12.7	4.7		0.0	22.0	0.8	1.7		8.5
Shen *et al.* [59]	1995	20–40	54	15	32	33.3	56.3	6.3			0.0	12.5	3.1			3.1
Steinberger *et al.* [60]	1996	1–21	50		40	20.0	0.0	15.0				35.0	30.0			20.0
Corrado *et al.* [61]	2001	<35	273		163	27.8	27.4	9.1	0.0	13.7			20.8	15.7		7.1
Wisten *et al.* [62]	2002	15–35	181		181	21.0	17.7	10.5	39.8	6.6		10.5	14.4	2.2	1.7	3.3
Puranik *et al.* [63]	2005	5–35	427	186	241	29.0	27.8	5.8	28.9	0.0	2.9	11.6	5.4			12.0
Fabre *et al.* [64]	2006	<35	223		223	53.4	Excluded*	6.7	11.2	2.7	4.9	7.6	2.2			5.8
Totals			1837	226	1499	20.9	36.5	6.8	2.5	2.7	5.5	8.3	8.2	4.0	0.2	9.5

Unresolved depicts the number of patients with normal cardiac findings at autopsy as a percentage of the total number of included patients minus the noncardiac deaths. ARVD, arrhythmogenic right ventricular cardiomyopathy; DCM, dilated cardiomyopathy; HCM, hypertrophic cardiomyopathy; LVH, left ventricular hypertrophy; *N*, total number of included patients; *N* NC, number of noncardiac sudden deaths (if empty then these were excluded by study design);*N* SCD, number of sudden cardiac death patients. *Excluded in the totals, as patients with coronary artery disease were excluded in this study.

testing, lipid screening, and DNA testing, could identify the underlying disease in 17 out of 43 families (40%) in which one SUD <40 years old had occurred. DNA testing could confirm the diagnosis in 23% of families [24]. Once the genetic basis of SCD is known within a family, DNA testing can be used as a screening tool. In conclusion, examination of relatives of young SCD victims has a high diagnostic and therapeutic yield and should be strongly advised in those concerned.

Multigenetic disease

Above 40 years of age, the prevalence of coronary artery disease rises sharply. Thereby, the cause of SCD in these patients is primarily atherosclerosis related. The question arises of whether genetics plays a role in the development of ventricular arrhythmias in this age group as well. Two case–control and one cohort study suggest genetic risk factors for SCD. A family history for sudden death turned out to be one of the most important risk factors, suggesting that gene variants or polymorphisms contribute to SCD risk.

The Paris Prospective Study included 7746 men employed by the city of Paris who were followed for 23 years. During this period 118 sudden cardiac deaths and 192 fatal myocardial infarctions occurred. The authors analyzed the role of traditional risk factors in these deaths. After correction for other risk factors, parental history of sudden death was independently related to the occurrence of sudden death [relative risk (RR) 1.80; 95% confidence interval (CI) 1.11–2.88), but was not associated with the occurrence of fatal myocardial infarction. In 19 patients in whom both parents died suddenly the risk was much higher (RR 9.44; $P = 0.01$), as would be expected when genetic factors are causally involved [25]. In a case–control study by Friedlander *et al.* [26] a selection of 235 cases of out-of-hospital primary cardiac arrest attended by paramedics in King County, Washington, were compared with 374 healthy controls from the general population. In this study there was a relative risk of 1.56 (95% CI 1.15–2.11) for sudden death if one parent died of sudden death. In our own Primary VF study, 330 primary VF survivors (cases) and 372 patients with a first ST-elevation myocardial infarction without VF (controls) were compared. Familial sudden death occurred significantly more frequently among cases than among controls (43.1% and 25.1%, respectively) resulting in an odds ratio of 2.72 (95% CI 1.84–4.03) [27].

Clearly, gene polymorphisms contribute to SCD risk and over recent years many polymorphisms have been related to SCD risk (Table 6.3). Lanfear *et al.* [28] prospectively studied 597 patients with an acute coronary syndrome who were treated with beta-blockers. They found that the risk of sudden cardiac death in this group was dependent on the *ADRB2* genotype, but not on the *ADRB1* genotype. The risk ranged from 6% in the GG/79GC group to 46% in the AA/79 CC group, possibly reflecting beta-blocker resistance in the latter.

Table 6.3 An overview of gene polymorphisms that have been related to risk of sudden cardiac death

Gene studied	Study type	Study group	Risk factor	Higher risk	Reference	OMIM
GP1BA	Case–control, autopsy	288 SCD vs 272 VD	1	(HPA-2 Met haplotype more prevalent in young SCD, but not on group level)	[31]	606672
F5, G20210A	Case–control	168 SCD vs 606 healthy controls	1	–	[65]	227400
KCNJ11	Case–control	86 SCD vs 84 with ⩾3 MIs	1	–	[66]	600937
SCN5A	Case–control	67 SCD vs 91 CAD patients	1	–	[36]	600163
ITGA2B	Case–control	94 SCD survivors vs 160 CAD patients	1	–	[67]	607759
SCN5A	Case–control	182 SCD vs 107 noncardiac SD; all black	1	RR 8.4 for Y1102 in subgroup with unexplained arrhythmias	[35]	600163
ADRB2	Prospective cohort	4441 European American cohort (156 SCD) 808 African American cohort (39 SCD) Replicated in 155 SCD cases and 144 controls (European Americans)	1.2–1.6	Gln27 homozygous participants had a 58% higher SCD risk than participants with ⩾1 Glu27 alleles	[29]	109690

ACE	Cohort	479 HF patients of whom 82 ICD for arrhythmias	2.06	Survival worse in ACE-DD subjects	[68]	106180
PAI-I 4G/5G	Case–control	97 SCD survivors with ICD vs 113 CAD patients	3.6	4G/4G genotype	[32]	173360
ADRB1 ADRB2	Prospective cohort	597 ACS patients with beta-blockers whereof 84 died during follow-up	1 2.41–5.36	– Patients with beta-blocker and 46AA or 79CC polymorphism	[28]	109690
HL	Case–control, autopsy	288 SCD vs 404 non-SCD	3.0	HL C480T polymorphism	[69]	151670
GPIIIA	Case–control, autopsy	281 SCD vs 258 VD	6.6	Pl^{A2} positive genotype more prevalent in SCD < 50 years	[30]	173470

ACE, angiotensin-converting enzyme; ACS, acute coronary syndrome; ADRB, β-adrenoreceptor; CAD, coronary artery disease; F5, factor 5 Leiden; GPIIIA, glycoprotein IIIA; GP1BA, glycoprotein 1B alpha; HF, heart failure; HL, hepatic lipase; ITGA2B, integrin-alpha-2B; MI, myocardial infarction; PAI-I, plasminogen activator inhibitor type I; RR, relative risk; SCD, sudden cardiac death; VD, violent death.

Sotoodehnia *et al.* [29] performed a prospective cohort study of 4441 white and 808 black participants in which they tested only the *ADRB2* genotype for two common single nucleotide polymorphisms that result in amino acid substitutions: Gly16Arg and Gln27Glu. They found that Gln27 homozygous participants had a 58% higher SCD risk than participants with one or more Glu27 alleles (ethnicity-adjusted Hazard Ratio (HR) 1.56; 95% CI 1.17–2.09). Mikkelsson *et al.* [30] have studied glycoprotein receptors involved in thrombus formation in a case–control autopsy study in which victims of SCD and those of violent death were compared. They found that the PI^{A2} polymorphism of the glycoprotein IIIa receptor was more prevalent in SCD cases <50 years old. The HPA-2 Met haplotype was more prevalent in young SCD cases [31]. Anvari *et al.* [32] studied plasminogen activator inhibitor type I polymorphisms in a case–control study of SCD survivors with an ICD compared with patients with coronary artery disease without a history of malignant ventricular arrhythmias. They found that carriers of the plasminogen activator inhibitor type I (PAI-I) 4G/4G genotype had an increased risk of sudden death. Bedi *et al.* [66] studied angiotensin-converting enzyme (ACE) polymorphisms in a cohort study of 479 patients with heart failure of whom 82 received an ICD. In this study, the ACE-DD genotype was associated with a worse survival, which could not be improved by ICD placement, suggesting that this genotype is associated with death due to heart failure rather than arrhythmic sudden death. A genome-wide study identified NOS1AP (CAPON), a regulator of neuronal nitric oxide synthase, as a new target that modulates cardiac repolarization. It could explain up to 1.5% of QT interval variation in a population of 200 subjects at the extremes of a population of 3966 subjects from the German KORA cohort in which QT intervals were measured. [33] Finally, several groups have studied polymorphisms of the *SCN5A* gene as a potential source for SCD. This gene is of special interest as it is involved in several of the primary arrhythmia syndromes. Splawski *et al.* [34] found that the Y1102 polymorphism of the *SCN5A* gene was present in 56.5% of 23 African Americans with suspected ventricular arrhythmias and in 13% in 468 healthy controls. They added evidence for a possible role for the Y1102 allele in arrhythmogenesis by showing that it causes a shift in voltage dependence of the sodium channel when transfected in human embryonic kidney cells. Burke *et al.* [35] later confirmed these findings in a larger study. Stecker *et al.* [36] studied SCN5A polymorphisms in 67 SCD cases and 91 controls with coronary artery disease, but without arrhythmias or syncope. They found a low prevalence of amino acid-altering polymorphisms in both groups and could not significantly associate polymorphisms with SCD risk. Studies of polymorphisms in the genes encoding for KCNJ11, factor 5 Leiden, and integrin-alpha-2B did not find an association with SCD risk.

Some limitations apply to the interpretation of these data. All studies were performed in relatively small groups. Furthermore, the studies by Mikkelsson *et al.* [30], Reiner *et al.*, [65] and Burke *et al.* [35] compare deceased patients with controls without coronary artery disease. This makes it difficult to discern whether the polymorphisms found are related to SCD or to ischemia, which is itself related to SCD.

In conclusion, the risk of ventricular arrhythmias and sudden death in both younger and older patients can at least be partly explained by the genetic profile. Some of the genes that are involved in primary arrhythmia syndromes might play a role in SCD risk in the older population as well. Genes are associated with arrhythmias at an ever-increasing rate. Current knowledge of genetic profiles starts to guide risk stratification and therapy. Further development will come from genome-wide strategies in larger patient populations [37,38]. Over the coming years, results of these studies will become available.

References

1 ACC/AHA/ESC. 2006 Guidelines for management of patients with ventricular arrhythmias and the prevention of sudden cardiac death. Executive summary: a report of the American College of Cardiology/American Heart Association Task Force and the European Society of Cardiology Committee for Practice Guidelines (Writing Committee to Develop Guidelines for Management of Patients With Ventricular Arrhythmias and the Prevention of Sudden Cardiac Death). *Journal of the American College of Cardiology* 2006; **48**: 1064–1108.

2 Fox CS, Evans JC, Larson MG *et al.* Temporal trends in coronary heart disease mortality and sudden cardiac death from 1950 to 1999: The Framingham Heart Study. *Circulation* 2004; **110**: 522–527.

3 Bunch TJ, White RD. Trends in treated ventricular fibrillation in out-of-hospital cardiac arrest: ischemic compared to non-ischemic heart disease. *Resuscitation* 2005; **67**: 51–54.

4 Goraya TY, Jacobsen SJ, Kottke TE *et al.* Coronary heart disease death and sudden cardiac death: a 20-year population-based study. *American Journal of Epidemiology* 2003; **157**: 763–770.

5 Quaglini S, Rognoni C, Spazzolini C *et al.* Cost-effectiveness of neonatal ECG screening for the long QT syndrome. *European Heart Journal* 2006; **27**: 1824–1832.

6 Priori SG, Napolitano C, Schwartz PJ. Low penetrance in the long-QT syndrome: clinical impact. *Circulation* 1999; **99**: 529–533.

7 Moss AJ, Shimizu W, Wilde AAM *et al.* Clinical aspects of type-1 long-QT syndrome by location, coding type, and biophysical function of mutations involving the KCNQ1 gene. *Circulation* 2007; **115**: 2481–2489.

8 Schwartz PJ, Priori SG, Spazzolini C *et al.* Genotype-phenotype correlation in the long-QT syndrome: gene-specific triggers for life-threatening arrhythmias. *Circulation* 2001; **103**: 89–95.

9 Priori SG, Schwartz PJ, Napolitano C *et al.* Risk stratification in the long-QT syndrome. *New England Journal of Medicine* 2003; **348**: 1866–1874.

10 Zareba W, Moss AJ, Schwartz PJ *et al.* Influence of genotype on the clinical course of the long-QT syndrome. International Long-QT Syndrome Registry Research Group. *New England Journal of Medicine* 1998; **339**: 960–965.

11 Gussak I, Brugada P, Brugada J *et al*. Idiopathic short QT interval: a new clinical syndrome? *Cardiology* 2000; **94**: 99–102.

12 Gussak I, Bjerregaard P. Short QT syndrome: 5 years of progress. *Journal of Electrocardiology* 2005; **38**: 375–377.

13 Giustetto C, Di Monte F, Wolpert C *et al*. Short QT syndrome: clinical findings and diagnostic-therapeutic implications. *European Heart Journal* 2006; **27**: 2440–2447.

14 Van Norstrand DW, Valdivia CR, Tester DJ *et al*. Molecular and functional characterization of novel glycerol-3-phosphate dehydrogenase 1 like gene (GPD1-L) mutations in sudden infant death syndrome. *Circulation* 2007; **116**: 2253–2259.

15 Antzelevitch C, Wilde A, Eckardt L *et al*. Diagnostic and genetic aspects of the Brugada and other inherited arrhythmias syndromes. *Journal of Electrocardiology* 2007; **40** (1 Suppl): S11–S14.

16 Wilde AA, Antzelevitch C, Borggrefe M *et al*. Proposed diagnostic criteria for the Brugada syndrome. *European Heart Journal* 2002; **23**: 1648–1654.

17 Sarkozy A, Boussy T, Kourgiannides G *et al*. Long-term follow-up of primary prophylactic implantable cardioverter-defibrillator therapy in Brugada syndrome. *European Heart Journal* 2007; **28(3)**:. 334–344.

18 Paul M, Gerss J, Schulze-Bahr E *et al*. Role of programmed ventricular stimulation in patients with Brugada syndrome: a meta-analysis of worldwide published data. *European Heart Journal* 2007; **28(3)**:. 334–344.

19 Gehi AK, Duong TD, Metz LD *et al*. Risk stratification of individuals with the brugada electrocardiogram: a meta-analysis. *Journal of Cardiovascular Electrophysiology* 2006; **17**: 577–583.

20 Epstein AE, DiMarco JP, Ellenbogen KA *et al*. ACC/AHA/HRS 2008 Guidelines for device-based therapy of cardiac rhythm abnormalities: a report of the American College of Cardiology/American Heart Association Task Force on Practice Guidelines (Writing Committee to Revise the ACC/AHA/NASPE 2002 Guideline Update for Implantation of Cardiac Pacemakers and Antiarrhythmia Devices) developed in collaboration with the American Association for Thoracic Surgery and Society of Thoracic Surgeons. *Journal of the American College of Cardiology* 2008; **51**: e1–62.

21 Priori SG, Napolitano C, Tiso N *et al*. Mutations in the cardiac ryanodine receptor gene (hRyR2) underlie catecholaminergic polymorphic ventricular tachycardia. *Circulation* 2001; **103**: 196–200.

22 Lahat H, Pras E, Olender T *et al*. A missense mutation in a highly conserved region of CASQ2 is associated with autosomal recessive catecholamine-induced polymorphic ventricular tachycardia in Bedouin families from Israel. *American Journal of Human Genetics* 2001; **69**: 1378–1384.

23 Behr ER, Dalageorgou C, Christiansen M *et al*. Sudden arrhythmic death syndrome: familial evaluation identifies inheritable heart disease in the majority of families. *European Heart Journal* 2008; **29**: 1670–1680.

24 Tan HL, Hofman N, van Langen IM *et al*. Sudden unexplained death: heritability and diagnostic yield of cardiological and genetic examination in surviving relatives. *Circulation* 2005; **112**: 207–213.

25 Jouven X, Desnos M, Guerot C, Ducimetiere P. Predicting sudden death in the population: the Paris Prospective Study I. *Circulation* 1999; **99**: 1978–1983.

26 Friedlander Y, Siscovick DS, Weinmann S *et al*. Family history as a risk factor for primary cardiac arrest. *Circulation* 1998; **97**: 155–160.

27 Dekker LRC, Bezzina CR, Henriques JPS *et al.* Familial sudden death is an important risk factor for primary ventricular fibrillation: a case–control study in acute myocardial infarction patients. *Circulation* 2006; **114**: 1140–1145.

28 Lanfear DE, Jones PG, Marsh S *et al.* β2-Adrenergic receptor genotype and survival among patients receiving β-blocker therapy after an acute coronary syndrome. *JAMA: The Journal of the American Medical Association* 2005; **294**: 1526–1533.

29 Sotoodehnia N, Siscovick DS, Vatta M *et al.* Beta2-adrenergic receptor genetic variants and risk of sudden cardiac death. *Circulation* 2006; **113**: 1842–1848.

30 Mikkelsson J, Perola M, Laippala P *et al.* Glycoprotein IIIa Pl(A1/A2) polymorphism and sudden cardiac death. *Journal of the American College of Cardiology* 2000; **36**: 1317–1323.

31 Mikkelsson J, Perola M, Penttila A, Karhunen PJ. Platelet glycoprotein Ibalpha HPA-2 Met/VNTR B haplotype as a genetic predictor of myocardial infarction and sudden cardiac death. *Circulation* 2001; **104**: 876–880.

32 Anvari A, Schuster E, Gottsauner-Wolf M *et al.* PAI-I 4G/5G polymorphism and sudden cardiac death in patients with coronary artery disease. *Thrombosis Research* 2001; **103**: 103–107.

33 Arking DE, Pfeufer A, Post W *et al.* A common genetic variant in the NOS1 regulator NOS1AP modulates cardiac repolarization. *Nature Genetics* 2006; **38**: 644–651.

34 Splawski I, Timothy KW, Tateyama M *et al.* Variant of SCN5A sodium channel implicated in risk of cardiac arrhythmia. *Science* 2002; **297**: 1333–1336.

35 Burke A, Creighton W, Mont E *et al.* Role of SCN5A Y1102 polymorphism in sudden cardiac death in blacks. *Circulation* 2005; **112**: 798–802.

36 Stecker EC, Sono M, Wallace E *et al.* Allelic variants of SCN5A and risk of sudden cardiac arrest in patients with coronary artery disease. *Heart Rhythm* 2006; **3**: 697–700.

37 Spooner PM, Albert C, Benjamin EJ *et al.* Sudden cardiac death, genes, and arrhythmogenesis : consideration of new population and mechanistic approaches from a national heart, lung, and blood institute workshop, part I. *Circulation* 2001; **103**: 2361–2364.

38 Spooner PM, Albert C, Benjamin EJ *et al.* Sudden cardiac death, genes, and arrhythmogenesis: consideration of new population and mechanistic approaches from a National Heart, Lung, and Blood Institute workshop, part II. *Circulation* 2001; **103**: 2447–2452.

39 Wilde AAM, Dekker LRC. Is there a genetic basis for malignant ventricular arrhythmias? *Heart Rhythm* 2005; **2**: 1145–1147.

40 Chen Q, Kirsch GE, Zhang D *et al.* Genetic basis and molecular mechanism for idiopathic ventricular fibrillation. *Nature* 1998; **392**: 293–296.

41 Antzelevitch C, Pollevick GD, Cordeiro JM *et al.* Loss-of-function mutations in the cardiac calcium channel underlie a new clinical entity characterized by ST-segment elevation, short QT intervals, and sudden cardiac death. *Circulation* 2007; **115**: 442–449.

42 Splawski I, Timothy KW, Vincent GM *et al.* Molecular basis of the long-QT syndrome associated with deafness. N Engl J Med. 1997; **336(22):** 1562–1567.

43 Splawski I, Tristani-Firouzi M, Lehmann MH *et al.* Mutations in the hminK gene cause long QT syndrome and suppress IKs function. *Nature Genetics* 1997; **17**: 338–340.

44 Wang Q, Curran ME, Splawski I *et al.* Positional cloning of a novel potassium channel gene: KVLQT1 mutations cause cardiac arrhythmias. *Nature Genetics* 1996; **12**: 17–23.

45 Curran ME, Splawski I, Timothy KW *et al.* A molecular basis for cardiac arrhythmia: HERG mutations cause long QT syndrome. *Cell* 1995; **80**: 795–803.
46 Mohler PJ, Schott JJ, Gramolini AO *et al.* Ankyrin-B mutation causes type 4 long-QT cardiac arrhythmia and sudden cardiac death. *Nature* 2003; **421**: 634–639.
47 Shalaby FY, Levesque PC, Yang WP *et al.* Dominant-negative KvLQT1 mutations underlie the LQT1 form of long QT syndrome. *Circulation* 1997; **96**: 1733–1736.
48 Abbott GW, Sesti F, Splawski I *et al.* MiRP1 forms IKr potassium channels with HERG and is associated with cardiac arrhythmia. *Cell* 1999; **97**: 175–187.
49 Plaster NM, Tawil R, Tristani-Firouzi M *et al.* Mutations in Kir2.1 cause the developmental and episodic electrical phenotypes of Andersen's syndrome. *Cell* 2001; **105**: 511–519.
50 Splawski I, Timothy KW, Decher N *et al.* Severe arrhythmia disorder caused by cardiac L-type calcium channel mutations. *Proceedings of the National Academy of Sciences of the USA* 2005; **102**: 8089–8096.
51 Vatta M, Ackerman MJ, Ye B *et al.* Mutant caveolin-3 induces persistent late sodium current and is associated with long-QT syndrome. *Circulation* 2006; **114**: 2104–2112.
52 Domingo AM, Kaku T, Tester DJ *et al.* AB16-6: sodium channel β4 subunit mutation causes congenital long QT syndrome. *Heart Rhythm* 2006; **3** (5, Suppl 1): S34.
53 Chen L, Marquardt ML, Tester DJ *et al.* Mutation of an A-kinase-anchoring protein causes long-QT syndrome. *Proceedings of the National Academy of Sciences of the USA* 2007; **104**: 20990.
54 Brugada R, Hong K, Dumaine R *et al.* Sudden death associated with short-QT syndrome linked to mutations in HERG. *Circulation* 2004; **109**: 30–35.
55 Bellocq C, van Ginneken AC, Bezzina CR *et al.* Mutation in the KCNQ1 gene leading to the short QT-interval syndrome. *Circulation* 2004; **109**: 2394–2397.
56 Priori SG, Pandit SV, Rivolta I *et al.* A novel form of short QT syndrome (SQT3) is caused by a mutation in the KCNJ2 gene. *Circulation Research* 2005; **96**: 800–807.
57 Burke AP, Farb A, Virmani R *et al.* Sports-related and non-sports-related sudden cardiac death in young adults. *American Heart Journal* 1991; **121** (2 Pt 1): 568–575.
58 Drory Y, Turetz Y, Hiss Y *et al.* Sudden unexpected death in persons less than 40 years of age. *American Journal of Cardiology* 1991; **68**: 1388–1392.
59 Shen WK, Edwards WD, Hammill SC *et al.* Sudden unexpected nontraumatic death in 54 young adults: a 30-year population-based study. *American Journal of Cardiology* 1995; **76**: 148–152.
60 Steinberger J, Lucas V, Edwards JE, Titus JL. Causes of sudden unexpected cardiac death in the first two decades of life. *American Journal of Cardiology* 1996; **77**: 992–995.
61 Corrado D, Basso C, Thiene G. Sudden cardiac death in young people with apparently normal heart. *Cardiovascular Research* 2001; **50**: 399–408.
62 Wisten A, Forsberg H, Krantz P, Messner T. Sudden cardiac death in 15–35-year olds in Sweden during 1992–99. *Journal of Internal Medicine* 2002; **252**: 529–536.
63 Puranik R, Chow CK, Duflou JA *et al.* Sudden death in the young. *Heart Rhythm* 2005; **2**: 1277–1282.
64 Fabre A, Sheppard MN. Sudden adult death syndrome and other non-ischaemic causes of sudden cardiac death. *British Heart Journal* 2006; **92**: 316–320.
65 Reiner AP, Rosendaal FR, Reitsma PH *et al.* Factor V Leiden, prothrombin G20210A, and risk of sudden coronary death in apparently healthy persons. *American Journal of Cardiology* 2002; **90**: 66–68.

66 Jeron A, Hengstenberg C, Holmer S *et al.* KCNJ11 polymorphisms and sudden cardiac death in patients with acute myocardial infarction. *Journal of Molecular and Cellular Cardiology* 2004; **36**: 287–293.
67 Anvari A, Janisiw M, T'rel Z *et al.* Platelet glycoprotein Ia gene dimorphism a2-807 in malignant arrhythmia in coronary artery disease. *Thrombosis Research* 2000; **98**: 281–286.
68 Bedi MS, Postava LA, Murali S *et al.* Interaction of implantable defibrillator therapy with angiotensin-converting enzyme deletion/insertion polymorphism. *Journal of Cardiovascular Electrophysiology* 2004; **15**: 1162–1166.
69 Fan YM, Lehtimki T, Rontu R *et al.* Age-dependent association between hepatic lipase gene C-480T polymorphism and the risk of pre-hospital sudden cardiac death: The Helsinki Sudden Death Study. *Atherosclerosis* 2007; **192**: 421–427.

Chapter 7

Hypertrophic cardiomyopathy and other forms of hypertrophy

Carolyn Y. Ho

Introduction

The study of inherited cardiomyopathies has illuminated distinct genetic defects which can give rise to the common phenotype of cardiac hypertrophy. Diverse pathways have been identified, implicating involvement of contractile proteins, intracellular calcium handling, and myocardial energetics in causing disease. Determining the fundamental mechanisms that link underlying gene mutations to clinical disease will provide important insights into pathogenesis, diagnosis, and treatment.

Hypertrophic cardiomyopathy: a disease of the sarcomere

Hypertrophic remodeling most commonly occurs in response to left ventricular pressure overload; however, unexplained left ventricular hypertrophy (LVH), which develops in the absence of such stimuli, indicates a primary myocardial process and is a defining feature of hypertrophic cardiomyopathy (HCM). HCM is a genetic cardiovascular disorder with autosomal dominant inheritance. Family linkage studies in the 1980s and 1990s led to the discovery of causal mutations in genes encoding different components of the contractile apparatus [1–3] and established the paradigm that HCM is a disease of the sarcomere (Fig. 7.1).

Clinical phenotype of hypertrophic cardiomyopathy

Natural history and clinical manifestations

HCM exhibits remarkable heterogeneity in clinical course, age of onset, degree and pattern of LVH, severity of symptoms, presence or absence of obstructive

Cardiovascular Genetics and Genomics. Edited by Dan Roden. © 2009 American Heart Association, ISBN: 978-14051-7540-1.

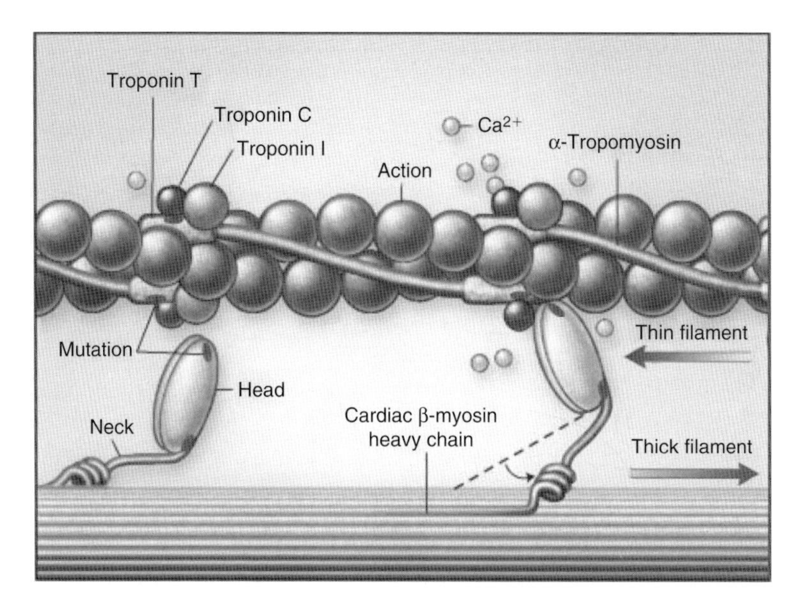

Fig. 7.1 The sarcomere is composed of interdigitating thick and thin filaments. Force is generated by cyclical crossbridge formation between actin and myosin. Hypertrophic cardiomyopathy is a disease of the sarcomere, caused by dominantly inherited mutations in contractile genes—most commonly β-myosin heavy chain, myosin binding protein C, and cardiac troponins T and I. Reprint from Kamisago M, *et al. N Engl J Med* 2000; 343: 1688–96, with permission, copyright 2000 Massachusetts Medical Society. All rights reserved.

physiology, and risk for sudden cardiac death (SCD) [4]. Clinical evaluation may be triggered in response to symptoms suggestive of HCM, or in asymptomatic individuals to investigate a systolic murmur, ECG abnormalities, or during family screening.

The histopathologic hallmarks of HCM are myocyte hypertrophy with disarray and fibrosis (Fig. 7.2). HCM is usually diagnosed by identifying unexplained LVH on cardiac imaging. Asymmetric septal hypertrophy is the most common morphologic pattern; however, any pattern, including concentric, apical, and isolated segmental hypertrophy, can be seen [5]. Rarely, patients may progress to the "burnt-out" or end-stage phase of HCM, marked by left ventricular systolic dysfunction, worsening symptoms, and occasionally progressive left ventricular (LV) wall thinning and chamber enlargement. Although only ~3–5% of patients develop this complication, the prognosis is less favorable than in typical HCM [6,7].

Estimates of annual mortality rates for HCM range from 4–6% in referral-based populations to 1–2% in community-based studies [8]. Sudden cardiac death (accounting for approximately half of HCM-related deaths), progressive

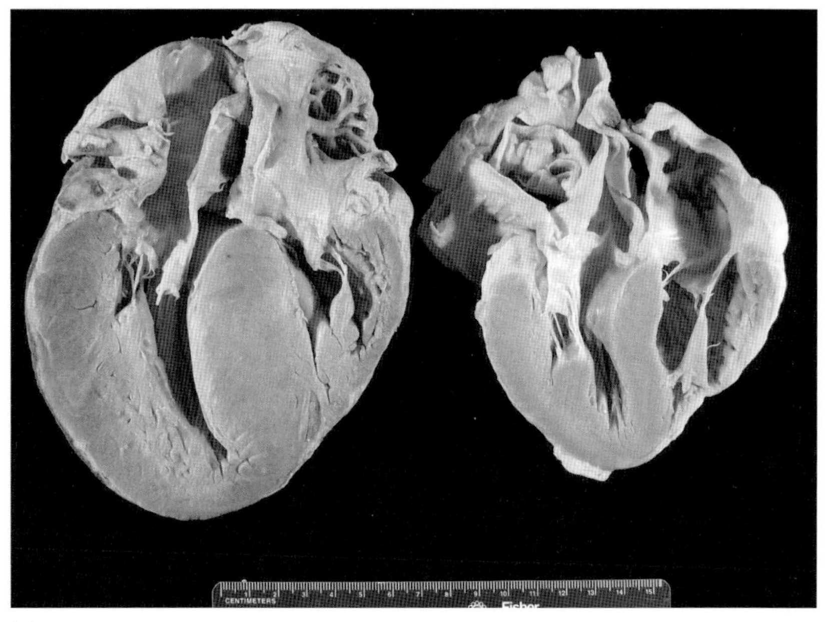

(a)

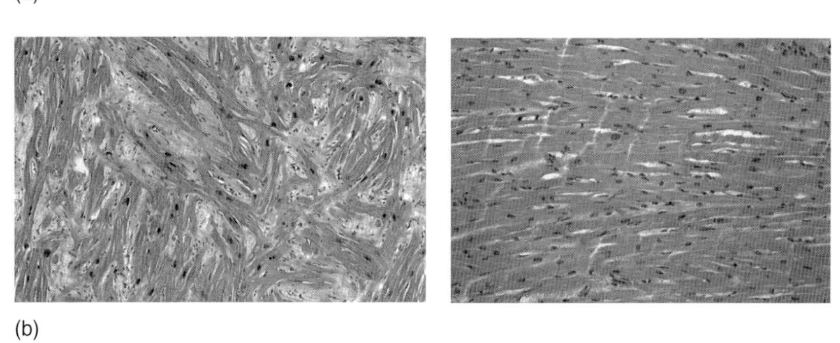

(b)

Fig. 7.2 (a) Gross pathology showing the markedly increased LV mass and left ventricular hypertrophy characteristic of hypertrophic cardiomyopathy (HCM) (left) compared with normal cardiac morphology (right). (b) Histologic sections stained with hematoxylin and eosin demonstrate the pathognomonic features of HCM with myocyte disarray and fibrosis (left) in contrast to the orderly arrangement of myocytes characteristic of normal myocardium (right). (Courtesy of Dr. Robert Padera, Department of Pathology, Brigham and Women's Hospital, Boston, MA, USA.)

heart failure, atrial fibrillation, and stroke are leading causes of the morbidity and mortality associated with HCM.

Management

Strategies to prevent disease progression in asymptomatic patients are not yet available; therefore, current treatment focuses on symptom management and

Table 7.1 Standard management strategies for hypertrophic cardiomyopathy

All patients	Family screening
	Genetic counseling
	Periodic assessment for SCD risk
	Education on recommended exercise restrictions
Mild to moderate symptoms (exercise intolerance, SOB, CP)	Beta-blockers or Calcium channel blockers (diltiazem or verapamil)
Symptomatic volume overload	Add diuretics (caution: hypovolemia may worsen obstructive physiology)
Persistent or worsening symptoms + obstructive physiology	Consider adding disopyramide
Medically refractory symptoms + obstructive physiology	Septal myectomy or Alcohol septal ablation
Heart failure/end-stage HCM	Diuretics as needed for volume overload
	ACE inhibitors/angiotensin receptor blockers
	Beta-blockers
	Consider cardiac transplantation

ACE, angiotensin-converting enzyme; CP, Chest pain; HCM, hypertrophic cardiomyopathy; LV, left ventricular; SCD, sudden cardiac death; SOB, shortness of breath.

assessment for risk of SCD, as summarized in Table 7.1. Medical therapy is first line, typically utilizing beta-blockers or L-type calcium channel blockers (verapamil or diltiazem) to increase diastolic filling time and reduce intracavitary gradients. Disopyramide may also be beneficial to reduce obstructive physiology via its negative inotropic effects. If symptoms of obstructive physiology are refractory to medical management, invasive approaches such as ethanol septal ablation or surgical myectomy may be used to mechanically reduce outflow tract obstruction [9–11]. Patients with end-stage HCM should be managed with standard therapy for advanced heart failure and may ultimately require cardiac transplantation.

HCM is associated with an increased risk of sudden cardiac death and is the leading cause of SCD in adolescents and competitive athletes in the United States. [9–12]. Therefore, assessment of SCD risk and determination of appropriate therapy are important, but challenging, components of management. Clinical predictors of increased SCD risk include a family history of sudden death, unexplained syncope, hypotensive blood pressure response to exercise, significant, spontaneous ventricular ectopy on Holter monitoring, and extreme LVH

(.30 mm). Implantable cardioverter defibrillator (ICD) therapy has been shown to be effective and should be considered for primary prevention of SCD in the appropriate setting [9,10,13,14]. But because the positive predictive value of these predictors individually is low, typically 20–30%, accurate identification of patients at increased risk is difficult [10,13,15]. Decision-making is guided by the number and nature of risk factors, as well as clinical judgment. Individuals who have survived cardiac arrest or have sustained ventricular tachycardia are at high risk for recurrent events and should receive ICDs for secondary prevention.

Genetics of hypertrophic cardiomyopathy

Distribution and prevalence of causal genes

The prevalence of unexplained LVH in the general population is estimated to be 1 in 500 [16,17]. The proportion accounted for by sarcomere mutations is unclear, but estimated at ~60% [18–20]. As such, HCM is the most common genetic cardiovascular disorder and the leading cause of sudden death among competitive athletes in the USA [21].

HCM demonstrates substantial allelic and nonallelic heterogeneity. Over 800 mutations have been identified in 11 different contractile genes, with no specific racial or ethnic predilections. Causal genes are summarized in Table 7.2 and updated data are available at http://cardiogenomics.med.harvard.edu. In addition to the genes listed in Table 7.2, other sarcomere-associated genes have been described in HCM, including cardiac troponin C (*TNNC1*), telethonin (*TCAP*), and muscle LIM protein (*CRP3*) [22–24]. Mutations in these genes are rare and the strength of evidence for causing disease is not as well established.

Currently, the majority of mutations identified (~60% in *MYBPC3* and *MYH7*) are novel sequence variants—not previously reported as disease causing [19,20,25,26]. Because of the high incidence of novel mutations and the degree of allelic heterogeneity, genetic testing should involve analysis of the full sequence of sarcomere genes, rather than trying to selectively target known mutations. Furthermore, when novel sequence variants are identified, family analysis to assess for cosegregation is valuable to assist in determination of their pathogenicity. A relatively high 3–5% rate of compound and double heterozygosity has also been observed in which two sarcomere mutations are present in a single individual with HCM [20,27].

Mutations in the genes encoding cardiac β-myosin heavy chain (*MYH7*), cardiac myosin binding protein C (*MYBPC3*), cardiac troponin T (*TNNT2*), and cardiac troponin I (*TNNI3*) combined account for almost 90% of described cases of HCM.

Cardiac β-myosin heavy chain (MYH7, β-MHC)

In 1989, the first mutation associated with HCM was identified in *MYH7* through linkage analysis of a large French Canadian family [1,28]. Since then, ~200

Table 7.2 Sarcomere mutations in hypertrophic cardiomyopathy

Protein	Gene	Chromosome	No. of mutations	Prevalence	Function	Comments
Cardiac β-myosin heavy chain*	*MYH7*	14q1	~200	~40%	Thick filament-force generation	Younger onset is typical
Cardiac myosin binding protein C*	*MYBPC3*	11q1	~150	~40%	?Structural support	Association with later-onset LVH
Cardiac troponin T*	*TNNT2*	1q3	~31	~5%	Thin filament-regulation	Increased SCD risk in some
Cardiac troponin I*	*TNNI3*	19p1	~27	~5%	Thin filament-regulation	
α-Tropomyosin*	*TPM1*	15q2	~11	~2%	Thin filament-regulation	
Myosin essential* and regulatory* light chains	*MYL2, MYL3*	3p, 12q	~15	~1%	Thick filament	
Actin*	*ACTC*	11q	~7	~1%	Thin filament-force generation	
Titin	*TTN*	2q3	2	Rare		
Myozenin	*MYOZ2*	4q26	2	Rare	Z-disk	
α-Myosin heavy chain	*MYH6*	14q1	1	Rare	Thick filament-force generation	

*Clinical genetic testing available.

LVH, left ventricular hypertrophy; SCD, sudden cardiac death.

different *MYH7* mutations have been reported in both familial and sporadic disease, accounting for ~30–40% of all cases of HCM [19,25,26] (http://cardiogenomics.med.harvard.edu).

Myosin heavy chains (MHCs) have two functional domains: an amino-terminal globular head that interacts with actin to generate force, and a carboxy-terminal rod which interacts with the myosin light chains [29]. HCM-causing mutations are almost exclusively missense (resulting in amino acid substitution) and clustered within the globular head or head–rod junction.

Cardiac myosin binding protein C (MYPBC3, cMyBPC)

Cardiac myosin binding protein C is thought to provide structural integrity to the sarcomere (binding MHC and titin), play a role in sarcomeric assembly [30], and may modulate myosin ATPase activity and cardiac contractility in response to adrenergic stimulation [31]. Missense mutations occur; however, splice site and small deletion/insertion mutations are common, leading to a truncated protein or null allele [20]. Approximately 150 mutations have been reported to date, accounting for ~30–40% of cases of HCM [19,25,26].

Cardiac troponin T (TNNT2, cTnT)

Troponin T links the troponin complex to α-tropomyosin and plays a central role in the regulation of contractility. Alternative splicing results in multiple isoforms of troponin T, including a cardiac-specific isoform. To date, ~30 missense, splice site, and deletion mutations have been reported in *TNNT2*, accounting for approximately 5% of cases of HCM [20] (http://cardiogenomics.med.harvard.edu).

Genotype–phenotype correlations

Although genotype certainly influences phenotype, most mutations are individually rare and not consistently benign or malignant. There is marked variation in symptoms, extent and location of LVH, and sudden death risk, even among family members who have inherited the same causal mutation. Consequently, robust genotype–phenotype correlations have not emerged. In most cases, the exact identity of the causal gene mutation is not highly predictive of outcome; however, a small number of specific point mutations have recurred and have demonstrated more stereotypical phenotypes in unrelated families. For example, the clinical course of *MYH7* mutations Arg403Gln, Arg719Trp, and Arg719Gln has been severe, associated with an increased risk of sudden death or development of end-stage heart failure. Certain *TNNT2* mutations (Arg92Trp, Arg92Gln, Ile79Asn) have been associated with mild LVH but an increased risk of sudden death in some families [3,26,30,32].

Genotype appears to play a role in influencing the age of onset of LVH and LV morphology. Most *MYH7* mutation carriers have demonstrable LVH by the second decade of life. In contrast, mutations in *MYBPC3* may not result in clinically evident hypertrophy until the fourth or fifth decade of life, and mutations in this gene have been associated with elderly-onset HCM (Fig. 7.3) [33,34]. A rare form of familial apical HCM has been associated with a Glu101Lys mutation in the cardiac actin gene [35]. However, caution must be used in generalizing these specific observations to other patients and families, as exceptions are well documented. The ultimate phenotype resulting from inherited sarcomere mutations reflects multiple factors, including genetic background and modifier genes as well as environmental factors, such as comorbid illnesses and lifestyle. Integration of genotype information with comprehensive clinical assessment and review of family history is necessary for optimal patient management.

Penetrance

Although history, physical findings, and ECG abnormalities may provide supportive evidence, identifying unexplained LVH on cardiac imaging is the current standard for establishing a clinical diagnosis of HCM. However, it is clear that LVH is not an infallible marker for genetic status or risk of disease-related complications, particularly early in life [36,37]. Although the causal sarcomere

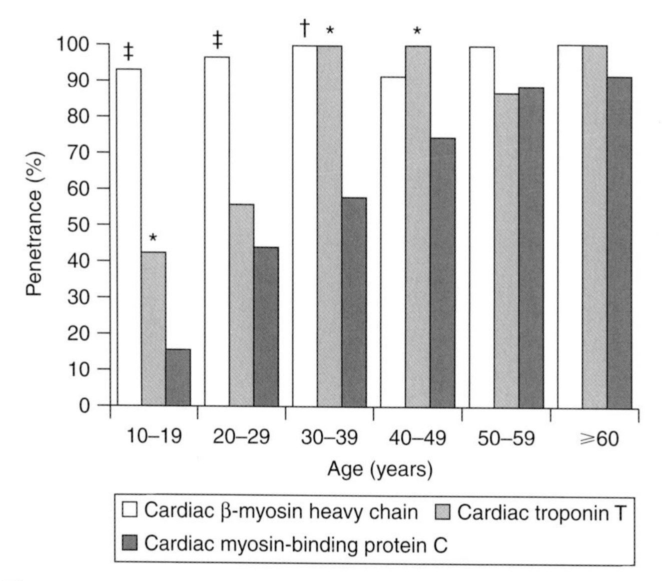

Fig. 7.3 The penetrance of left ventricular hypertrophy in hypertrophic cardiomyopathy (HCM) is dependent on age and influenced by the underlying sarcomere mutation. HCM caused by mutations in the b-myosin heavy chain is typically associated with demonstrable LVH early in life, with near universal expression by the age 20 years. In contrast, HCM due to mutations in the myosin binding protein C gene may not show clinically evident LVH until middle age or later. Asterisks denote $p<0.05$, dagger $p<0.0005$, and double dagger $p<0.001$. (Adapted from Niimura *et al. New England Journal of Medicine* 1998; **338**: 1248–1257. *With permission. Copyright 1998 Massachusetts Medical Society. All rights reserved.*)

mutation is inherited or introduced at the time of fertilization, it is unusual for obvious manifestations of HCM to be detected in infancy or early childhood. LVH more commonly becomes evident in adolescence, in conjunction with the pubertal growth spurt.

Because the penetrance of LVH is age-dependent and incomplete, a sarcomere mutation and attendant risk of developing HCM and related complications, including SCD, may be present with any degree of LVH, even normal wall thickness. Longitudinal studies which include apparently healthy preclinical mutation carriers will help to more accurately determine the true penetrance of sarcomere mutations, to identify more sensitive and specific markers of disease, and to describe the full spectrum of the HCM phenotype.

Implications of genetic discoveries: refining the phenotype of hypertrophic cardiomyopathy

Systolic function

Although it seems predictable that mutations in sarcomere proteins will perturb contractile function, the precise functional consequences are not fully understood and important details remain unresolved despite intense laboratory study [38,39]. Some contradictory results have been observed however the bulk of experimental evidence suggests that sarcomere mutations in HCM exert a predominantly activating effect. *In vitro* models have shown enhanced motor activity, as reflected by increased actin-activated ATPase activity, sliding filament velocity, and calcium sensitivity, and *in vivo* models have suggested enhanced systolic function and ejection fraction [40–44].

Diastolic dysfunction

Abnormal diastolic function is a common feature of overt HCM and may largely account for symptoms of pulmonary congestion and exercise intolerance. Moreover, animal and human studies indicate that diastolic dysfunction is an intrinsic feature of the HCM phenotype, present early the evolution of in disease development and prior to the development of LVH. Invasive hemodynamic studies on a genetically modified knock-in mouse model of HCM in which a heterozygous myosin heavy chain Arg403Gln missense mutation is introduced (aMHC403/1) have shown that diastolic abnormalities develop well in advance of gross or histopathologic LVH, fibrosis, and disarray [45,46]. Impaired relaxation in these animals has been related to alterations in intracellular calcium handling and slowed actin–myosin dissociation kinetics [47–49]. A TNNT2 I79N transgenic mouse model also develops hypercontractile systolic function but increased diastolic stiffness in the absence of significant hypertrophy or fibrosis [44].

More recently, tissue Doppler echocardiographic studies on genotyped human subjects have similarly demonstrated that individuals with sarcomere gene mutations have impaired LV relaxation early in disease, prior to the development of LVH [50,51]. These studies suggest that diastolic abnormalities are a primary manifestation of the underlying sarcomere mutation, rather than merely a secondary consequence of altered myocardial compliance characteristics due to the LVH, fibrosis, and disarray present in established disease.

Alteration of intracellular calcium handling

Myocardial contraction is coordinated by the orchestrated cycling of calcium from the cytoplasm, sarcoplasmic reticulum (SR), and sarcomere through excitation–contraction coupling (Fig. 7.4). Biochemical studies using the $\alpha MHC^{403/+}$ mouse model of HCM indicate that altered intracellular Ca^{2+} handling (present at 4 weeks of age) is one of the earliest detectable manifestations of sarcomere mutations, preceding histologic changes (age ~20 weeks) and development of diastolic dysfunction (age ~6 weeks) [49,52].

Furthermore, the identification of these early biochemical changes suggests that targeting intracellular Ca^{2+} handling may provide a means to modify

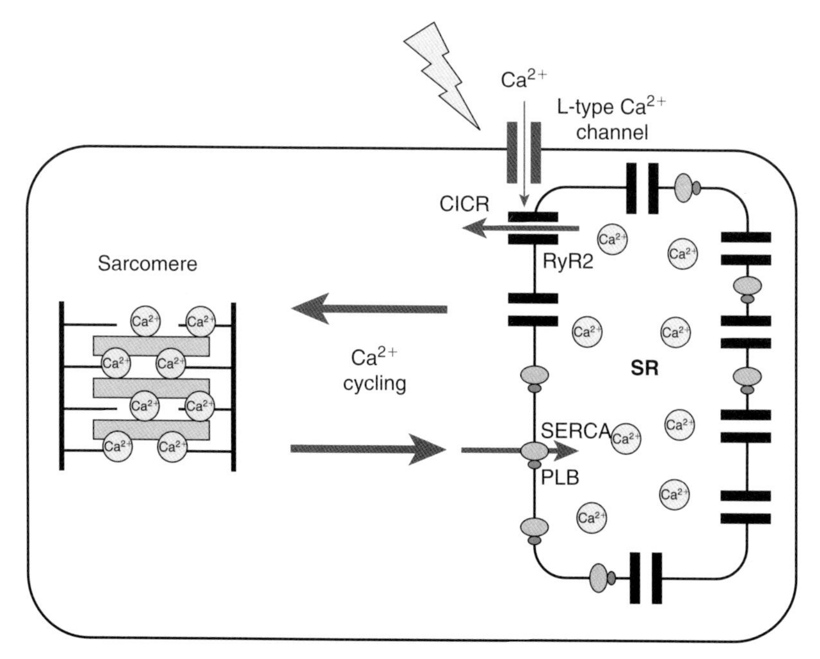

Fig. 7.4 Excitation–contraction coupling and intracellular calcium cycling. Membrane depolarization by the action potential opens voltage-gated L-type calcium channels on the cardiac myocyte membrane. The resultant influx of Ca^{2+} leads to a greater calcium-induced calcium release (CICR) from stores in the sarcoplasmic reticulum (SR). Ca^{2+} binds to the sarcomere, allowing actin–myosin crossbridge formation and generation of the power stroke. Calcium is then taken back up into the SR via the SERCA pump (SR calcium ATPase). (Adapted from Semsarian *et al.* [52], with permission)

the phenotype of HCM. Pharmacological studies on young (prehypertrophic) $\alpha MHC^{403/+}$ HCM mice demonstrated that treatment with the L-type calcium channel blocker diltiazem resulted in less hypertrophy and improved intracellular Ca^{2+} handling than placebo [52]. There was no demonstrable benefit if drug administration was initiated after the development of LVH. These data have intriguing implications for future clinical management of HCM, suggesting that early pharmacologic intervention to counteract biochemical abnormalities, given in advance of obvious disease expression, may attenuate the expression of the underlying sarcomere gene mutation.

Arrhythmias

The determinants of SCD and ventricular arrhythmias in HCM remain incompletely defined and are likely complex and multifactorial. Focal ischemia, abnormalities of intramural arteries, abnormalities of calcium signaling, and changes in myocardial architecture have all been implicated in arrhythmogenicity. Because myocardial fibrosis and disarray are prominent and characteristic features of HCM, they have been hypothesized to be the anatomic substrate for electrical instability, triggering ventricular tachycardia (VT) and SCD [53]. However, direct evidence linking fibrosis, disarray, and arrhythmias is limited. Studies on the $\alpha MHC^{403/+}$ mouse model have demonstrated that the extent, location, and pattern of fibrosis and disarray are highly variable. There was no clear correlation between these parameters and susceptibility to inducible arrhythmias on programmed stimulation. In contrast, increasing degrees of LVH and increased contractility correlated with inducible arrhythmias [54]. Although preliminary, these results suggest that a common pathway, governed by the sarcomere mutation, connects hypertrophy and arrhythmias.

Increased susceptibility to arrhythmias may also be linked to alterations in calcium signaling, both because calcium handling is directly perturbed in HCM and because increased contractility has been associated with increased Ca^{2+} cycling [54,55].

Abnormalities in myocardial energetics

Impaired myocardial energetics has been proposed as a unifying mechanism by which sarcomere mutations may result in both cardiac hypertrophy and heart failure [47,56,57]. ^{31}P magnetic resonance spectroscopy (MRS) studies on the $\alpha MHC^{403/+}$ mouse have demonstrated that less force is generated per molecule of ATP hydrolyzed, resulting in reduced mechanical efficiency and, potentially, compensatory hypertrophy due to myocardial energy depletion [47]. *In vivo* MRS studies on a genotyped human population demonstrated impaired myocardial energetics in prehypertrophic sarcomere mutation carriers as well as subjects with overt disease, further suggesting a primary role of energy deficiency in the pathogenesis of HCM [56]. Energy depletion may provide a common mechanistic basis for the shared phenotype of cardiac hypertrophy seen in mutations which alter myocardial metabolism (reviewed below) and mitochondrial disease.

Other paradigms of genetic cardiac hypertrophy

Sarcomere mutations are not identified in ~30–50% of individuals with a clinical diagnosis of HCM. This incomplete detection rate is partially explained by methodologic limitations. Although DNA sequencing technology is highly robust and reliable, in-frame deletions and promoter mutations will not be detected by current candidate gene sequencing strategies. Indirect methods such as denaturing high-performance liquid chromatography (DHPLC) or single-strand conformation polymorphism (SSCP) analysis are occasionally used as an initial screening step, but are less sensitive than direct sequencing and may lead to a higher false-negative rate. Furthermore, not all sarcomere genes known to cause HCM are routinely tested nor have all causal genes been identified.

Metabolic cardiomyopathies

Apart from these methodological limitations, phenocopies of HCM have been identified, in which LVH is caused by mutations in nonsarcomere proteins (Table 7.3). Genetic studies of families and sporadic cases of unexplained LVH with conduction abnormalities (progressive atrioventricular block, atrial fibrillation, ventricular preexcitation) have identified a distinct category of metabolic cardiomyopathies: genetic cardiac hypertrophy caused by mutations in *PRKAG2,* encoding the $\gamma 2$ regulatory subunit of adenosine monophosphate-activated protein kinase (AMPK), as well as mutations in the X- linked lysosome-associated membrane protein (*LAMP2*) gene. Mutations in these genes may be present in roughly 2–12% of individuals who carry a clinical diagnosis of HCM and over 40% of individuals with combined features of LVH and preexcitation [58–61].

PRKAG2

AMP kinase is a heterotrimeric enzyme that is involved in the regulation of energy stores and metabolism, including glycolysis, and functions as a cellular fuel gauge. Normally inactive, AMPK is activated in response to increased energy demands or decreased energy stores [62]. Mutations in its regulatory subunit, *PRKAG2,* have led to constitutive activation of AMPK and myocardial glycogen accumulation [60,62]. Up to 60% of individuals with *PRKAG2* mutations have preexcitation and over 30% have required permanent pacemaker implantation for progressive atrioventricular (AV) block [60]. The high prevalence of conduction abnormalities and preexcitation can help to discriminate disease caused by *PRKAG2* mutations from HCM caused by sarcomere mutations.

LAMP2

LAMP2 encodes a lysosome-associated membrane protein involved in lysosomal glycogen degradation. X-linked LAMP2 mutations may be distinguished from HCM by male predominance, earlier age of presentation, ventricular preexcitation, and more striking ECG and echocardiographic manifestations of LVH. Early-onset LVH (often in childhood) with rapid progression of heart

Table 7.3 Phenocopies of hypertrophic cardiomyopathy

Protein	Gene	Chromosome	Associated disease	Comments
γ-Subunit, AMP-kinase	*PRKAG2*	7q3		Preexcitation and conduction disease
Lysosome-associated membrane protein	*LAMP2*	Xq2	Danon disease	Cardiomyopathy, skeletal myopathy, and mental retardation; preexcitation on ECG; rapid progression in adolescence, particularly males
α-Galactosidase	*GLA*	X	Fabry disease	Assess plasma or lymphocyte α-Gal activity (males); consider enzyme replacement therapy
Transthyretin	*TTR*	18q12	Familial amyloidosis	

failure and a poor prognosis are characteristic [61]. Affected males typically die from cardiovascular disease or require cardiac transplantation by late adolescence. LAMP2 mutations are the genetic etiology of Danon disease, a multisystem disorder with cardiac, neurologic, skeletal muscle (manifest as increased serum creatinine kinase (CK) level), and hepatic involvement (manifest by increased serum alanine aminotransaminase (ALT) level). The cardiomyopathy tends be the dominant feature and has been described in carrier females [63].

Histopathologically, *PRKAG2* and *LAMP2* mutations do not display either the myocardial disarray or interstitial fibrosis pathognomonic for HCM, but instead are characterized by prominent myocardial vacuolization with glycogen and amylopectin (Fig. 7.5). Animal models of *PRKAG2* cardiomyopathy suggest that glycogen-filled cardiac myocytes disrupt the annulus fibrosis and may account for AV-nodal block and bypass tracts which lead to preexcitation. [62]. Although incompletely defined, the molecular pathways triggered by *PRKAG2* and *LAMP2* mutations (Fig. 7.6) are likely distinct from sarcomere gene mutations. As such, management tenets for HCM may not be applicable to metabolic cardiomyopathies. Genetic testing for both *PRKAG2* and *LAMP2* is available and may be considered when unexplained LVH is accompanied by preexcitation, or if marked LVH is present in young males (*LAMP2*). If a mutation in *LAMP2* is identified, important prognostic information is gained given the uniformly poor outcome in affected males. In this setting, more aggressive follow up and management may be appropriate.

Storage and infiltrative disorders

Although storage and infiltrative disorders may be familial and result in cardiac hypertrophy, multisystem involvement is typically apparent and allows distinction from HCM. However, with the increasing recognition that HCM may present late in life when other confounding medical comorbidities may be present, and that cardiac-predominant phenotypes of other conditions are

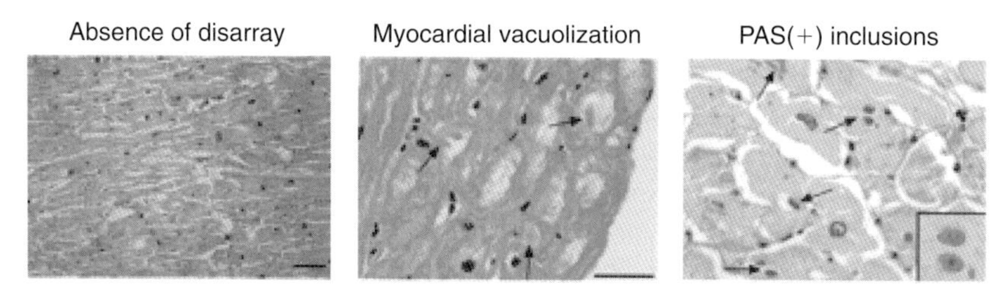

Fig. 7.5 The histopathology of metabolic cardiomyopathies caused by mutations in PRKAG2 and LAMP2 is distinct from HCM and characterized by glycogen-filled vacuoles without significant disarray, fibrosis, or myocyte hypertrophy. (Courtesy of Christine Seidman, MD, Harvard Medical School and Brigham and Women's Hospital, Boston, MA.)

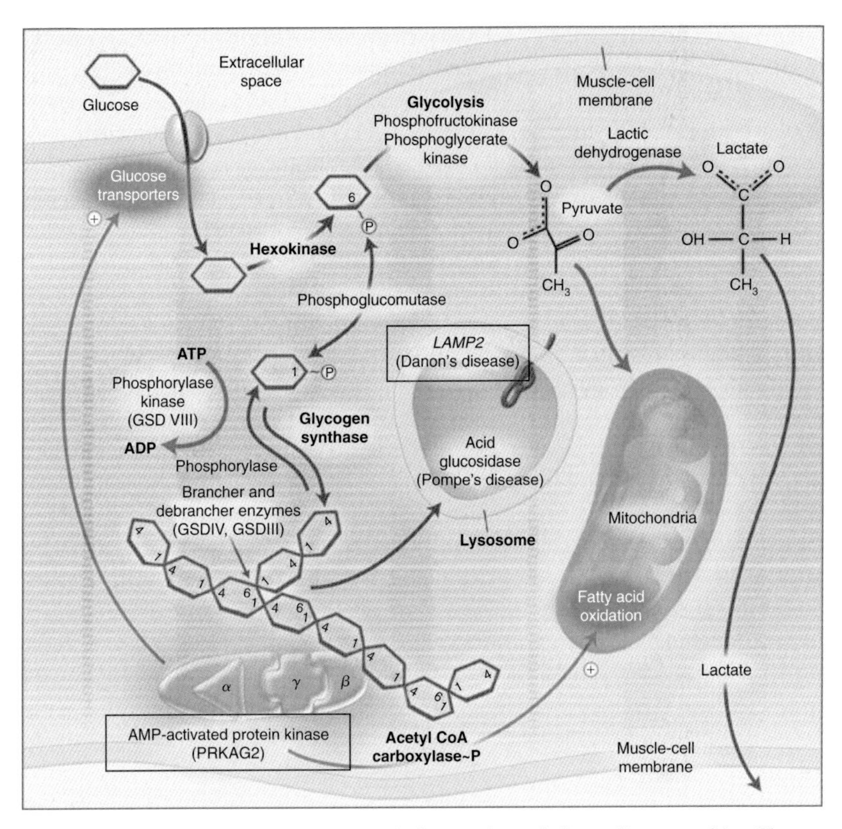

Fig. 7.6 Pathways of myocyte glucose metabolism and metabolic cardiomyopathies. Glucose enters the myocyte via membrane transporters and is directed to pathways for glycolysis (for immediate energy needs) or glycogen synthesis (for energy storage). Glycogen metabolism is influenced by AMP-kinase and lysosome activity. Mutations in PRKAG2 and LAMP2 may result in glycogen accumulation leading to cardiac hypertrophy and electrophysiological abnormalities. (Reprinted from Arad, *et al. N Engl J Med* 2005;352:362–372, *with permission. Copyright 2005 Massachusetts Medical Society. All rights reserved.*)

present, there is potential for overlap, particularly with more recognized disorders such as Fabry disease and amyloidosis (Table 7.3).

Fabry disease

Fabry disease is an X-linked recessive disorder caused by mutations in the gene encoding the lysosomal hydrolase a-galactosidase (GLA), resulting in enzyme deficiency and glycosphingolipid accumulation in the heart, kidneys, nervous system, and skin. Classic Fabry disease occurs at a prevalence of ,1/40 000 and usually presents in childhood or adolescence. A cardiac-predominant variant of Fabry disease has been described and typically presents later in life.

Studies suggest that roughly of unexplained LVH in adult men may be due to underlying Fabry disease [64,65]. Measuring plasma or leukocyte a-galactosidase activity can reliably diagnose males. GLA mutation testing is also available and is particularly helpful to diagnose hemizygous heterozygous female carriers who may have normal a-galactosidase activity. Identifying patients with Fabry disease is important owing to the availability of effective a-galactosidase enzyme replacement therapy [66].

Cardiac amyloidosis

This Cardiac involvement in amyloidosis can also result in cardiac hypertrophy owing to myocardial infiltration and accumulation of amyloidogenic protein. The prognosis and type of amyloidosis (primary/AL, familial, or senile) is determined by the underlying amyloidogenic protein. AL (primary) amyloidosis results from a plasma cell dyscrasia and is composed of monoclonal immunoglobulin light chains.Typically, there is associated renal involvement with ,5% of patients having isolated cardiac involvement [67]. Overall, prognosis is poor and, without treatment, median survival is 6 months after the onset of symptomatic heart failure [67]. Transthyretin (prealbumin) can be deposited either as a mutant (familial amyloidosis) or wild-type (senile amyloidosis) protein. Both carry a more favorable prognosis and renal involvement is less prominent than in AL amyloidosis. Accurate diagnosis can be made by detecting excess light chains in serum or urine, or by histologic analysis of a biopsy specimen with differential staining for light chains or transthyretin. Genetic testing for familial amyloidosis can be performed by evaluating the gene encoding transthyretin (TTR).

The algorithm presented in Fig. 7.7 may assist in the diagnosis of unexplained cardiac hypertrophy.

From bench to bedside: integrating genetic information into clinical practice

Incorporating genetic information into clinical practice will be increasingly important to refine diagnosis and prognosis, to optimally manage families with inherited disease, and to improve understanding of disease pathogenesis.

Family screening: clinical evaluation

HCM follows autosomal dominant inheritance; therefore, clinical screening of first-degree relatives of affected individuals is recommended, incorporating history, physical examination, 12-lead ECG, and echocardiography. Since the penetrance of LVH is age dependent, the lack of diagnostic clinical findings on initial assessment does not exclude the possibility of future disease development or the presence of an underlying sarcomere mutation, particularly in children. Longitudinal follow-up of apparently healthy HCM family members is required to avoid potential false-negative results with standard clinical

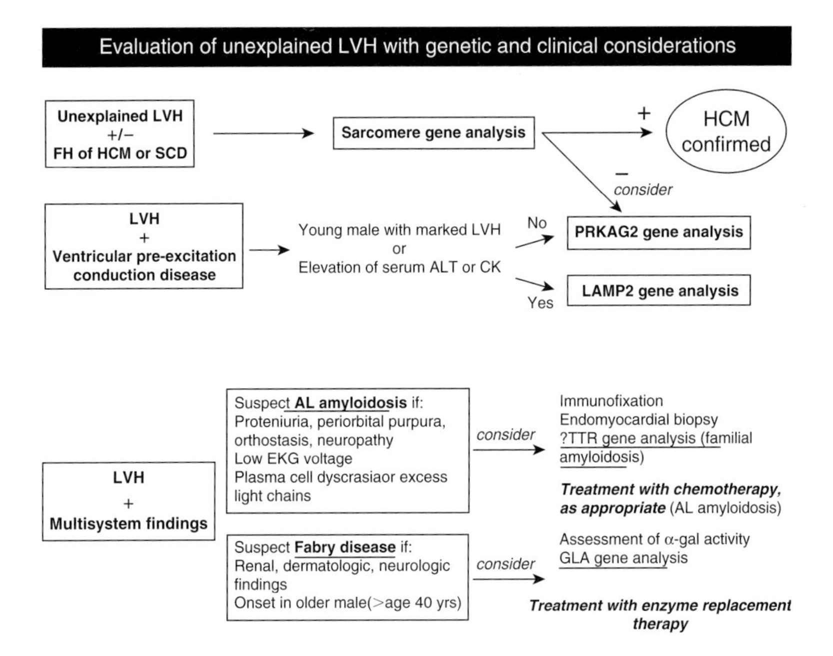

Fig. 7.7 Evaluating unexplained cardiac hypertrophy. ALT, alanine aminotransferase; CK, creatinine kinase; FH, family history; LVH, left ventricular hypertrophy; HCM, hypertrophic cardiomyopathy; SCD, sudden cardiac death.

screening. The strategy outlined in Fig. 7.8 has been proposed for screening members of families with HCM [37].

Genetic testing

The identification of a sarcomere gene mutation, in the appropriate clinical setting, can provide a definitive diagnosis of HCM, establish the exact genetic etiology of disease, and allow for more accurate diagnosis, prognosis, and management of patients and their families. Testing can be highly fruitful in the context of familial disease, since a sarcomere mutation is likely to be found in ~60% of probands, and 50% of their first-degree relatives are predicted to carry the mutation. A substantial advantage of genetic testing is that, once the family-specific mutation is identified, family members at risk for disease can be definitively identified. This allows longitudinal clinical follow-up to be appropriately focused and relieves the anxiety associated with the otherwise uncertain future risk of disease development. Family members who have not inherited the mutation can be reassured and do not require serial clinical evaluation. Family members who have inherited the causal mutation require serial clinical follow-up as well as counseling regarding the risk of transmission to offspring.

Genetic testing can also help to resolve uncertain clinical situations such as differentiating athlete's heart or hypertensive heart disease from HCM.

Recommended clinical screening of family members:
Physical examination, Echocardiography and Electrocardiogram

<12 years old	Optional unless: Severe family history of early HCM-related death, early development of LV hypertrophy, or other adverse complications Competitive athlete in intense training Onset of symptoms
12–22 years old	Repeat evaluation every 12–18 months
>22 years old	Repeat evaluation approximately every 5 years, or in response to symptoms. Tailor evaluation if there is a family pattern of late-onset LVH or HCM-related complications
If genetic results are available:	**Genotype (+)** family members: Serial clinical evaluation as above **Genotype (−)** family members: Reassurance; no need for further testing

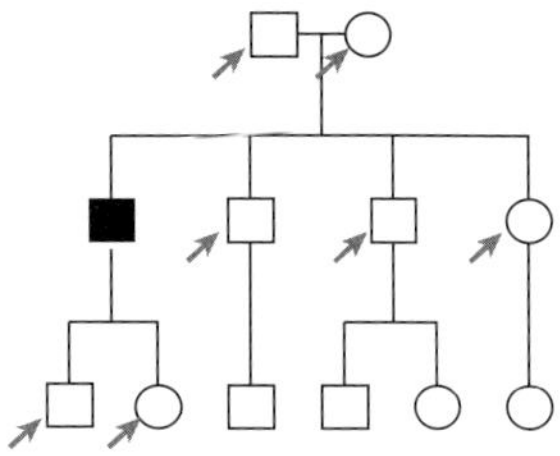

The proband is the solid square, here indicating a male with a diagnosis of HCM. Clinical evaluation is recommended for 1st degree relatives, designated indicated by the arrows.

Fig. 7.8 Screening strategy for the detection of clinical hypertrophic cardiomyopathy in family members. [37]

Distinction is important owing to the significant implications for lifestyle, family members, and prognosis associated with a diagnosis of HCM. Furthermore, specific treatment may be required if phenocopies of HCM are identified.

Currently, genetic testing relies on DNA sequence analysis, and an important caveat to this strategy is that the failure to identify a causal mutation via candidate gene sequencing is an inconclusive result and does not exclude the possibility of rare genetic causes of HCM or other types of inherited LVH. As advances in more rapid, high-throughput methods for mutation detection emerge, genetic testing will become increasingly affordable and feasible.

Conclusions

Studying the genetic basis of inherited cardiac hypertrophy will provide important insights into the myriad of mechanisms involved in hypertrophic remodeling of the heart. Understanding the pathways leading from gene mutation to clinical disease will improve the practical management of our patients by enabling precise diagnosis, definitive identification of at-risk family members individuals, determination of early markers of disease, and ultimately the development of novel treatment paradigms designed to change the natural history of disease.

References

1 Jarcho JA, McKenna W, Pare JA *et al.* Mapping a gene for familial hypertrophic cardiomyopathy to chromosome 14q1. *The New England Journal of Medicine* 1989; **321**: 1372–1378.

2 Thierfelder L, Watkins H, MacRae C *et al.* Alpha-tropomyosin and cardiac troponin T mutations cause familial hypertrophic cardiomyopathy: a disease of the sarcomere. *Cell* 1994; **77**: 701–712.
3 Watkins H, McKenna WJ, Thierfelder L *et al.* Mutations in the genes for cardiac troponin T and alpha-tropomyosin in hypertrophic cardiomyopathy. *The New England Journal of Medicine* 1995; **332**: 1058–1064.
4 Maron BJ, McKenna WJ, Danielson GK *et al.* American College of Cardiology/European Society of Cardiology clinical expert consensus document on hypertrophic cardiomyopathy. A report of the American College of Cardiology Foundation Task Force on Clinical Expert Consensus Documents and the European Society of Cardiology Committee for Practice Guidelines. *Journal of the American College of Cardiology* 2003; **42**: 1687–1713.
5 Klues HG, Schiffers A, Maron BJ. Phenotypic spectrum and patterns of left ventricular hypertrophy in hypertrophic cardiomyopathy: morphologic observations and significance as assessed by two-dimensional echocardiography in 600 patients. *Journal of the American College of Cardiology* 1995; **26**: 1699–1708.
6 Harris KM, Spirito P, Maron MS *et al.* Prevalence, clinical profile, and significance of left ventricular remodeling in the end-stage phase of hypertrophic cardiomyopathy. *Circulation* 2006; **114**: 216–225.
7 Biagini E, Coccolo F, Ferlito M *et al.* Dilated-hypokinetic evolution of hypertrophic cardiomyopathy: prevalence, incidence, risk factors, and prognostic implications in pediatric and adult patients. *Journal of the American College of Cardiology* 2005; **46**: 1543–1550.
8 Maron BJ, Casey SA, Hauser RG, Aeppli DM. Clinical course of hypertrophic cardiomyopathy with survival to advanced age. *Journal of the American College of Cardiology* 2003; **42**: 882–888.
9 Maron BJ. Hypertrophic cardiomyopathy: a systematic review. *JAMA: The Journal of the American Medical* 2002; **287**: 1308–1320.
10 McKenna WJ, Behr ER. Hypertrophic cardiomyopathy: management, risk stratification, and prevention of sudden death. *Heart* 2002; **87**: 169–176.
11 Elliott P, McKenna WJ. Hypertrophic cardiomyopathy. *Lancet* 2004; **363**: 1881–1891.
12 Nishimura RA, Holmes DR, Jr. Clinical practice. Hypertrophic obstructive cardiomyopathy. *The New England Journal of Medicine* 2004; **350**: 1320–1327.
13 Elliott PM, Poloniecki J, Dickie S *et al.* Sudden death in hypertrophic cardiomyopathy: identification of high risk patients. *Journal of the American College of Cardiology* 2000; **36**: 2212–2218.
14 Elliott PM, Gimeno Blanes JR, Mahon NG *et al.* Relation between severity of left-ventricular hypertrophy and prognosis in patients with hypertrophic cardiomyopathy. *Lancet* 2001; **357**: 420–424.
15 Zipes DP, Camm AJ, Borggrefe M *et al.* ACC/AHA/ESC 2006 Guidelines for Management of Patients with Ventricular Arrhythmias and the Prevention of Sudden Cardiac Death: a report of the American College of Cardiology/American Heart Association Task Force and the European Society of Cardiology Committee for Practice Guidelines (Writing Committee to Develop Guidelines for Management of Patients with Ventricular Arrhythmias and the Prevention of Sudden Cardiac Death): developed in collaboration with the European Heart Rhythm Association and the Heart Rhythm Society. *Circulation* 2006; **114**: e385–484.

16 Maron BJ, Gardin JM, Flack JM *et al.* Prevalence of hypertrophic cardiomyopathy in a general population of young adults-echocardiographic analysis of 4111 subjects in the CARDIA study. *Circulation* 1995; 92: 785–789.
17 Zou Y, Song L, Wang Z *et al.* Prevalence of idiopathic hypertrophic cardiomyopathy in China: a population-based echocardiographic analysis of 8080 adults. *American Journal of Medicine* 2004; **116**: 14–18.
18 Van Driest SL, Ellsworth EG, Ommen SR *et al.* Prevalence and spectrum of thin filament mutations in an outpatient referral population with hypertrophic cardiomyopathy. *Circulation* 2003; **108**: 445–451.
19 Richard P, Charron P, Carrier L *et al.* Hypertrophic cardiomyopathy: distribution of disease genes, spectrum of mutations, and implications for a molecular diagnosis strategy. *Circulation* 2003; **107**: 2227–2232.
20 Richard P, Villard E, Charron P, Isnard R. The genetic bases of cardiomyopathies. *Journal of the American College of Cardiology* 2006; **48** (9 Suppl): A79–89.
21 Maron BJ. Sudden death in young athletes. *The New England Journal of Medicine* 2003; **349**: 1064–1075.
22 Bos JM, Poley RN, Ny M *et al.* Genotype–phenotype relationships involving hypertrophic cardiomyopathy-associated mutations in titin, muscle LIM protein, and telethonin. *Molecular Genetics and Metabolism* 2006; **88**: 78–85.
23 Geier C, Perrot A, Ozcelik C *et al.* Mutations in the human muscle LIM protein gene in families with hypertrophic cardiomyopathy. *Circulation* 2003; **107**: 1390–1395.
24 Osio A, Tan L, Chen SN *et al.* Myozenin 2 is a novel gene for human hypertrophic cardiomyopathy. *Circulation Research* 2007; **100**: 766–768.
25 Seidman JG, Seidman C. The genetic basis for cardiomyopathy: from mutation identification to mechanistic paradigms. *Cell* 2001; **104**: 557–567.
26 Marian AJ, Roberts R. The molecular genetic basis for hypertrophic cardiomyopathy. *Journal of Molecular and Cellular Cardiology* 2001; **33**: 655–670.
27 Van Driest SL, Vasile VC, Ommen SR *et al.* Myosin binding protein C mutations and compound heterozygosity in hypertrophic cardiomyopathy. *Journal of the American College of Cardiology* 2004; **44**: 1903–1910.
28 Geisterfer-Lowrance AA, Kass S, Tanigawa G *et al.* A molecular basis for familial hypertrophic cardiomyopathy: a beta cardiac myosin heavy chain gene missense mutation. *Cell* 1990; **62**: 999–1006.
29 Rayment I, Holden HM, Whittaker M *et al.* Structure of the actin–myosin complex and its implications for muscle contraction. *Science* 1993; **261**: 58–65.
30 Tardiff JC. Sarcomeric proteins and familial hypertrophic cardiomyopathy: linking mutations in structural proteins to complex cardiovascular phenotypes. *Heart Failure Reviews* 2005; **10**: 237–248.
31 Freiburg A, Gautel M. A molecular map of the interactions between titin and myosin-binding protein C. Implications for sarcomeric assembly in familial hypertrophic cardiomyopathy. *European Journal of Biochemistry* 1996; **235**: 317–323.
32 Moolman JC, Corfield VA, Posen B *et al.* Sudden death due to troponin T mutations. *Journal of the American College of Cardiology* 1997; **29**: 549–55.
33 Niimura H, Bachinski LL, Sangwatanaroj S *et al.* Mutations in the gene for cardiac myosin-binding protein C and late-onset familial hypertrophic cardiomyopathy [see comments]. *The New England Journal of Medicine* 1998; **338**: 1248–1257.

34 Niimura H, Patton KK, McKenna WJ *et al.* Sarcomere protein gene mutations in hypertrophic cardiomyopathy of the elderly. *Circulation* 2002; **105**: 446–451.
35 Arad M, Penas-Lado M, Monserrat L *et al.* Gene mutations in apical hypertrophic cardiomyopathy. *Circulation* 2005; **112**: 2805–2811.
36 Charron P, Heron D, Gargiulo M *et al.* Genetic testing and genetic counselling in hypertrophic cardiomyopathy: the French experience. *Journal of Medical Genetics* 2002; **39**: 741–746.
37 Maron BJ, Seidman JG, Seidman CE. Proposal for contemporary screening strategies in families with hypertrophic cardiomyopathy. *Journal of the American College of Cardiology* 2004; **44**: 2125–2132.
38 Marian AJ, Zhao G, Seta Y *et al.* Expression of a mutant (Arg92Gln) human cardiac troponin T, known to cause hypertrophic cardiomyopathy, impairs adult cardiac myocyte contractility. *Circulation Research* 1997; **81**: 76–85.
39 Fatkin D, Graham RM. Molecular mechanisms of inherited cardiomyopathies. *Physiology Reviews* 2002; **82**: 945–980.
40 Tyska MJ, Hayes E, Giewat M *et al.* Single-molecule mechanics of R403Q cardiac myosin isolated from the mouse model of familial hypertrophic cardiomyopathy. *Circulation Research* 2000; **86**: 737–744.
41 Palmiter KA, Tyska MJ, Haeberle JR *et al.* R403Q and L908V mutant beta-cardiac myosin from patients with familial hypertrophic cardiomyopathy exhibit enhanced mechanical performance at the single molecule level. *Journal of Muscle Research and Cell Motility* 2000; **21**: 609–620.
42 Lowey S. Functional consequences of mutations in the myosin heavy chain at sites implicated in familial hypertrophic cardiomyopathy. *Trends in Cardiovascular Medicine* 2002; **12**: 348–354.
43 Palmer BM, Fishbaugher DE, Schmitt JP *et al.* Differential cross-bridge kinetics of FHC myosin mutations R403Q and R453C in heterozygous mouse myocardium. *American Journal of Physiology* 2004; **287**: H91–99.
44 Westermann D, Knollmann BC, Steendijk P *et al.* Diltiazem treatment prevents diastolic heart failure in mice with familial hypertrophic cardiomyopathy. *European Journal of Heart Failure* 2006; **8**: 115–121.
45 Geisterfer-Lowrance AA, Christe M, Conner DA *et al.* A mouse model of familial hypertrophic cardiomyopathy. *Science* 1996; **272**: 731–734.
46 Georgakopoulos D, Christe ME, Giewat M *et al.* The pathogenesis of familial hypertrophic cardiomyopathy: early and evolving effects from an alpha-cardiac myosin heavy chain missense mutation [see comments]. *Nature Medicine* 1999; **5**: 327–330.
47 Spindler M, Saupe KW, Christe ME *et al.* Diastolic dysfunction and altered energetics in the alphaMHC403/+ mouse model of familial hypertrophic cardiomyopathy. *The Journal of Clinical Investigation* 1998; **101**: 1775–1783.
48 Blanchard E, Seidman C, Seidman JG *et al.* Altered crossbridge kinetics in the alphaMHC403/+ mouse model of familial hypertrophic cardiomyopathy. *Circulation Research* 1999; **84**: 475–483.
49 Fatkin D, McConnell BK, Mudd JO *et al.* An abnormal Ca(2+) response in mutant sarcomere protein-mediated familial hypertrophic cardiomyopathy. *The Journal of Clinical Investigation* 2000; **106**: 1351–1359.
50 Nagueh SF, Bachinski LL, Meyer D *et al.* Tissue Doppler imaging consistently detects myocardial abnormalities in patients with hypertrophic cardiomyopathy and provides

a novel means for an early diagnosis before and independently of hypertrophy. *Circulation* 2001; **104**: 128–130.
51 Ho CY, Sweitzer NK, McDonough B *et al.* Assessment of diastolic function with Doppler tissue imaging to predict genotype in preclinical hypertrophic cardiomyopathy. *Circulation* 2002; **105**: 2992–2997.
52 Semsarian C, Ahmad I, Giewat M *et al.* The L-type calcium channel inhibitor diltiazem prevents cardiomyopathy in a mouse model. *The Journal of Clinical Investigation* 2002; **109**: 1013–1020.
53 Varnava AM, Elliott PM, Mahon N *et al.* Relation between myocyte disarray and outcome in hypertrophic cardiomyopathy. *American Journal of Cardiology* 2001; **88**: 275–279.
54 Wolf CM, Moskowitz IP, Arno S *et al.* Somatic events modify hypertrophic cardiomyopathy pathology and link hypertrophy to arrhythmia. *Proceedings of the National Academy of Sciences of the USA* 2005; **102**: 18123–18128.
55 London B, Baker LC, Lee JS *et al.* Calcium-dependent arrhythmias in transgenic mice with heart failure. *American Journal of Physiology* 2003; **284**: H431–441.
56 Crilley JG, Boehm EA, Blair E *et al.* Hypertrophic cardiomyopathy due to sarcomeric gene mutations is characterized by impaired energy metabolism irrespective of the degree of hypertrophy. *Journal of the American College of Cardiology* 2003; **41**: 1776–1782.
57 Ashrafian H, Watkins H. Reviews of translational medicine and genomics in cardiovascular disease: new disease taxonomy and therapeutic implications cardiomyopathies: therapeutics based on molecular phenotype. *Journal of the American College of Cardiology* 2007; **49**: 1251–1264.
58 Blair E, Redwood C, Ashrafian H *et al.* Mutations in the gamma(2) subunit of AMP-activated protein kinase cause familial hypertrophic cardiomyopathy: evidence for the central role of energy compromise in disease pathogenesis. *Human Molecular Genetics* 2001; **10**: 1215–1220.
59 Gollob MH, Green MS, Tang AS *et al.* Identification of a gene responsible for familial Wolff-Parkinson-White syndrome. *The New England Journal of Medicine* 2001; **344**: 1823–1831.
60 Arad M, Benson DW, Perez-Atayde AR *et al.* Constitutively active AMP kinase mutations cause glycogen storage disease mimicking hypertrophic cardiomyopathy. *The Journal of Clinical Investigation* 2002; **109**: 357–362.
61 Arad M, Maron BJ, Gorham JM *et al.* Glycogen storage diseases presenting as hypertrophic cardiomyopathy. *The New England Journal of Medicine* 2005; **352**: 362–372.
62 Arad M, Seidman CE, Seidman JG. AMP-activated protein kinase in the heart: role during health and disease. *Circulation Research* 2007; **100**: 474–488.
63 Sugie K, Yamamoto A, Murayama K *et al.* Clinicopathological features of genetically confirmed Danon disease. *Neurology* 2002; **58**: 1773–1778.
64 Nakao S, Takenaka T, Maeda M *et al.* An atypical variant of Fabry's disease in men with left ventricular hypertrophy. *The New England Journal of Medicine* 1995; **333**: 288–293.
65 Sachdev B, Takenaka T, Teraguchi H *et al.* Prevalence of Anderson-Fabry disease in male patients with late onset hypertrophic cardiomyopathy. *Circulation* 2002; **105**: 1407–1411.
66 Banikazemi M, Bultas J, Waldek S *et al.* Agalsidase-beta therapy for advanced Fabry disease: a randomized trial. *Annals of Internal Medicine* 2007; **146**: 77–86.
67 Falk RH. Diagnosis and management of the cardiac amyloidoses. *Circulation* 2005; **112**: 2047–2060.

Genetics and genomics of dilated cardiomyopathy

Jeffrey A. Towbin and Matteo Vatta

Introduction

Cardiomyopathies are not uncommon causes of morbidity and mortality and, over the past 20 years, limited improvements in outcome have been reported. However, improvement in the understanding of the major forms of cardiomyopathy has occurred over that time, in large part due to advances in genetics and genomics. In addition, new forms of cardiomyopathy have been described and classified over that time frame, in large part due to our improved genetic-based understanding of heart muscle disease. Further, the improved understanding gained in heart muscle disease has led to understanding of similarities and differences in heart and skeletal muscle and their often overlapping clinical presentations.

Dilated cardiomyopathy (DCM) is the most common form of cardiomyopathy, accounting for approximately 55% of cases [1]. Mortality in the United States due to cardiomyopathy is greater than 25,000 as the underlying cause or over 51,000 when cardiomyopathy listed anywhere in the death certificate is accounted for [2]. The total cost of healthcare in the USA focused on cardiomyopathies is in the billions of dollars and only limited success has been achieved. In order to achieve improved care and outcomes in children and adults, understanding of the causes of these disorders has been sought.

Dilated cardiomyopathy has become a popular target of research over the past 10–15 years, with multiple genes identified during that time period. These genes appear to encode two major subgroups of proteins, cytoskeletal and sarcomeric proteins [3]. The cytoskeletal proteins identified to date include

Cardiovascular Genetics and Genomics. Edited by Dan Roden. © 2009 American Heart Association, ISBN: 978-14051-7540-1.

dystrophin, desmin, lamin A/C, δ-sarcoglycan, β-sarcoglycan, and metavinculin. In the case of sarcomere-encoding genes, the same genes identified for hypertrophic cardiomyopathy (HCM) appear to be culprits, and include β-myosin heavy chain, myosin binding protein C, actin, α-tropomyosin, and cardiac troponin T. A new group of sarcomeric genes, those encoding Z-disk proteins, have also been identified and include cypher/ZASP [4], muscle LIM protein, and α-actinin-2 [5]. In addition, phospholamban and G4.5/tafazzin have also been reported. Another form of DCM, the acquired disorder viral myocarditis, has the same clinical features as DCM including heart failure, arrhythmias, and conduction block [6]. The most common causes of myocarditis are viral, including the enteroviruses (coxsackieviruses and echovirus), adenoviruses, and parvovirus B19, among other cardiotropic viruses [6]. Evidence exists that suggests that viral myocarditis and DCM (genetic) have similar mechanisms of disease based on the proteins targeted.

In order to understand the mechanisms responsible for the development of the clinical phenotype, an understanding of normal cardiac structure is necessary.

Normal cardiac structure

Cardiac muscle fibers are composed of separate cellular units (myocytes) connected in series [7]. In contrast to skeletal muscle fibers, cardiac fibers do not assemble in parallel arrays but bifurcate and recombine to form a complex three-dimensional network. Cardiac myocytes are joined at each end to adjacent myocytes at the intercalated disk, the specialized area of interdigitating cell membrane (Fig. 8.1). The intercalated disc contains gap junctions (containing connexins), and mechanical junctions, composed of adherens junctions (containing N-cadherin, catenins, and vinculin) and desmosomes (containing desmin, desmoplakin, desmocollin, desmoglein). Cardiac myocytes are surrounded by a thin membrane (sarcolemma) and the interior of each myocyte contains bundles of longitudinally arranged myofibrils. The myofibrils are formed by repeating sarcomeres, the basic contractile units of cardiac muscle composed of interdigitating thin (actin) and thick (myosin) filaments (Fig. 8.1) that give the muscle its characteristic striated appearance [8,9]. The thick filaments are composed primarily of myosin but additionally contain myosin binding proteins C, H, and X. The thin filaments are composed of cardiac actin, α-tropomyosin (α-TM), and troponins T, I, and C (cTnT, cTnI, cTnC). In addition, myofibrils contain a third filament formed by the giant filamentous protein titin, which extends from the Z-disk to the M-line and acts as a molecular template for the layout of the sarcomere. The Z-disk at the borders of the sarcomere is formed by a lattice of interdigitating proteins that maintain myofilament organization by crosslinking antiparallel titin and thin filaments from adjacent sarcomeres (Fig. 8.2). Other proteins in the Z-disk include α-actinin, nebulette, telethonin/T-cap, capZ, MLP, myopalladin, myotilin, Cypher/ZASP, filamin, and FATZ [8–10].

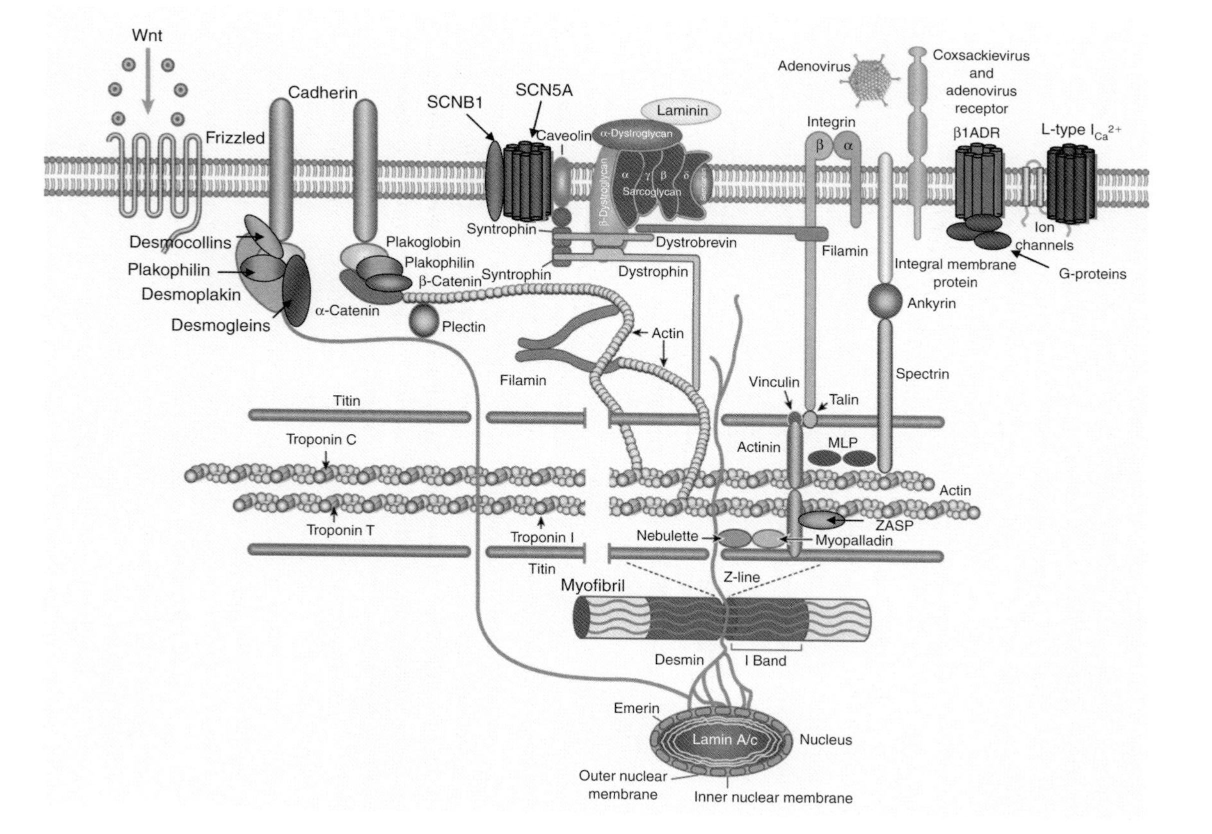

Fig. 8.1 Cardiac myocyte cytoarchitecture. The interactions between dystrophin and the dystrophin-associated proteins in the sarcolemma and intracellular cytoplasm (dystroglycans, sarcoglycans, syntrophins, dystrobrevin, sarcospan) at the C-terminal end of the dystrophin. The integral membrane proteins interact with the extracellular matrix via α-dystroglycan–α_2-laminin connections. The amino-terminus of dystrophin binds actin and connects dystrophin with the sarcomere intracellularly, the sarcolemma and extracellular matrix. MLP, muscle LIM protein.

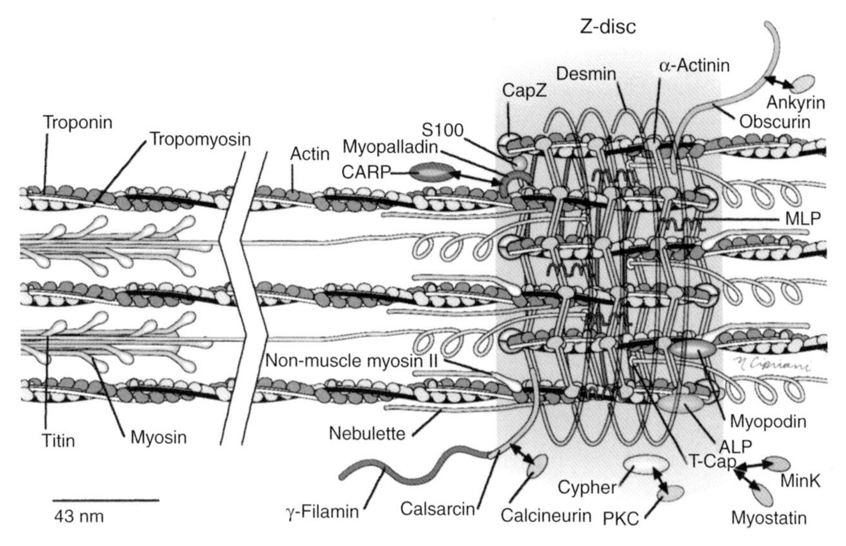

Fig. 8.2 Z-disk architecture. The Z-disk of the sarcomere is composed of multiple interacting proteins that anchor the sarcomere. MLP, muscle LIM protein. (Reproduced with permission from Pyle and Solaro [63].)

Finally, the extrasarcomeric cytoskeleton, a complex network of proteins linking the sarcomere with the sarcolemma and the extracellular matrix (ECM), provides structural support for subcellular structures and transmits mechanical and chemical signals within and between cells. The extrasarcomeric cytoskeleton has intermyofibrillar and subsarcolemmal components, with the intermyofibrillar cytoskeleton composed of intermediate filaments (IFs), microfilaments, and microtubules [11,12]. Desmin IFs form a three-dimensional scaffold throughout the extrasarcomeric cytoskeleton with desmin filaments surrounding the Z-disk, allowing for longitudinal connections to adjacent Z-disks and lateral connections to subsarcolemmal costameres [12]. Microfilaments composed of nonsarcomeric actin (mainly γ-actin) also form complex networks linking the sarcomere (via α-actinin) to various components of the costameres. Costameres are subsarcolemmal domains located in a periodic, grid-like pattern, flanking the Z-disks and overlying the I-bands, along the cytoplasmic side of the sarcolemma. These costameres are sites of interconnection between various cytoskeletal networks linking sarcomere and sarcolemma and are thought to function as anchor sites for stabilization of the sarcolemma and for integration of pathways involved in mechanical force transduction. Costameres contain three principal components: the focal adhesion-type complex, the spectrin-based complex, and the dystrophin/dystrophin-associated protein complex (DAPC) [13,14]. The focal adhesion-type complex, composed of cytoplasmic proteins (i.e., vinculin, talin, tensin, paxillin, zyxin), connect with cytoskeletal actin filaments and with the transmembrane proteins α-, β-dystroglycan, α-, β-, γ-, δ-sarcoglycans, dystrobrevin, and syntrophin. Several actin-associated proteins are located at sites of attachment of cytoskeletal actin filaments with costameric complexes, including α-actinin and the muscle LIM protein (MLP). The C-terminus of dystrophin binds β-dystroglycan (Fig. 8.1), which in turn interacts with α-dystroglycan to link to the ECM (via α-2-laminin). The N-terminus of dystrophin interacts with actin. Also notable, voltage-gated sodium channels colocalize with dystrophin, β-spectrin, ankyrin, and syntrophins (Fig. 8.1), while potassium channels interact with the sarcomeric Z-disk and intercalated discs [15,16] (Fig. 8.2). Since arrhythmias and conduction system diseases are common in children and adults with DCM, this could play an important role. Hence, disruption of the links from the sarcolemma to ECM at the dystrophin C-terminus and those to the sarcomere and nucleus via N-terminal dystrophin interactions could lead to a "domino effect" disruption of systolic function and development of arrhythmias.

Clinical genetics of dilated cardiomyopathy

Dilated cardiomyopathy was initially believed to be inherited in a small percentage of cases until Michels *et al.* [17] showed that approximately 20% of probands had family members with echocardiographic evidence of DCM when family screening was performed, including a dilated left ventricle and systolic dysfunction (typically described by depressed ejection fraction or shortening fraction) (Fig. 8.3). More recently, inherited, familial DCM (FDCM) has been shown to occur in 30–40% of cases [18], with autosomal dominant inheritance being the predominant pattern of transmission; X-linked, autosomal recessive, and mitochondrial inheritance is less common.

Molecular genetics of dilated cardiomyopathy

Over the past decade, progress has been made in the understanding of the genetic etiology of FDCM (Table 8.1). Initial progress was made studying families with X-linked forms of DCM, with the autosomal dominant forms of DCM beginning to unravel over the past few years. In the case of X-linked forms of DCM, two disorders have been well characterized: X-linked cardiomyopathy (XLCM), which presents in adolescence and young adults, and Barth syndrome, which is most frequently identified in infancy [19,20].

X-linked cardiomyopathies

X-linked dilated cardiomyopathy

First described in 1987 by Berko and Swift [19] as DCM occurring in males in the teen years and early twenties with rapid progression from congestive

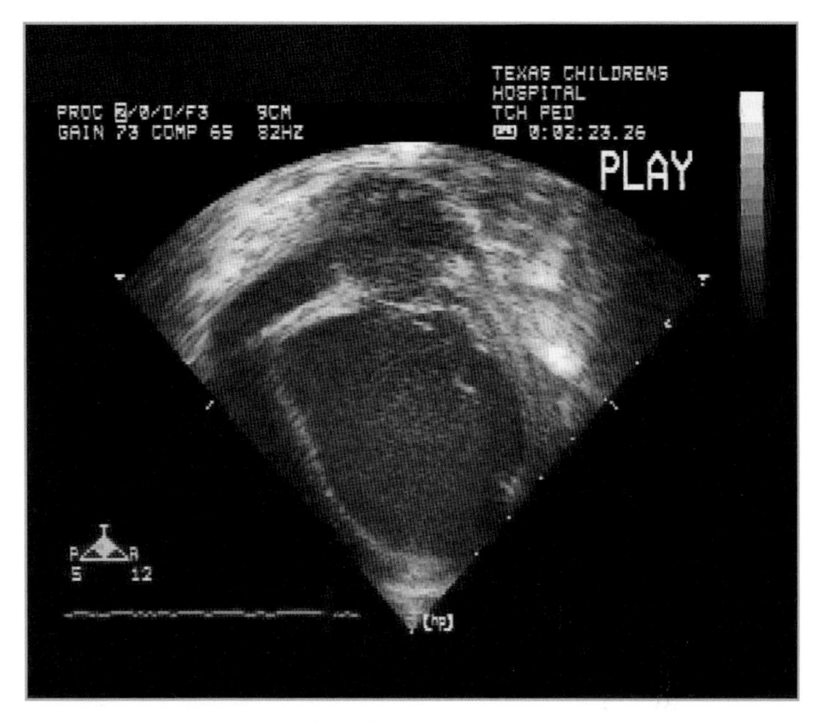

Fig. 8.3 Echocardiography in dilated cardiomyopathy. Apical four chamber view demonstrating a severely dilated left ventricle.

heart failure (CHF) to death due to ventricular tachycardia (VT)/ventricular fibrillation (VF) or transplantation, these patients are distinguished by elevated serum creatine kinase muscle isoforms (CK-MM) Female carriers tend to develop mild to moderate DCM in the fifth decade and the disease is slowly progressive. Towbin and colleagues [21] were the first to identify the disease-causing gene and characterize the functional defect. In this report, the dystrophin gene was shown to be responsible for the clinical abnormalities, and protein analysis by immunoblotting demonstrated severe reduction or absence of dystrophin protein in the heart of these patients. These findings were later confirmed by Muntoni *et al.* [22] when a mutation in the muscle promoter and exon 1 of dystrophin was identified in another family with XLCM. Subsequently, multiple mutations have been identified in dystrophin in patients with XLCM.

Dystrophin is a cytoskeletal protein which provides structural support to the myocyte by creating a lattice-like network to the sarcolemma [23]. In addition, dystrophin plays a major role in linking the sarcomeric contractile apparatus to the sarcolemma and extracellular matrix [23–26]. Furthermore, dystrophin is

Table 8.1 Dilated cardiomyopathy (DCM) genetics

Chromosome locus	Gene	Protein
Xp21.2	*DYS*	Dystrophin
Xq28	*G4.5*	Tafazzin
1q21	*LMNA*	Lamin A/C
1q32	*TNNT2*	Cardiac troponin T
1q42–43	*ACTN*	α-Actinin
2q31	*TTN*	Titin
2q35	*DES*	Desmin
5q33	*SGCD*	δ-Sarcoglycan
6q22.1	*PLN*	Phospholamban
10q22.3–23.2	*LDB3/ZASP/Cypher*	ZASP
10q22–q23	*VCL*	Metavinculin
11p11	*MYBPC3*	Myosin binding protein C
11p15.1	*MLP*	Muscle LIM protein
14q12	*MYH7*	β-Myosin heavy chain
15q14	*ACTC*	Cardiac actin
15q22	*TPM1*	α-Tropomyosin

involved in cell signaling, particularly through its interactions with nitric oxide synthase. The dystrophin gene is responsible for Duchenne and Becker muscular dystrophy (DMD/BMD) when mutated as well [27]. These skeletal myopathies present early in life (DMD is diagnosed before age 12 years whereas BMD is seen in teenage males older than 16 years of age) and the vast majority of patients develop DCM before their 25th birthday. In most patients, CK-MM is elevated similar to that seen in XLCM; in addition, manifesting female carriers develop disease late in life, similar to XLCM. Furthermore, immunohistochemical analysis demonstrates reduced levels (or absence) of dystrophin, similar to that seen in the hearts of patients with XLCM.

Murine models of dystrophin deficiency demonstrate abnormalities of muscle physiology based on membrane structural support abnormalities [28]. In addition to the dysfunction of dystrophin, mutations in dystrophin secondarily affect proteins which interact with dystrophin. At the amino-terminus (N-terminus), dystrophin binds to the sarcomeric protein actin, a member of the thin filament of the contractile apparatus. At the carboxy-terminus (C-terminus), dystrophin interacts with α-dystroglycan, a dystrophin-associated membrane-bound protein which is involved in the function of the DAPC, which includes β-dystroglycan, the sarcoglycan subcomplex (α-, β-, γ-, δ-, and ε-sarcoglycan), syntrophins, and dystrobrevins [29–31] (Fig. 8.1). In turn, this complex interacts with α_2-laminin and the extracellular matrix [32]. Like dystrophin, mutations in these genes lead to muscular dystrophies with or without cardiomyopathy, supporting the contention that this group of proteins are important to the normal function of the myocytes of the heart and skeletal muscles [32,33]. In both cases, mechanical stress [28] appears to play a significant role in the age-onset-dependent dysfunction of these muscles. The information gained from the studies on XLCM, DMD, and BMD led us to hypothesize that DCM is a disease of the cytoskeleton/sarcolemma which affects the sarcomere [34], a "final common pathway" of DCM [35]. We also have suggested that dystrophin mutations play a role in idiopathic DCM in males. This was supported when we showed that three out of 22 boys with DCM had dystrophin mutations and all were later found to have elevated CK-MM as well [36]. In addition, eight families with DCM and possible X-linked inheritance were also screened and, in three out of eight families, dystrophin mutations were noted. Again, CK-MM was elevated in all subjects carrying mutations [37].

Barth syndrome

Initially described as X-linked cardioskeletal myopathy with abnormal mitochondria and neutropenia by Neustein *et al.* [38] and Barth *et al.* [39], this disorder typically presents in male infants as CHF associated with neutropenia (cyclic) and 3-methylglutaconic aciduria [40]. Mitochondrial dysfunction is noted on electron microscopy (EM) and electron transport chain biochemical analysis. Recently, abnormalities in cardiolipin have been noted [41]. Echocardiographically these infants typically have left ventricular dysfunction with left ventricular dilation, endocardial fibroelastosis, or a dilated hypertrophic left ventricle. In some cases these infants succumb due to CHF/sudden death VT/VF, or sepsis due to leukocyte dysfunction. The majority of these children survive infancy and do well clinically, although DCM usually persists. In some cases, cardiac transplantation has been performed. Histopathologic evaluation typically demonstrates the features of DCM, although endocardial fibroelastosis may be prominent and the mitochondria are abnormal in shape and abundance.

The genetic basis of Barth syndrome was first described by Bione *et al.* [42], who cloned the disease-causing gene, G4.5. This gene encodes a novel protein called tafazzin, whose gene product is an acyltransferase and results in cardiolipin abnormalities [41]. Mutations in G4.5 result in a wide clinical spectrum, which includes apparent classic DCM, hypertrophic DCM, endocardial fibroelastosis (EFE), or left ventricular noncompaction [3,43].

Autosomal dominant dilated cardiomyopathy

The most common form of inherited DCM is the autosomal dominant form of disease [3]. These patients present as classic "pure" DCM or DCM associated with conduction system disease (CDDC). In the latter case, patients usually present in the third decade of life with mild conduction system disease which can progress to complete heart block over decades. DCM usually presents late in the course but is out of proportion to the degree of conduction system disease [44]. The echocardiographic and histologic findings in both subgroups are classic for DCM, although the conduction system may be fibrotic in patients with CDDC. In both groups of DCM patients, VT, VF, and torsades de pointest (TdP) occur and may result in sudden death.

Genetic heterogeneity exists for autosomal dominant DCM with more than 15 loci mapped for pure DCM and five loci for CDDC [3]. In the case of pure DCM, 10 genes have been identified to date, including three by our group (δ-sarcoglycan, α-actinin-2, ZASP) [3,5,45], as well as actin, desmin, troponin T, β-myosin heavy chain, titin, metavinculin, myosin binding protein C, α-tropomyosin, MLP, β-sarcoglycan and phospholamban [3,46,47] (Table 8.1).

The majority of genes identified to date encode either cytoskeletal or sarcomeric proteins. In the case of cytoskeletal proteins (desmin, δ-sarcoglycan, metavinculin, MLP), defects of force transmission are considered to result in the DCM phenotype, while defects of force generation have been speculated to cause sarcomeric protein-induced DCM [3,34].

Cardiac actin is a sarcomeric protein that is a member of the sarcomeric thin filament interacting with tropomyosin and the troponin complex. As previously noted, actin plays a significant role in linking the sarcomere to the sarcolemma via its binding to the N-terminus of dystrophin, and the mutations in actin which resulted in DCM as described by Olson *et al.* [48] appear to be directly involved in the binding of dystrophin. The DCM-causing mutations are believed to result by causing force transmission abnormalities. Further, actin interacts in the sarcomere with TnT and β-MHc, two other genes resulting in either DCM or HCM depending on the position of the mutation [49]. In the case of TnT and β-MHC, force generation abnormalities have been speculated as the responsible mechanism.

Desmin is a cytoskeletal protein that forms intermediate filaments specific for muscle [12]. This muscle-specific 53 kDa subunit of class III intermediate filaments forms connections between the nuclear and plasma membranes of cardiac, skeletal, and smooth muscle. Desmin is found at the Z lines and intercalated disk of muscle and its role in muscle function appears to involve attachment or stabilization of the sarcomere. Mutations in this gene appear to cause abnormalities of force and signal transmission similar to that believed to occur with actin mutations [50].

Another DCM-causing gene, δ-sarcoglycan, is a member of the sarcoglycan subcomplex of the DAPC [45,51]. This gene encodes for a protein involved in stabilization of the myocyte sarcolemma as well as signal transduction. Mutations identified in familial and sporadic cases resulted in reduction of the protein within the myocardium. In the absence of δ-sarcoglycan, the remaining sarcoglycans (δ, β, γ, ε) cannot assemble properly in the endoplasmic reticulum [52]. Mouse models of δ-sarcoglycan deficiency demonstrate dilated, hypertrophic cardiomyopathy, sarcolemmal fragility, and disrupted vasculin smooth muscle which leads to vascular spasm, including coronary spasm [53,54]. In addition, mutations in this gene lead to the phenotype of the cardiomyopathic Syrian hamster [55]. Other human mutations in δ-sarcoglycan cause a form of autosomal recessive limb girdle muscular dystrophy (LGMD2F), which rarely is associated with heart disease.

The final cytoskeletal protein-encoding gene, metavinculin, encodes vinculin and its splice variant metavinculin. Vinculin is ubiquitously expressed and metavinculin is coexpressed with vinculin in heart, skeletal, and smooth muscle, with this protein complex localized to subsarcolemmal costameres in the heart where they interact with α-actinin, talin, and γ-actin to form a microfilamentous network linking cytoskeleton and sarcolemma. In addition, these proteins are present in adherens junctions in intercalated disks and participate in cell–cell adhesion. Mutations in metavinculin have been shown to disrupt the intercalated disks and alter actin filament crosslinking [56,57].

Mutations in the sarcomere may produce hypertrophic cardiomyopathy or dilated cardiomyopathy. In the latter case, abnormalities in force generation or transmission are thought to contribute to the development of this phenotype [49]. In addition to mutations in the thin filament protein actin, mutations in the thick filament protein-encoding gene β-myosin heavy chain have been shown to cause DCM with associated sudden death in at least one infant, as well as DCM in older children and adults [49,58]. Mutations in this gene are thought to perturb the actin–myosin interaction and force generation or alter crossbridge movement during contraction. Mutations in cardiac troponin T, a thin filament protein, have been speculated to disrupt calcium-sensitive troponin C binding [49,58]. Mutations in phospholamban [59,60] have also been identified which further support calcium handling as a potentially important mechanism in the development of DCM. Interestingly, Haghighi *et al.* [60] identified homozygous mutations causing dilated cardiomyopathy and heart failure, while heterozygotes had cardiac hypertrophy. Recessive mutation in troponin I is thought to impair the interaction with troponin T, while α-tropomyosin mutations have also been identified and were predicted to alter the surface charge of the protein leading to impaired interaction with actin [61,62].

A recent area of interest for evaluation at the molecular level is the Z-disk [63]. Knoll *et al.* [64] identified mutations in MLP and demonstrated that this results in defects in the interaction with telethonin [64]. Using mouse models, they also demonstrated that MLP acts as a stretch sensor and that mutant MLP causes defects in this activity. More recently, Mohapatra *et al.* [5] demonstrated mutations in MLP in families and sporadic cases and identified abnormalities in the T-tubule system and Z-disk architecture by electron microscopy, which correlates with the histopathology seen in MLP-knockout mice [65]. This was further supported by the finding of reduced expression of MLP in chronic human heart failure [66,67]. In addition, mutations in α-actinin-2, which is involved in crosslinking actin filaments and shares a common actin-binding domain with dystrophin, were also identified in familial DCM, which disrupt its binding to MLP [5]. Vatta *et al.* [4] identified mutations in the Z-band alternatively spliced PDZ-motif protein ZASP, the human homolog of the mouse cypher gene which when disrupted leads to DCM [68]. Multiple mutations in this gene were identified in families and sporadic cases of DCM and with left ventricular (LV) noncompaction. This protein, which interacts with α-actinin-2, disrupts the actin cytoskeleton when mutated. Another gene, titin, which encodes the giant sarcomeric cytoskeletal protein titin that contributes to the maintenance of the sarcomere organization and myofibrillar elasticity, interacts with these proteins at the Z-disk/I-band transition zone [69]. Mutations have been identified in familial DCM as well [70].

As seen in pure autosomal dominant DCM, genetic heterogeneity also exists for CDDC. To date, CDDC genes have been mapped to chromosomes 1p1–1q1, 2q14–21, 3p25–22, and 6q23. The only gene thus far identified was reported to be lamin A/C on chromosome 1q21, which encodes a nuclear envelope intermediate filament protein [71,72].

Lamin A/C

The lamins are located in the nuclear lamina at the nucleoplasmic side of the inner nuclear membrane, and lamin A and C are expressed in heart and skeletal muscle [73]. Mutations in this gene were initially reported to cause the autosomal dominant form of Emery–Dreifuss muscular dystrophy (EDMD) [74,75], which has skeletal myopathy associated with DCM and conduction system disease. It has also been found to cause a form of autosomal dominant limb girdle muscular dystrophy (LGMD1B), which is also associated with conduction system disease [76]. Multiple mutations have been identified in patients with DCM and conduction system disease which, in some cases, had mildly elevated creatine kinase. This gene defect appears to be relatively common in patients with CDDC. The mechanism(s) responsible for the development of DCM and conduction system abnormalities and skeletal myopathy are being determined [77]. Understanding may be aided by knowledge of how other genes that encode interacting proteins result in disease, such as thymopoietin [78].

Muscle is muscle: cardiomyopathy and skeletal myopathy genes overlap

Interestingly, nearly all of the genes identified for inherited DCM are also known to cause skeletal myopathy in humans and/or mouse models. In the case of dystrophin, mutations cause DMD and BMD while δ-sarcoglycan mutations cause limb girdle muscular dystrophy (LGMD2F). Lamin A/C has been shown to cause autosomal dominant EDMD and LGMD1B, while actin mutations are associated with nemaline myopathy. Desmin, G4.5, α-dystrobrevin, Cypher/ZASP, MLP, α-actinin-2, titin, and β-sarcoglycan mutations also have associated skeletal myopathy, suggesting that cardiac and skeletal muscle function is interrelated and that possibly the skeletal muscle fatigue seen in patients with DCM with and without CHF may be due to primary skeletal muscle disease and not only related to the cardiac dysfunction. It also suggests that the function of these muscles has a "final common pathway" and that both cardiologists and neurologists should consider evaluation of both sets of muscles.

Further support for this concept comes from studies of animal models. Mutations in δ-sarcoglycan in hamsters results in cardiomyopathy while mutations in all sarcoglycan subcomplex genes in mice cause skeletal and cardiac muscle disease. Mutations in other DAPC genes as well as dystrophin in murine models consistently demonstrate abnormalities of skeletal and cardiac muscle function. Arber *et al.* [65] also produced a mouse deficient in MLP, a structural protein that links the actin cytoskeleton to the contractile apparatus. The resultant mice develop severe DCM, CHF, and disruption of cardiac myocyte cytoskeletal architecture. Murine mutations in titin, cypher, α-dystrobrevin, desmin, and others all demonstrate cardiac and skeletal muscle disease. Finally, Badorff *et al.* [79] has shown that the DCM that develops after viral myocarditis has a mechanism similar to the inherited forms. Using coxsackievirus B3 (CVB3) infection of mice, the authors showed that the CVB3 genome encodes for a protease (enteroviral protease 2A) that cleaves dystrophin at the third hinge region of dystrophin, resulting in force transmission abnormalities and DCM (Fig. 8.4). In addition, Xiong *et al.* [80] showed that abnormal dystrophin increases susceptibility to viral infection and resultant myocarditis. Interestingly, a similar dystrophin mutation which affects the first hinge region of dystrophin in patients with XLCM was previously reported by our laboratory, demonstrating a consistent mechanism of DCM development and abnormalities of the cytoskeleton/sarcolemma and sarcomere. In addition, we have shown that N-terminal dystrophin is reduced or absent in hearts of patients with all forms of DCM (ischemic, acquired, genetic, idiopathic) and that reduction of mechanical stress by use of left ventricular assist devices results in reverse remodeling of dystrophin and of the heart itself [81,82].

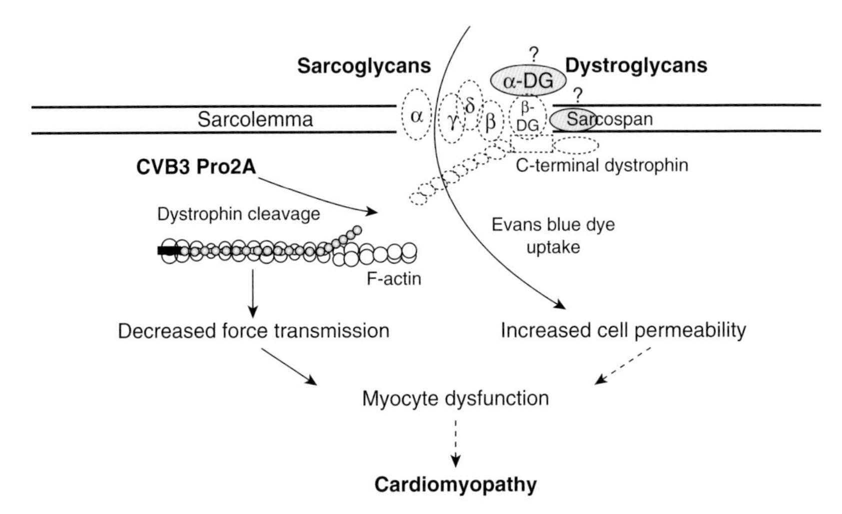

Fig. 8.4 Coxsackievirus B3 (CVB3) protease 2A cleaves dystrophin, resulting in dilated cardiomyopathy in viral myocarditis. (Reproduced with permission from Xiong *et al.* [80].)

Conclusions

Dilated cardiomyopathy results from disruption in the "final common pathway" linking the sarcomere and sarcolemma, and mutations in the affected genes are responsible for cardiac and skeletal muscle dysfunction. The mechanisms of disease, which include mechanical stress and stretch, are being elucidated. Many of the genes identified are now clinically available in fee-for-service laboratories. Novel therapies will likely result from the improved understanding of this clinical phenotype.

References

1 Report of the 1995 World Health Organization/International Society and Federation of Cardiology Task Force on the Definition and Classification of Cardiomyopathies. *Circulation* 1996; **93**: 841–842.

2 Rosamond W, Flegal K, Furie K *et al.* A+merican Heart Association Statistics Committee and Stroke Statistics Subcommittee. Heart disease and stroke statistics 2008 update: a report from the American Heart Association Statistics Committee and Stroke Statistics Subcommittee. *Circulation*; **117**: e25–e146, 2008. Epub 2007 Dec 17.

3 Towbin JA, Bowles NE. The failing heart. *Nature* 2002; **415**: 227–233.

4 Vatta M, Mohapatra B, Jimenez S, *et al.* Mutations in cypher/ZASP in patients with dilated cardiomyopathy and left ventricular non-compaction. *Journal of the American College of Cardiology* 2003; **42**: 2014–2027.

5 Mohapatra B, Jimenez S, Lin JH *et al.* Mutations in the muscle LIM protein and α-actinin-2 genes in dilated cardiomyopathy and endocardial fibroelastosis. *Molecular Genetics and Metabolism* 2003; **80**: 207–215.

6 Towbin JA. Myocarditis. In: Finberg L, Kleinman R, eds. *Saunders Manual of Pediatric Practice*, 2nd edn. W.B. Saunders Co., Philadelphia, PA, 2002: 660–663.
7 Schwartz SM, Duffy JY, Pearl JM, Nelson DP. Cellular and molecular aspects of myocardial dysfunction. *Critical Care Medicine* 2001; **29**: S214–S219.
8 Gregorio CC, Antin PB. To the heart of myofibril assembly. *Trends in Cellular Biology* 2000; **10**: 355–362.
9 Clark KA, McElhinny AS, Beckerle MC, Gregorio CC. Striated muscle cytoarchitecture: an intricate web of form and function. *Annual Review of Developmental Biology* 2002; **18**: 637–706.
10 Vigoreaux JO. The muscle Z band: lessons in stress management. *Journal of Muscle Research and Cell Motility* 1994; **15**: 237–255.
11 Barth AL, Nathke IS, Nelson WJ. Cadherins, catenins and APC protein; interplay between cytoskeletal complexes and signaling pathways. *Current Opinion in Cell Biology* 1997; **9**: 683–690.
12 Capetanaki Y. Desmin cytoskeleton: a potential regulator of muscle mitochondrial behaviour and function. *Trends in Cardiovascular Medicine* 2002; **12**: 339–348.
13 Sharp WW, Simpson DG, Borg TK *et al*. Mechanical forces regulate focal adhesion and costamere assembly in cardiac myocytes. *American Journal of Physiology* 1997; **273**: H546–556.
14 Straub V, Campbell KP. Muscular dystrophies and the dystrophin-glycoprotein complex. *Current Opinion in Neurology* 1997;**10**: 168–175.
15 Furukawa T, Ono Y, Tsuchiya H *et al*. Specific interaction of the potassium channel beta-subunit with the sarcomeric protein T-cap suggests a T-tubule-myofibril linking system. *Journal of Molecular Biology* 2001; **313**: 775–784.
16 Kucera JP, Rohr S, Rudy Y. Localization of sodium channels in intercalated disks modulates cardiac conduction. *Circulation Research* 2002; 91: 1176–1182.
17 Michels VV, Moll PP, Miller FA *et al*. The frequency of familial dilated cardiomyopathy in a series of patients with idiopathic dilated cardiomyopathy. *New England Journal of Medicine* 1992; **326**: 77–82.
18 Grunig E, Tasman JA, Kucherer H *et al*. Frequency and phenotypes of familial dilated cardiomyopathy. *Journal of the American College of Cardiology* 1998; **31**: 186–194.
19 Berko BA, Swift M. X-linked dilated cardiomyopathy. *New England Journal of Medicine* 1987; **316**: 1186–1191.
20 Towbin JA, Bowles KR, Bowles NE. Etiologies cardiomyopathy and heart failure. *Nature Medicine* 1999; **5**: 266–267.
21 Towbin JA, Hejtmancik JF, Brink P *et al*. X-linked dilated cardiomyopathy (XLCM): molecular genetic evidence of linkage to the Duchenne muscular dystrophy gene at the Xp21 locus. *Circulation* 1993; **87**: 1854–1865.
22 Muntoni F, Cau M, Ganau A *et al*. Brief report: deletion of the dystrophin muscle-specific promoter region associated with X-linked dilated cardiomyopathy. *New England Journal of Medicine* 1993; **329**: 921–925.
23 Cox GF, Kunkel LM. Dystrophies and heart disease. *Current Opinion in Cardiology* 1997; **12**: 329–343.
24 Hoffman EP, Brown RH, Kunkel LM. Dystrophin: the protein product of the Duchenne muscular dystrophy locus. *Cell* 1987; **51**: 919–928.
25 Meng H, Leddy JJ, Frank J *et al*. The association of cardiac dystrophin with myofibrils/z-discs regions in cardiac muscle suggests a novel role in the contractile apparatus. *Journal of Biological Chemistry* 1996; **271**: 12364–12371.

26 Kaprielian RR, Stevenson S, Rothery SM *et al*. Distinct patterns of dystrophin organization in myocyte sarcolemma and transverse tubules of normal and diseased human myocardium. *Circulation* 2000; **101**: 2586–2594.
27 Koenig M, Hoffman EP, Bertelson CJ *et al*. Complete cloning of the Duchenne muscular dystrophy (DMD) cDNA and preliminary genomic organization of the DMD gene in normal and affected individuals. *Cell* 1987; **50**: 509–517.
28 Petrof BJ, Shrager JB, Stedman HH *et al*. Dystrophin protects the sarcolemma from stresses developed during muscle contraction. *Proceedings of the National Academy of Sciences of the USA* 1993; **90**: 3710–3714.
29 Campbell KP. Three muscular dystrophies: loss of cytoskeleton-extracellular matrix linkage. *Cell* 1995; **80**: 675–679.
30 Klietsch R, Ervasti JM, Arnold W *et al*. Dystrophin-glycoprotein complex and laminin colocalize to the sarcolemma and transverse tubules of cardiac muscle. *Circulation Research* 1993; **72**: 349–360.
31 Ozawa E, Yoshida M, Suzuki A *et al*. Dystrophin-associated proteins in muscular dystrophy. *Human Molecular Genetics* 1995; **4**: 1711–1716.
32 Emery AE. The muscular dystrophies. *Lancet* 2002; **359**: 687–695.
33 Davies KE, Nowak KJ. Molecular mechanisms of muscular dystrophies: old and new players. *Nature Reviews Molecular and Cellular Biology* 2006; **7**: 762–773
34 Towbin JA. The role of cytoskeletal proteins in cardiomyopathies. *Current Opinion in Cell Biology* 1998; **10**: 131–139
35 Bowles NE, Bowles KR, Towbin JA. The "final common pathway" hypothesis and inherited cardiovascular disease: the role of cytoskeletal proteins in dilated cardiomyopathy. *Herz* 2000; **25**: 168–175.
36 Feng J, Yan J, Buzin CH *et al*. Mutations in the dystrophin gene are associated with sporadic dilated cardiomyopathy. *Molecular Genetics and Metabolism* 2002; **77**: 119–126.
37 Feng J, Yan J, Buzin CH *et al*. Comprehensive mutation scanning of the dystrophin gene in patients with nonsyndromic X-linked dilated cardiomyopathy. *Journal of the American College of Cardiology* 2002; **40**: 1120–1124.
38 Neustein HD, Lurie PR, Dahms B, Takahashi M. An X-linked recessive cardiomyopathy with abnormal mitochondria. *Pediatrics* 1979; **64**: 24–29.
39 Barth PG, Scholte HR, Berden JA *et al*. An X-linked mitochondrial disease affecting cardiac muscle, skeletal muscle and neutrophil leucocytes. *Journal of the Neurological Sciences* 1983; **62**: 327–355.
40 Kelley RI, Cheatham JP, Clark BJ *et al*. X-linked dilated cardiomyopathy with neutropenia, growth retardation, and 3-methylglutaconic aciduria. *Journal of Pediatrics* 1991; **119**: 738–747.
41 Schlame M, Towbin JA, Heerdt PM *et al*. Deficiency of tetralinoleoyl-cardiolipin in Barth syndrome. *Annals of Neurology* 2002; **51**: 634–637.
42 Bione S, D'Adamo P, Maestrini E *et al*. A novel X-linked gene, G4.5, is responsible for Barth syndrome . *Nature Genetics* 1996; **12**: 385–389.
43 Bleyl SB, Mumford BR, Thompson V *et al*. Neonatal, lethal noncompaction of the left ventricular myocardium is allelic with Barth syndrome. *American Journal of Human Genetics* 1997; **61**: 868–872.
44 Graber HL, Unverferth DV, Baker PB *et al*. Evolution of hereditary cardiac conduction and muscle disorder: a study involving a family with 6 generations affected. *Circulation* 1986; **74**: 21–35.

45 Tsubata S, Bowles KR, Vatta M *et al.* Mutations in the human delta-sarcoglycan gene in familial and sporadic dilated cardiomyopathy. *Journal of Clinical Investigation* 2000; **106**: 655–662.
46 Karkkainen S, Peuhkurinen K. Genetics of dilated cardiomyopathy. *Annals of Medicine* 2007; **32**: 91–107.
47 Towbin JA, Bowles NE. Dilated cardiomyopathy: a tale of the cytoskeleton and beyond. *Journal of Cardiovascular Electrophysiology* 2006; **17**: 919–926.
48 Olson TM, Michels VV, Thibodeau SN *et al.* Actin mutations in dilated cardiomyopathy, a heritable form of heart failure. *Science* 1998; **280**: 750–752.
49 Kamisago M, Sharma SD, DePalma SR *et al.* Mutations in sarcomere protein genes as a cause of dilated cardiomyopathy. *New England Journal of Medicine* 2000; **343**: 1688–1696.
50 Li D, Tapscott T, Gonzalez O *et al.* Desmin mutations responsible for idiopathic dilated cardiomyopathy. *Circulation* 1999; **100**: 461–464.
51 Fatkin D, Graham RM. Molecular mechanisms of inherited cardiomyopathies. *Physiology Reviews* 2002; **82**: 945–980.
52 Ozawa E, Mizumo Y, Hagiwara Y *et al.* Molecular and cellular biology of the sarcoglycan complex. *Muscle and Nerve* 2005; **32**: 563–576.
53 Coral-Vazquez R, Cohn RD, Moore SA *et al.* Disruption of the sarcoglycan-sarcospan complex in vascular smooth muscle: a novel mechanism for cardiomyopathy and muscular dystrophy. *Cell* 1999; **98**: 465–474.
54 Wheeler MT, Allikian MJ, Heydemann A *et al.* Smooth muscle cell-extrinsic vascular spasms arise from cardiomyocyte degeneration in sarcoglycan-deficient cardiomyopathy. *Journal of Clinical Investigation* 2004; **113**: 668–675.
55 Sakamoto A, Ono K, Abe M *et al.* Both hypertrophic and dilated cardiomyopathies are caused by mutation of the same gene, delta-sarcoglycan, in hamster: an animal model of disrupted dystrophin-associated glycoprotein complex. *Proceedings of the National Academy of Sciences of the USA* 1997; **94**: 13873–13878.
56 Olson TM, Illenberger S, Kishimoto NY *et al.* Metavinculin mutations alter actin interaction in dilated cardiomyopathy. *Circulation* 2002; **105**: 431–437.
57 Maeda M, Holder E, Lowes B *et al.* Dilated cardiomyopathy associated with deficiency of the cytoskeletal protein metavinculin. *Circulation* 1997; **95**: 17–20.
58 Chang AN, Potter JD. Sarcomeric protein mutations in dilated cardiomyopathy. *Heart Failure Reviews* 2005; **10**: 225–235.
59 Schmitt JP, Kamisago M, Asahi M *et al.* 2003; Dilated cardiomyopathy and heart failure caused by a mutation in phospholamban. *Science* **299**: 1410–1413.
60 Haghighi K, Kolokathis F, Pater L *et al.* Human phospholamban null results in lethal dilated cardiomyopathy revealing a critical difference between mouse and human. *Journal of Clinical Investigation* 2003; **111**: 869–876.
61 Murphy RT, Mogensen J, Shaw A *et al.* Novel mutation in cardiac troponin I in recessive idiopathic dilated cardiomyopathy. *Lancet* 2004; **363**: 371–372.
62 Olson TM, Kishimoto NY, Whitby FG, Michels VV. Mutations that alter the surface charge of alpha-tropomyosin are associated with dilated cardiomyopathy. *Journal of Molecular and Cellular Cardiology* 2001; **33**: 723–732.
63 Pyle WG, Solaro RJ. At the crossroads of myocardial signaling: the role of Z-discs in intracellular signaling and cardiac function. *Circulation Research* 2004; **94**: 296–305.

64 Knoll R, Hoshijima M, Hoffman HM *et al.* The cardiac mechanical stretch sensor machinery involves a Z disc complex that is defective in a subset of human dilated cardiomyopathy. *Cell* 2002; **11**: 943–955.

65 Arber S, Hunter JJ, Ross J Jr. *et al.* MLP-deficient mice exhibit a disruption of cardiac cytoarchitectural organization, dilated cardiomyopathy, and heart failure. *Cell* 1997; **88**: 393–403.

66 Zolk O, Caroni P, Bohm M. Decreased expression of the cardiac LIM domain protein MLP in chronic human heart failure. *Circulation* 2000; **101**: 2674–2677.

67 Katz AM. Cytoskeletal abnormalities in the failing heart. Out on a LIM? *Circulation* 2000; **101**: 2672–2673.

68 Zhou Q, Chu PH, Huang C *et al.* Ablation of cypher, a PDZ-LIM domain Z-line protein, causes a severe form of congenital myopathy. *Journal of Cell Biology* 2001; **155**: 605–612.

69 Granzier H, Labeit S. The grant protein titin: A major player in myocardial mechanics, signaling, and disease. *Circulation Research* 2004; **94**: 284–295.

70 Gerul B, Gramlich M, Atherton J *et al.* Mutations of TTN encoding the giant muscle filament titin, cause familial dilated cardiomyopathy. *Nature Genetics* 2002; **30**: 201–204.

71 Fatkin D, MacRae C, Sasaki T *et al.* Missense mutations in the rod domain of the lamin A/C gene as causes of dilated cardiomyopathy and conduction-system disease. *New England Journal of Medicine* 1999; **34**: 1715–1724.

72 Brodsky GL, Muntoni F, Miocic S *et al.* Lamin A/C gene mutation associated with dilated cardiomyopathy with variable skeletal muscle involvement. *Circulation* 2000; **101**: 473–476.

73 Stuurman N, Heins S, Aebi U. Nuclear lamins: their structure, assembly and interactions. *Journal of Structural Biology* 1998; **122**: 42–66.

74 Bonne G, DiBarletta MR, Varnous S *et al.* Mutations in the gene encoding lamin A/C cause autosomal dominant Emery-Dreifuss muscular dystrophy. *Nature Genetics* 1999; **21**: 285–288.

75 Di Barletta R, Ricci E, Galluzzi G *et al.* Different mutations in the LMNA gene cause autosomal dominant and autosomal recessive Emery-Dreifuss muscular dystrophy. *American Journal of Human Genetics* 2000; **66**: 1407–1412.

76 Muchir A, Bonne G, van der Kooi AJ *et al.* Identification of mutations in the gene encoding lamin A/C in autosomal dominant limb girdle muscular dystrophy with atrioventricular conduction disturbance (LGMD1B). *Human Molecular Genetics* 2000; **9**: 1453–1459.

77 Decostre V, Ben Yaou R, Bonne G. Laminopathies affecting skeletal and cardiac muscles: clinical and pathological aspects. *Acta Myologica* 2005; **24**: 104–109.

78 Taylor MR, Slavov D, Gajewski A *et al.* Thymopoietin (lamina-associated polypeptide 2) gene mutation associated with dilated cardiomyopathy. *Human Mutation* 2005; **26**: 566–574.

79 Badorff C, Lee G-H, Lamphear BJ *et al.* Enteroviral protease 2A cleaves dystrophin: Evidence of cytoskeletal disruption in an acquired cardiomyopathy. *Nature Medicine* 1999; **5**: 320–326.

80 Xiong D, Lee GH, Badorff C *et al.* Dystrophin deficiency markedly increases enterovirus-induced cardiomyopathy: A genetic predisposition to viral heart disease. *Nature Medicine* 2002; **8**: 872–877.

81 Vatta M, Stetson SJ, Perez-Verdra A *et al.* Molecular remodeling of dystrophin in patients with end-stage cardiomyopathies and reversal for patients on assist device therapy. *Lancet* 2000; **359**: 936–941.
82 Vatta M, Stetson SJ, Jimenez S *et al.* Molecular normalization of dystrophin in the failing left and right ventricle of patients treated with either pulsatile or continuous flow-type ventricular assist devices. *Journal of the American College of Cardiology* 2004; **43**: 811–817.

Chapter 9

Arrhythmogenic right ventricular cardiomyopathy

Srijita Sen-Chowdhry, Petros Syrris, and William J. McKenna

Introduction

Arrhythmogenic right ventricular cardiomyopathy (ARVC) is a genetically determined heart muscle disorder that may result in arrhythmia, sudden cardiac death (SCD), or, less commonly, heart failure. With the advent of the implantable cardioverter defibrillator (ICD), prevention of arrhythmic death has become achievable but remains dependent upon timely diagnosis and optimal risk stratification, both of which may pose significant clinical challenges.

Initial descriptions of ARVC highlighted the cardinal findings of ventricular tachycardia of right ventricular origin, right precordial T-wave inversion, and isolated right heart failure in the absence of pulmonary hypertension [1,2]. The underlying pathological features are progressive myocyte loss and fibroadipose replacement. These changes may be localized and show an early predilection for the so-called "triangle of dysplasia": the inflow, outflow, and apical regions of the right ventricle. Aneurysm formation is typical. Diffuse myocardial involvement leads to global right ventricular dilation and dysfunction. Fibroadipose substitution of the left ventricle is a recognized end-stage complication; the posterolateral wall is preferentially affected [3], with relative sparing of the septum. Patchy inflammatory infiltrates may be present in areas of myocardial damage [4]. Biventricular pump failure ultimately ensues [1].

Cardiovascular Genetics and Genomics. Edited by Dan Roden. © 2009 American Heart Association, ISBN: 978-14051-7540-1.

This traditional perspective on the natural history of ARVC is, however, based primarily on clinical–pathologic correlation studies of SCD victims and medium-term follow-up studies of symptomatic index cases—the severe end of the disease spectrum. Unbiased representation of an inherited disorder requires *in vivo* assessment of families. A family history of ARVC is present in 30–50% of reported cases, but this is likely to be a conservative estimate of the true prevalence of familial disease [5]. Since the disease is often clinically silent, elucidation of the family history alone is insufficient; relatives should be encouraged to undergo cardiac evaluation. Another major factor is the incomplete penetrance that often accompanies autosomal dominant inheritance; the penetrance of ARVC in some kindreds may be as low as 20–30% [5]. Evaluation of small families in clinical practice may therefore create the false impression of sporadic disease. Finally, relatives may show mild, nonspecific phenotypes, contributing to underrecognition of familial disease [6,7].

Familial studies confirm that stepwise progression from regional to global right ventricular dysfunction, followed by left ventricular involvement, occurs in a proportion of individuals with ARVC, notably probands [8]. This "classic" phenotype is not ubiquitous, however, and two additional patterns of disease expression have been identified [8]. The "biventricular" form is characterized by early and parallel involvement of both ventricles, initially localized but progressing to biventricular dilation and/or dysfunction, with arrhythmia of both right and left ventricular origin [8]. The "left-dominant" phenotype has been recognized by pathologists in SCD victims with predominant fibrofatty atrophy of the left ventricle, often with septal involvement [9,10]; clinical manifestations include lateral T-wave inversion, arrhythmia of left ventricular (LV) origin, and isolated LV dilation or systolic impairment [8,9], mirroring the clinical profile of ARVC [5].

Recognition of variants of ARVC with early and/or predominant LV involvement have prompted proposal of the broader term arrhythmogenic cardiomyopathy [8,10,12]. The issue of differentiation from dilated cardiomyopathy (DCM) has also become pertinent, since right ventricular preponderance can no longer be considered a major point of distinction [5,8]. Prominent regional involvement and aneurysms on imaging raise suspicion of arrhythmogenic cardiomyopathy rather than DCM [8,9]. The defining clinical characteristic of arrhythmogenic cardiomyopathy is, however, a propensity towards ventricular arrhythmia and SCD in the absence of overt ventricular dysfunction [8,9]. While SCD accounts for at least 30% of the overall mortality in DCM [50], it is seldom the mode of presentation. In contrast, SCD is the first clinical manifestation of the disease in more than 50% of index cases with ARVC [6,7]. Equally, ventricular arrhythmia is a relatively common finding in DCM but rare in the absence of significant ventricular dilation and impairment. Arrhythmogenic cardiomyopathy is well known to manifest a "concealed" phase, during which lack of clinical abnormalities may belie a significant risk of SCD [1,5].

Elucidation of the genetic basis of the disease in the past decade has shed light on the molecular mechanisms underlying its unique arrhythmic potential and provided a powerful tool for facilitating early diagnosis.

Genetics of recessive and syndromic ARVC

Although arrhythmogenic cardiomyopathy is commonly inherited as an autosomal dominant trait, the molecular studies that led to identification of the first disease-causing gene were performed on a recessive variant known as Naxos disease. One of the major syndromic forms of ARVC, Naxos disease is characterized by nonepidermolytic palmoplantar keratoderma and woolly hair, features that facilitated recognition of affected subjects. In 1998, Coonar *et al.* [13] mapped the genetic locus to 17q21. Two years later, McKoy *et al.* [14] isolated a 2 base pair deletion in the gene for junctional plakoglobin (JUP), resulting in frameshift and premature termination of the protein. The cutaneous phenotype is penetrant in homozygotes with Naxos disease from infancy. Children may also develop ventricular arrhythmia and ECG changes, but symptom onset is typically delayed until adolescence. The annual mortality thereafter is around 3%, marginally higher than that observed in dominant forms of ARVC [15].

Plakoglobin is a major constituent of cell adhesion junctions, and its isolation in Naxos disease paved the way for a search for related genes. Gene identification studies were already ongoing for another recessive cardiocutaneous syndrome, consisting of a triad of woolly hair, epidermolytic palmoplantar keratoderma, and apparent DCM. First recognized by Rao *et al.* [16] in 1996 in India, it was subsequently described in several Ecuadorian families by Carvajal-Huerta [17]. The cardiac phenotype of Carvajal syndrome, originally reported as DCM, shows closer resemblance to arrhythmogenic cardiomyopathy. ECG abnormalities in the Ecuadorian families are typical of ARVC, with inverted T waves in V1–V3 or beyond. Frequent and complex ventricular arrhythmia has been documented in the majority of patients with Carvajal syndrome, and may precede the onset of heart failure [18]. Pathological examination of the heart from a patient with Carvajal syndrome revealed aneurysms in the posterior and anteroseptal walls of the markedly dilated left ventricle, and at the triangle of dysplasia in the modestly dilated right ventricle [19].

Within months of the identification of plakoglobin in Naxos disease, Norgett *et al.* [20] reported homozygous a deletion in desmoplakin (DSP) as the causative mutation in Carvajal syndrome. This mutation is predicted to cause truncation of the C-terminal domain in the tail end of the protein. Alcalai *et al.* [21] subsequently isolated a recessive missense mutation in the C-terminus of desmoplakin in an Arab family with recessive ARVC, woolly hair, and a pemphigous-like skin disorder. While both mutations are located in exon 24 of the desmoplakin gene, Carvajal syndrome shows a left-dominant pattern, while the phenotype in the Arab family appears to be classic ARVC [5].

Genetics of dominant ARVC

Desmoplakin was also the first gene implicated in autosomal dominant ARVC, when Rampazzo *et al.* [22] reported a missense mutation in a large Italian family with the classic right ventricular phenotype. The resulting amino acid substitution modifies a putative phosphorylation site in the N-terminal plakoglobin-binding domain. Norman *et al.* [11] subsequently isolated a single adenine insertion in the N-terminal of desmoplakin in a family with left-dominant arrhythmogenic cardiomyopathy. This frameshift mutation is predicted to introduce a premature stop codon, resulting in truncation of the rod and C-terminal domains.

Two years after the identification of desmoplakin, Gerull and colleagues [23] reported a 27% prevalence of heterozygous mutations in plakophilin-2 (PKP2) in a series of 120 unrelated index cases with ARVC. The proportion was still higher in the US cohort described by Dalal and coworkers [24], in which 25 of 58 unrelated ARVC probands had PKP2 mutations. van Tintelen *et al.* [25] reported a similar 43% frequency of PKP2 mutations in their series of 56 ARVC index cases in The Netherlands. A key finding in the Dutch study was that 16 out of 23 (70%) probands with demonstrable familial disease had mutations in PKP2, suggesting that plakophilin-2 is the major determinant of familial ARVC in The Netherlands [25]. Dalal *et al.* [24] did not find common haplotypes among individuals with identical PKP2 mutations in the US study. In the Dutch cohort, however, haplotype analysis of index cases with four apparently recurrent PKP2 mutations revealed allele sharing, consistent with founder effects [25]. Founder mutations have previously been recognized in the Dutch population in conjunction with a number of other diseases [25].

Two additional desmosomal genes implicated in the disease are desmoglein-2 (DSG2) [26], which has an estimated prevalence of 7–10% among index cases [8,26], and desmocollin-2 (DSC2), which appears to play a lesser role [27].

Of the three additional genes linked with ARVC, the cardiac ryanodine receptor (RyR2) causes a distinct clinical entity, ARVD2, characterized by juvenile SCD and effort-induced polymorphic ventricular tachycardia [28]. The typical electrocardiographic features of ARVC do not arise, and structural abnormalities are limited to mild regional wall motion abnormalities of the right ventricle, with preservation of global systolic function. As such, the phenotype of ARVD2 bears closer resemblance to familial catecholaminergic polymorphic ventricular tachycardia, which is also linked with mutations in RyR2 Transmembrane protein 43 (TMEM43) has recently been linked to ARVD5, which is associated with early and prominent LV involvement [29]. The TMEM43 gene contains a response element for PPAR-gamma, an adipogenic transcription factor that is also involved in epithelial cell differentiation; at this juncture, however, an association with desmosomal development and function remains speculative [9,29].

A third extradesmosomal gene implicated in ARVC is transforming growth factor beta-3 (TGF-β3), which stimulates production of components of the extracellular matrix. Mutations in the untranslated regions of TGF-β3, predicted to result in overexpression, have been isolated in one large family and an unrelated proband with ARVD1 linkage [30]. That two ARVD1 kindreds lacked mutations in TGF-β3 is a caveat in gauging its overall contribution to the genetic profile of ARVC [5,31]. Nevertheless, *in vitro* studies suggest that TGF-β may modulate expression of desmosomal genes, lending further support to the hypothesis that impaired desmosomal function is the "final common pathway" in ARVC [32]. Elucidating the pathogenesis of arrhythmogenic cardiomyopathy is dependent on understanding the function and interplay of the cell adhesion proteins implicated.

The intercellular junction: a simplified model

Rather than forming a multinucleated syncytium like skeletal myofibers, cardiac myocytes rely on specialized structures known as intercalated disks for both mechanical and electrical coupling. Intercalated disks contain three distinct types of cell–cell connection: gap junctions, adherens junctions, and desmosomes. Gap junction channels, of which connexin-43 is a major constituent, mediate intercellular ion transfer. Transmission of contractile force is accomplished by cardiac adherens junctions, which comprise a transmembrane component (the Ca^{2+}-dependent glycoprotein N-cadherin), attached at its cytoplasmic tail to β-catenin and plakoglobin (γ-catenin), both of which bind α-catenin, which interacts with actin microfilaments within the sarcomere [5].

Desmosomes provide mechanical coupling between the cytoplasmic membranes of adjacent cells, with their intracellular components linking directly with intermediate filaments, mainly desmin. Proteins from three separate families assemble to form desmosomes: the desmosomal cadherins, armadillo proteins, and plakins. The genes encoding the desmosomal cadherins are clustered on chromosome 18q12.1. Four desmogleins (DSG1–4) and three desmocollins (DSC1–3) are recognized. The desmosomal cadherins constitute the transmembrane component of the desmosomal complex. Their extracellular domains interface directly with their counterparts on neighboring cells (Fig. 9.1) [5]. Besides their role in cell adhesion, the desmosomal cadherins may function as regulators of morphogenesis.

The intracellular portions of the desmosomal cadherins interact with proteins of the armadillo family: plakoglobin and plakophilin. Binding sites for both plakoglobin and plakophilin are situated in the N-terminal domain of desmoplakin. At its C-terminal, desmoplakin anchors desmin intermediate filaments to the cell surface. Another member of the plakin family, plectin, is also present in desmosomes. While its absence does not alter the ultrastructure

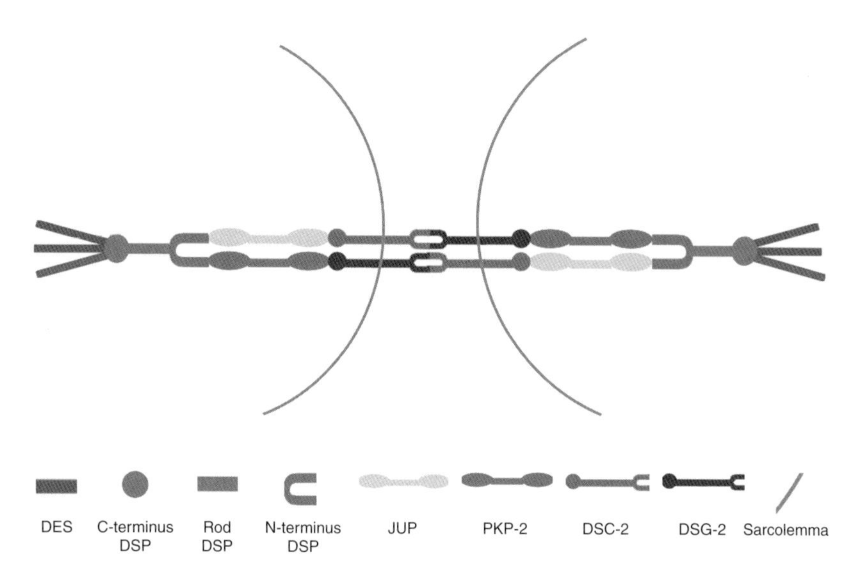

Fig. 9.1 Desmosomal structure. The desmosomal cadherins, desmoglein-2 (DSG-2) and desmocollin-2 (DSC-2), constitute the transmembrane component of the desmosomal complex. Their extracellular domains interface directly with their counterparts on neighboring cells. The intracellular portions of the desmosomal cadherins interact with proteins of the armadillo family: junctional plakoglobin (JUP) and plakophilin-2 (PKP-2), which in turn bind to the N-terminal domain of desmoplakin (DSP). At its C-terminal, DSP anchors desmin (DES) intermediate filaments to the cell surface. (Modified from Sen-Chowdhry *et al.* [8,51].)

of desmosomes, plectin appears to contribute significantly to the mechanical strengthening of cells [5].

Pathogenesis of ARVC: the desmosomal model

Desmosomes are most prevalent in tissues exposed to frictional and shear stress, such as myocardium and epithelium, where they play a key role in imparting mechanical strength through formation of a three-dimensional network. Defects in components of desmosomes may compromise their function, predisposing to myocyte detachment and death. Significant myocyte loss may be accompanied by an inflammatory response. The regenerative capacity of the myocardium is limited, necessitating repair by fibrofatty substitution. Both wall thickness and shear stress are heterogeneous, resulting in regional disease expression and aneurysm formation. Progressive myocyte loss and fibrotic repair cause gradual ventricular dilation [5].

Since desmosomal genes are expressed in both ventricles, there is no inherent reason why a mutation should preferentially affect one side of the heart. The molecular basis of the distinct patterns of disease expression in arrhythmogenic cardiomyopathy therefore warrants further exploration. Early work suggests that chain-termination mutations, particularly in desmoplakin, may be associated with prominent LV involvement [8]. Myocytes in the high-pressure left ventricle may be particularly vulnerable to mutations that impair intermediate filament function. Truncation of the C-terminus of desmosomal proteins is liable to result in disruption of intermediate filament binding, thereby generating a phenotype with marked or dominant LV disease [8,32]. In contrast, the increased distensibility of the thin-walled right ventricle, an adaptation to wide variations in preload in the normal state, may confer vulnerability to mutations that affect cell adhesion [8, 9]. Nevertheless, coexistence of distinct disease patterns within families, termed phenotypic discordance, suggests a key role for modifier genes in determining the ultimate phenotype [5,8].

The desmosomal model offers a molecular basis for age-related penetrance, which appears to be characteristic of ARVC [33], and may be related to progressive exposure to mechanical stress. Long-term endurance athletes appear to have structurally severe forms of the disease [8], a finding supported by animal studies in which endurance training hastened the development of right ventricular dysfunction and arrhythmia in heterozygous plakoglobin-deficient mice [34]. The disease may progress more slowly in individuals leading a sedentary life, with myocardial injury accumulating as part of the aging process.

The extramyocardial manifestations of syndromic ARVC are also explicable in terms of desmosomal dysfunction under conditions of mechanical stress. Cutaneous disease may be particularly conspicuous in the areas most exposed to pressure and/or abrasion: the palmar and plantar surfaces and knees [21]. Martini *et al.* [35] reported on a patient with ARVC and mitral valve prolapse, a link that was subsequently highlighted in a postmortem series [36]. It can be speculated that disruption of normal cell–cell adhesion predisposes to myxomatous degeneration of the mitral valve. Chronic aortic dissection has also been reported in the setting of ARVC. Autopsy revealed degenerative changes in the media of the aorta [37]. Whether this was coincidental or true pleiotropy remains unresolved; the history of hypertension was a major confounder. Nevertheless, disruption of the internal elastic lamina, accompanied by intimal and medial hyperplasia, has been observed in the arteries of patients with ARVC [38]. Fontaine *et al.* [39] have cited this finding as one possible explanation for the atypical chest pain often reported by these patients. Intimal hyperplasia is widely held to be a response to endothelial cell injury, to which vessels with cell adhesion defects may naturally be more susceptible. Recessive ARVC and anterior polar cataracts have been described in a consanguineous family from Argentina [40]. Fibrotic changes and abnormal accumulation of crystallins are observed in the lens epithelial cells of patients with anterior polar cataracts. Crystallins are essential determinants of lens transparency that may undergo modification in response to aging or stress [41]. A common undercurrent of stress-induced damage to cell surfaces is therefore evident.

Garcia-Gras *et al.* [42] have proposed an alternative molecular mechanism for the pathogenesis of ARVC. Besides their importance in cell–cell adhesion, desmosomes appear to have a role in signaling networks, including the evolutionarily conserved Wnt/β-catenin pathway. The pivotal events in the canonical Wnt pathway are accumulation of β-catenin in the cytoplasm, which promotes its translocation to the nucleus, where it interacts with the T cell factor/lymphoid enhancer factor (Tcf/Lef) family of transcription factors to promote specific gene expression. Inhibition of Wnt/β-catenin signaling stimulates adipogenesis, fibrogenesis, and apoptosis.

Suppression of desmoplakin expression in atrial myocyte cell lines leads to nuclear translocation of plakoglobin, a twofold reduction in canonical Wnt/β-catenin signaling through Tcf/Lef1 transcription factors, increased expression of adipogenic and fibrogenic genes, and accumulation of fat droplets [42]. Loss of desmoplakin is postulated to free plakoglobin from desmosomes. Plakoglobin (γ-catenin) has structural and functional similarities to β-catenin, and may act as a competitive antagonist, disrupting the Wnt/β-catenin axis and resulting in a shift from myocyte fate to adipocyte fate, even in the heart. As predicted, heterozygous desmoplakin-deficient mice demonstrated increased myocyte apoptosis and accumulation of adipocytes and fibrous tissue in the myocardium [42]. It is less easy, however, to reconcile this mechanism with the occurrence of a similar phenotype in plakoglobin-deficient mice and indeed in Naxos disease in man [43].

Mechanisms underlying arrhythmia

At least four distinct mechanisms may underlie ventricular arrhythmia in ARVC. Sustained monomorphic ventricular tachycardia in the overt stage is traditionally ascribed to reentrant circuits arising from fibrofatty substitution of the myocardium. Less easy to account for is the phenomenon of "hot phases," during which previously stable patients with mild disease may have unheralded arrhythmic events or even die suddenly. The disease is thought to remain quiescent for long periods, until an unknown stimulus triggers myocyte loss and inflammation in hitherto unaffected regions of the myocardium. The resulting bouts of myocarditis provide the substrate for transient electrical instability [5].

Recent studies have also shed light on the basis for arrhythmia in "concealed" ARVC. Kaplan *et al.* [44] examined cardiac tissue from four patients with Naxos disease, and reported reduced localization of connexin-43 to intercalated disks. Smaller and fewer gap junctions were observed [44]. Gap junctions have a high protein content, which renders the normally fluid cytoplasmic membrane rigid and prone to rupture. Their close proximity to desmosomes at the intercalated disks may protect them from mechanical stress. Destabilization of cell adhesion complexes will inhibit preservation of normal numbers of gap junctions. The resultant heterogeneous conduction may be a significant contributor to arrhythmogenesis.

Of particular interest was reduced expression of connexin-43 in the heart of a 7 year old child homozygous for the Naxos mutation [44]. Prior cardiac evaluation had revealed >14000 ventricular extrasystoles of predominantly right ventricular origin in a 24 hour period, and typical ECG features, including QRS prolongation (from 80 to 110ms) in leads V1–3 with a right bundle branch block pattern, epsilon waves, and T-wave inversion. Following her death from leukemia, histological examination of her heart showed no evidence of fibrofatty replacement, leukemic infiltrates, or chemotherapy-related damage [44].

The critical importance of this case is in illustrating that both ventricular arrhythmia and typical ECG abnormalities may arise in ARVC in the absence of fibroadipose replacement. Furthermore, it appears that gap junction remodeling may account for arrhythmogenesis in the so-called "concealed" phase. Whether this mechanism has the potential to produce lethal tachyarrhythmia is unresolved. As Kaplan *et al.* [44] suggest, however, superimposition of even mild myocardial abnormalities could impart a marked propensity towards arrhythmic events.

Equally remarkable are the findings of Kirchhof and colleagues [34], who reported increased right ventricular volumes, reduced right ventricular function, and spontaneous ventricular ectopy in 10 month old heterozygous plakoglobin-deficient mice, abnormalities which were accelerated by endurance training. Spontaneous ventricular tachycardia of right ventricular origin was observed in isolated, perfused plakoglobin-positive or -negative hearts, which also demonstrated prolonged right ventricular conduction times compared with wild type. Histology and electron microscopy failed to identify either fibrofatty replacement or reduced expression of connexin-43 [34], implying that impaired desmosomal function *per se* may be sufficient to cause right ventricular dilation and dysfunction, conduction delay, and ventricular arrhythmia, perhaps via mechanoelectric feedback.

Feasibility of genetic testing in clinical practice

Although genetic studies have provided important insights into the pathogenesis of ARVC, rapid integration of genotyping into clinical practice is impeded by a number of practical considerations. First, the clinical feasibility of genetic testing is dependent in large part on its success rate in the target population. In a UK referral center sample, mutation screening of the five desmosomal genes so far implicated in ARVC in 69 unrelated individuals allowed successful genotyping of 20 (~30%) [8]. No mutations were identified in plakoglobin. In a contemporaneous

Italian series, mutation screening of the "big three" ARVC genes (namely desmoplakin, plakophilin-2, and desmoglein-2, in order of frequency) allowed successful genotyping of 32 out of 80 unrelated index cases (40%). Inclusion of TGF-β3 effected a modest increase in the detection rate to 42.5% [26,45].

A key departure from the UK–Italian experience in other published cohorts has been the frequency of mutations in PKP2, which ranges from 27% to 43% in reports from Gerull *et al.* [23], Dalal *et al.* [24] in the USA, and van Tintelen *et al.* [25] in The Netherlands. While founder effects were apparent in the Dutch population, this was not the case in the original study from Gerull *et al.* or the subsequent American series, requiring that an alternative explanation be sought for the discrepancy in the prevalence of PKP2 mutations [23–25]. Differences in subject selection may be at least partly responsible. At most referral centers, individuals with symptomatic arrhythmias of right ventricular origin account for the majority of index cases. In comparison, the UK cohort included a much higher proportion of cases identified by familial evaluation following the death of the proband from pathologically proven ARVC [8]. It has also been suggested that some of the numerous missense changes may be pathogenic only when accompanied by additional genetic polymorphisms [8].

Gene identification in ARVC remains an active area of research, with additional components of the desmosome-intermediate filament complex and associated proteins as the primary candidates. Comprehensive screening of all known and candidate genes is likely to place the detection rate in the 40–50% [51] range, sufficient to justify clinical application in the near to immediate future, if technical challenges can be overcome.

The main technical obstacle to implementation of genotyping in clinical practice is the prohibitive cost of performing sequence analysis of a genomic region exceeding 40 kb. Marked allelic heterogeneity appears to be the rule for the main ARVC genes. Furthermore, while the number of mutations so far reported in desmocollin-2 and plakoglobin is too small to allow comment, current experience indicates a preponderance of private mutations in the "big three" genes in ARVC. Neither do there appear to be any mutational hotspots in the "big three" genes, with defects occurring in the N-terminus, rod, and C-terminus of desmoplakin, every exon of PKP2, and spread through the functional domains of DSG2. The result of this is that, in attempting to genotype patients with ARVC, no shortcut can obviate the need for systematic sequencing of the desmosomal genes, although it may be prudent to begin the search with PKP2, DSP, and DSG2.

An additional corollary of frequent private mutations is a substantial likelihood of isolating a novel mutation, with no information available regarding its pathogenicity. In general, it may be safe to assume a causative role for deletions, frameshift mutations, and nonsense mutations, but the same does not apply to single amino acid substitutions. Once a novel missense change has been identified, and its absence from ethnically matched control subjects verified, it becomes necessary to screen other family members and establish causality through correlation of clinical and genetic findings. Emerging data also suggest that an important minority of patients with ARVC are homozygous, double heterozygous, or compound heterozygous [8,46,47], underscoring the importance of screening every coding region of all known disease-causing genes, even after isolation of a putative pathogenic mutation.

Confirmatory and predictive testing in relatives with and without clinical features of the disease is more straightforward. Allelic diversity precludes any role for DNA probes, however, and although polymerase chain reaction restriction fragment length polymorphism (PCR-RFLP) analysis is relatively inexpensive, utility is limited to mutations that fall within restriction sites. Consequently, direct bidirectional sequencing of the exon containing the defect remains the preferred approach for known-mutation detection in ARVC, affording the highest diagnostic accuracy of any available technique.

Applications of genotyping in clinical practice

Presymptomatic diagnosis is the aspect of ARVC in which genotyping is most likely to find a niche. That SCD is the first clinical manifestation of the disease in over 50% of index cases may be the most compelling argument in favor of adopting a proactive approach to familial evaluation [6,7]. While presymptomatic diagnosis may be possible in a significant proportion of family members through standard, noninvasive clinical assessment, genetic analysis is invaluable in allowing cascade screening of families. The advantages are twofold: first, in affording a lifetime of reassurance to gene-negative relatives, who will constitute around 50% of those tested; and second, in allowing clinical resources to be targeted to proven gene carriers.

Mutation analysis may also be of value in allowing confirmatory testing to corroborate clinical suspicion of ARVC in index cases. Furthermore, identification of a desmosomal mutation may facilitate differentiation of dilated cardiomyopathy from "left-dominant" or "biventricular" forms of arrhythmogenic cardiomyopathy in late presenters [8,9]. In neither case, however, does a negative result exclude ARVC.

On the basis of currently available data, any attempt to gauge the potential influence of genotyping on risk stratification and therapy is likely to be premature. In accordance with the desmosomal model, it may be prudent for proven ARVC gene carriers to avoid highly strenuous activity, particularly endurance training. Without knowledge of the penetrance of a mutation, however, many are apt to consider such blanket recommendations unnecessarily restrictive. Similarly, the dual influences of incomplete penetrance and variable expressivity confound the adverse prognostic impact of carrying an ARVC mutation to the point where neither prenatal diagnosis nor proscriptive reproductive counseling are clinically justified, particularly as effective therapies are available.

A family history of premature sudden death does not appear to be a key indicator of adverse prognosis in ARVC, suggesting that the ultimate role of genotyping in risk stratification will be limited. Variations in disease expression between families carrying the same mutation, and among members of the same family, suggest that modifier genes contribute significantly to the overall phenotype in ARVC [8,48]; phenotypic differences between monozygotic twins imply that environmental influences also operate [33]. Nevertheless, mutations of the TMEM43 gene at the ARVD5 locus appear to be particularly malignant, and genotyping has been advocated to facilitate early diagnosis and prophylactic placement of ICDs [29,49]. Dalal *et al.* [24] compared ICD intervention rates in patients with ARVC with (n = 25) and without (n = 33) PKP2 mutations. Inducibility at electrophysiological study, spontaneous ventricular tachycardia, and diffuse right ventricular disease appeared to be predictors of increased risk among patients without PKP2 mutations, but did not influence the frequency of ICD interventions among PKP2-positive patients. The generalizability of these findings awaits validation in large-scale genotype–phenotype correlation studies.

Conclusion

Originally described as a developmental anomaly of the right ventricular myocardium, arrhythmogenic cardiomyopathy is now recognized to be a heart muscle disorder with a genetic basis that may occur as "left-dominant" and "biventricular" variants in addition to the "classic" right ventricular form. Causative mutations have been identified in components of the desmosome, the protein complex that anchors intermediate filaments to the cytoplasmic membrane in adjacent cells. A mutation in a desmosomal protein may, depending on its location, compromise cell adhesion or intermediate filament function, or both. The thin-walled, distensible right ventricle may be dependent on robust intercellular attachment, while the high-pressure left ventricle may require the support of an intact intermediate filament network. Modifier genes and environmental influences, particularly exposure to mechanical stress, may contribute significantly to the ultimate phenotype. There is growing evidence that ventricular arrhythmia may precede the development of the characteristic histological feature of fibrofatty replacement, highlighting the importance of early molecular diagnosis.

Clinical applications of genetic analysis in ARVC include cascade screening of families and confirmatory testing of index cases with a borderline diagnosis. The role of genotyping in predicting prognosis is limited at present, although the increased identification of individuals with early disease intensifies the need for definitive clinical risk stratification.

References

1 Corrado D, Fontaine G, Marcus FI *et al.* Arrhythmogenic right ventricular dysplasia/cardiomyopathy: need for an international registry. European Society of Cardiology

and the Scientific Council on Cardiomyopathies of the World Heart Federation. *Journal of Cardiovascular Electrophysiology* 2000; **11**: 827–832.

2 Marcus FI, Fontaine GH, Guiraudon G *et al.* Right ventricular dysplasia: a report of 24 adult cases. *Circulation* 1982; **65**: 384–398.

3 Corrado D, Basso C, Thiene G *et al.* Spectrum of clinicopathologic manifestations of arrhythmogenic right ventricular cardiomyopathy/dysplasia: a multicenter study. *Journal of the American College of Cardiology* 1997; **30**: 1512–1520.

4 Basso C, Thiene G, Corrado D *et al.* Arrhythmogenic right ventricular cardiomyopathy. Dysplasia, dystrophy, or myocarditis? *Circulation* 1996; **94**: 983–991.

5 Sen-Chowdhry S, Syrris P, McKenna WJ. Genetics of right ventricular cardiomyopathy. *Journal of Cardiovascular Electrophysiology* 2005; **16**: 927–935.

6 Nava A, Bauce B, Basso C *et al.* Clinical profile and long-term follow-up of 37 families with arrhythmogenic right ventricular cardiomyopathy. *Journal of the American College of Cardiology* 2000; **36**: 2226–2233.

7 Hamid MS, Norman M, Quraishi A *et al.* Prospective evaluation of relatives for familial arrhythmogenic right ventricular cardiomyopathy/dysplasia reveals a need to broaden diagnostic criteria. *Journal of the American College of Cardiology* 2002; **40**: 1445–1450.

8 Sen-Chowdhry S, Syrris P, Ward D *et al.* Clinical and genetic characterization of families with arrhythmogenic right ventricular dysplasia/cardiomyopathy provides novel insights into patterns of disease expression. *Circulation* 2007; **115**: 1710–1720.

9 Sen-Chowdhry S, Syrris P, Prasad SK, *et al.* Left-dominant arrhythmogenic cardiomyopathy: an under-recognized clinical entity. *Journal of the American College of Cardiology* 2008; **52**: 2175–2187.

10 Michalodimitrakis M, Papadomanolakis A, Stiakakis J, Kanaki K. Left side right ventricular cardiomyopathy. *Medicine Science and the Law* 2002; **42**: 313–317.

11 Norman M, Simpson M, Mogensen J *et al.* Novel mutation in desmoplakin causes arrhythmogenic left ventricular cardiomyopathy. *Circulation* 2005; **112**: 636–642.

12 Gallo P, d'Amati G, Pelliccia F. Pathologic evidence of extensive left ventricular involvement in arrhythmogenic right ventricular cardiomyopathy. *Human Pathology* 1992; **23**: 948–952.

13 Coonar AS, Protonotarios N, Tsatsopoulou A *et al.* Gene for arrhythmogenic right ventricular cardiomyopathy with diffuse nonepidermolytic palmoplantar keratoderma and woolly hair (Naxos disease) maps to 17q21. *Circulation* 1998; **97**: 2049–2058.

14 McKoy G, Protonotarios N, Crosby A *et al.* Identification of a deletion in plakoglobin in arrhythmogenic right ventricular cardiomyopathy with palmoplantar keratoderma and woolly hair (Naxos disease). *Lancet* 2000; **355**: 2119–2124.

15 Protonotarios N, Tsatsopoulou A, Anastasakis A *et al.* Genotype-phenotype assessment in autosomal recessive arrhythmogenic right ventricular cardiomyopathy (Naxos disease) caused by a deletion in plakoglobin. *Journal of the American College of Cardiology* 2001; **38**: 1477–1484.

16 Rao BH, Reddy IS, Chandra KS. Familial occurrence of a rare combination of dilated cardiomyopathy with palmoplantar keratoderma and curly hair. *Indian Heart Journal* 1996; **48**: 161–162.

17 Carvajal-Huerta L. Epidermolytic palmoplantar keratoderma with woolly hair and dilated cardiomyopathy. *Journal of the American Academy of Dermatology* 1998; **39**: 418–421.

18 Protonotarios N, Tsatsopoulou A. Naxos disease and Carvajal syndrome: cardiocutaneous disorders that highlight the pathogenesis and broaden the spectrum of arrhythmogenic right ventricular cardiomyopathy. *Cardiovascular Pathology* 2004; **13**: 185–194.

19 Kaplan SR, Gard JJ, Carvajal-Huerta L *et al.* Structural and molecular pathology of the heart in Carvajal syndrome. *Cardiovascular Pathology* 2004; **13**: 26–32.
20 Norgett EE, Hatsell SJ, Carvajal-Huerta L *et al.* Recessive mutation in desmoplakin disrupts desmoplakin-intermediate filament interactions and causes dilated cardiomyopathy, woolly hair and keratoderma. *Human Molecular Genetics* 2000; **9**: 2761–2766.
21 Alcalai R, Metzger S, Rosenheck S *et al.* A recessive mutation in desmoplakin causes arrhythmogenic right ventricular dysplasia, skin disorder, and woolly hair. *Journal of the American College of Cardiology* 2003; **42**: 319–327.
22 Rampazzo A, Nava A, Malacrida S *et al.* Mutation in human desmoplakin domain binding to plakoglobin causes a dominant form of arrhythmogenic right ventricular cardiomyopathy. *American Journal of Human Genetics* 2002; **71**: 1200–1206.
23 Gerull B, Heuser A, Wichter T *et al.* Mutations in the desmosomal protein plakophilin-2 are common in arrhythmogenic right ventricular cardiomyopathy. *Nature Genetics* 2004; **36**: 1162–1164.
24 Dalal D, Molin LH, Piccini J *et al.* Clinical features of arrhythmogenic right ventricular dysplasia/cardiomyopathy associated with mutations in plakophilin-2. *Circulation* 2006; **113**: 1641–1649.
25 van Tintelen JP, Entius MM, Bhuiyan ZA *et al.* Plakophilin-2 mutations are the major determinant of familial arrhythmogenic right ventricular dysplasia/cardiomyopathy. *Circulation* 2006; **113**: 1650–1658.
26 Pilichou K, Nava A, Basso C *et al.* Mutations in desmoglein-2 gene are associated with arrhythmogenic right ventricular cardiomyopathy. *Circulation* 2006; **113**: 1171–1179.
27 Syrris P, Ward D, Evans A *et al.* Arrhythmogenic right ventricular dysplasia/cardiomyopathy associated with mutations in the desmosomal gene desmocollin-2. *American Journal of Human Genetics* 2006; **79**: 978–984.
28 Tiso N, Stephan DA, Nava A *et al.* Identification of mutations in the cardiac ryanodine receptor gene in families affected with arrhythmogenic right ventricular cardiomyopathy type 2 (ARVD2). *Human Molecular Genetics* 2001; **10**: 189–194.
29 Merner ND, Hodgkinson KA, Haywood AF, *et al.* Arrhythmogenic right ventricular cardiomyopathy type 5 is a fully penetrant, lethal arrhythmic disorder caused by a missense mutation in the TMEM43 gene. *American Journal of Human Genetics* 2008; **82**: 809–821
30 Beffagna G, Occhi G, Nava A *et al.* Regulatory mutations in transforming growth factor-beta3 gene cause arrhythmogenic right ventricular cardiomyopathy type 1. *Cardiovascular Research* 2005; **65**: 366–373.
31 Nattel S, Schott JJ. Arrhythmogenic right ventricular dysplasia type 1 and mutations in transforming growth factor beta3 gene regulatory regions: a breakthrough? *Cardiovascular Research* 2005; **65**: 302–304.
32 Yang Z, Bowles NE, Scherer SE *et al.* Desmosomal dysfunction due to mutations in desmoplakin causes arrhythmogenic right ventricular dysplasia/cardiomyopathy. *Circulation Research* 2006; **99**: 646–655.
33 Dalal D, James C, Devanagondi R *et al.* Penetrance of mutations in plakophilin-2 among families with arrhythmogenic right ventricular dysplasia/cardiomyopathy. *Journal of the American College of Cardiology* 2006; **48**: 1416–1424.
34 Kirchhof P, Fabritz L, Zwiener M *et al.* Age- and training-dependent development of arrhythmogenic right ventricular cardiomyopathy in heterozygous plakoglobin-deficient mice. *Circulation* 2006; **114**: 1799–1806.

35 Martini B, Basso C, Thiene G. Sudden death in mitral valve prolapse with Holter monitoring-documented ventricular fibrillation: evidence of coexisting arrhythmogenic right ventricular cardiomyopathy. *International Journal of Cardiology* 1995; **49**: 274–278.

36 Corrado D, Basso C, Nava A *et al.* Sudden death in young people with apparently isolated mitral valve prolapse. *Giornale Italiano di Cardiologia* 1997; **27**: 1097–1105.

37 Merten M, Meinertz T, Willems S, Heinemann A. Arrhythmogenic right ventricular cardiomyopathy with left ventricular involvement and aortic dissection. *Pacing and Clinical Electrophysiology* 2004; **27**: 408–411.

38 Smith M, Kickuk MR, Ratliff NB. Clinical and pathologic study of two siblings with arrhythmogenic right ventricular cardiomyopathy. *Cardiovascular Pathology* 1999; **8**: 273–278.

39 Fontaine G, Fontaliran F, Frank R. Arrhythmogenic right ventricular cardiomyopathies: clinical forms and main differential diagnoses. *Circulation* 1998; **97**: 1532–1535.

40 Frances R, Rodriguez Benitez AM, Cohen DR. Arrhythmogenic right ventricular dysplasia and anterior polar cataract. *American Journal of Medical Genetics* 1997; **73**: 125–126.

41 Hwang KH, Lee EH, Jho EH *et al.* Accumulation and aberrant modifications of alpha-crystallins in anterior polar cataracts. *Yonsei Medical Journal* 2004; **45**: 73–80.

42 Garcia-Gras E, Lombardi R, Giocondo MJ *et al.* Suppression of canonical Wnt/beta-catenin signaling by nuclear plakoglobin recapitulates phenotype of arrhythmogenic right ventricular cardiomyopathy. *Journal of Clinical Investigation* 2006; **116**: 2012–2021.

43 MacRae CA, Birchmeier W, Thierfelder L. Arrhythmogenic right ventricular cardiomyopathy: moving toward mechanism. *Journal of Clinical Investigation* 2006; **116**: 1825–1828.

44 Kaplan SR, Gard JJ, Protonotarios N *et al*: Remodeling of myocyte gap junctions in arrhythmogenic right ventricular cardiomyopathy due to a deletion in plakoglobin (Naxos disease). *Heart Rhythm* 2004; **1**: 3–11.

45 Corrado D, Thiene G. Arrhythmogenic right ventricular cardiomyopathy/dysplasia: clinical impact of molecular genetic studies. *Circulation* 2006; **113**: 1634–1637.

46 Awad MM, Dalal D, Cho E *et al.* DSG2 mutations contribute to arrhythmogenic right ventricular dysplasia/cardiomyopathy. *American Journal of Human Genetics* 2006; **79**: 136–142.

47 Awad MM, Dalal D, Tichnell C *et al.* Recessive arrhythmogenic right ventricular dysplasia due to novel cryptic splice mutation in PKP2. *Human Mutation* 2006; **27**: 1157.

48 Kannankeril PJ, Bhuiyan ZA, Darbar D *et al.* Arrhythmogenic right ventricular cardiomyopathy due to a novel plakophilin 2 mutation: wide spectrum of disease in mutation carriers within a family. *Heart Rhythm* 2006; **3**: 939–944.

49 Hodgkinson KA, Parfrey PS, Bassett AS *et al.* The impact of implantable cardioverter-defibrillator therapy on survival in autosomal-dominant arrhythmogenic right ventricular cardiomyopathy (ARVD5). *Journal of the American College of Cardiology* 2005; **45**: 400–408.

50 Priori SG, Aliot E, Blomstrom-Lundgvist C *et al.* Task force on sudden Cardiac Death of the European Society of Cardiology. *European Heart Journal* 2001; **22**: 1374–1450.

51 Sen-Chowdhry S, Syrris P, McKenna WJ. Role of genetic analysis in the management of patients with arrhythmogenic right ventricular dysplasia/cardiomyopathy. *Journal of the American College of Cardiology* 2007; **50**: 1813–1821.

Chapter 10

Genetics of atherosclerosis

Robert Roberts, Ruth McPherson, and Alexandre F.R. Stewart

Prevalence and importance of atherosclerosis

The single most common cause of morbidity and mortality in the world is coronary heart disease (CAD) [1,2]. In 2005, it accounted for 18% of all deaths in the USA and approximately one-fifth of all deaths in the world [2]. The annual cost of CHD in the USA in 2008 was estimated to be $156.4 billion; 1.2 million Americans experience CHD annually. At birth, the lifetime chance of a cardiac event is 47% and, if combined with cerebral vascular disease, it is more than 60% [3]. The impact of CAD on morbidity and mortality worldwide and its massive economic implications make a compelling argument for the development of new treatment and prevention strategies. The fundamental pathology responsible for CAD is atherosclerosis, which with the superimposition of a thrombus impedes coronary blood flow to result in ischemia and myocardial infarction. Atherosclerosis is a generalized vascular disease that affects all organs, but the sequelae are most prevalent and devastating for organs such as the heart, brain, and the kidneys.

Gene identification, a prerequisite for comprehensive prevention and treatment in the era of personalized medicine

Atherosclerosis and its sequelae are preventable and could be markedly attenuated if not eliminated in this century [4]. However, this requires delineation of genetic as well as environmental risk. The prerequisite to identify the genes responsible for coronary atherosclerosis will enable personalized medicine based on the individual's genetic variants, which is seen as a future model for optimal prevention and treatment [5]. The genome sequence is 99.9%

Cardiovascular Genetics and Genomics. Edited by Dan Roden. © 2009 American Heart Association, ISBN: 978-14051-7540-1.

identical among humans, leaving the remaining 0.1% to account for all individual variations including predisposition or resistance to disease [6]. Thus, the major thrust of cardiovascular genomics and genetic research is to identify these genetic variants that predispose or protect the individual from coronary atherosclerosis.

While the discussion is directed to the phenotype of coronary atherosclerosis, the approach and implications are similar for atherosclerosis in other organs but they are discussed under separate chapters.

Evidence for genetic predisposition

Atherosclerosis and, in particular, CAD results from the interaction of environmental and genetic risk factors. About 50% of susceptibility to CAD is genetic and this includes polymorphisms affecting known and occult risk factors such as cholesterol, hypertension, and diabetes [7]. It is worthy of note that 10% of all heart disease is diagnosed before the age of 50 years [1], and the predominant risk factors in premature atherosclerosis are genetic rather than environmental. In a study of premature CAD only 38% (Box 10.1) had abnormal screening lipids [8]. Evidence indicating atherosclerosis has significant genetic predisposition will be discussed under the subsequent headings.

Familial aggregation studies

There is a clustering of susceptibility to atherosclerosis in families having risk factors associated with abnormalities such as lipid metabolism, hypertension, diabetes, and obesity indicating a genetic basis for these risk factors [8–10]. Population genetic studies have shown a twofold increase in CAD risk associated with a family history of CAD even after adjusting for all other traditional risk factors [1]. Genetic studies in twins—particularly the Danish twins registry, which includes over 8000 twin pairs—show a higher incidence of CAD and CAD deaths in monozygotic twins of subjects with CAD than in dizygotic twins of subjects with CAD (44% versus 14%) [11]. In a Swedish study of 21 004 twins followed longitudinally, if one twin died of CAD, the relative risk of fatal CAD developing in the second twin was 8.1 for monozygotic twins and 3.8 for dizygotic twins [12]. The earlier the onset of CAD in a particular individual, the greater the risk of relatives developing CAD [13]. In families with onset of CAD before age 45, heritability was estimated to be

Box 10.1 Genetic predisposition to atherosclerosis

- 50% of susceptibility to coronary artery disease is genetic
- Premature heart disease (only 38% have lipid abnormalities)

92–100%, whereas within families of older cases the heritability ranges from 15% to 30% [14]. Coronary artery disease occurring in the young reflects a multi-hit genetic inheritance and these individuals transmit an even greater genetic load to their offspring. A family history of CAD in a first-degree relative below the age of 60 is an independent risk factor for early myocardial infarction even after controlling for traditional risk factors [15]. The role of family history in heart disease is perhaps most dramatically reinforced by the observations in the state of Utah, where 14% of the population has a family history of heart disease; within this cohort 72% of all premature myocardial infarctions occur and 48% of all coronary events [16]. Similarly, approximately 11% of the population has a family history of cerebral vascular disease and, within this segment of the population, over 86% of all premature strokes occurred.

Rare Mendelian disorders cause premature atherosclerosis

Cholesterol, the pivotal etiological agent in atherosclerosis, is transported primarily in low-density lipoprotein (LDL) particles into the subendothelial space and, following oxidative modification, is engulfed by monocyte-derived macrophages, leading to foam cell formation. Lipid accumulation and the resulting inflammatory and cell proliferative response lead to atherosclerosis and narrowing of the vessel lumen. Plaque rupture predisposes to thrombosis, which obstructs coronary flow leading to myocardial ischemia and infarction. While many genes predispose to atherosclerosis, those responsible for lipid metabolism, particularly LDL and high-density lipoprotein (HDL), would be expected to predominate as causes for rare single-gene disorders. Although mutations in these proteins are rare (<1%) they induce a phenotype of premature CAD associated with early myocardial infarction, which facilitated their discovery. Such discoveries enhance the cholesterol hypothesis and support the role for hereditary factors in CAD.

Autosomal dominant hypercholesterolemia is the most common and well-recognized example of a single-gene disorder that increases the risk of CAD and myocardial infarction (Box 10.2). The underlying genetic effects include three different genes, the LDL receptor gene [17], the apolipoprotein B gene [18], and gain-of-function mutations in the *PCSK9* gene (proprotein convertase subtilisin/kexin type 9). The LDL receptor gene, located

Box 10.2 Familial hypercholesterolemia

- Low-density lipoprotein receptor gene
- Apolipoprotein B gene
- *PCSK9* gene

on chromosome 19 (19p13.2) [19], in the heterozygous form occurs in 1 in 500 individuals and over 700 mutations have been identified. This disorder accounts for 5% of all myocardial infarctions that occur in individuals below the age of 60.

Familial combined hyperlipidemia and hypertriglyceridemia is even more common, affecting 1–2% of the Western population [20]. While linkage studies have mapped three loci responsible for this disorder, 1q21–23, 11p14, and 16q22–24 [17,21], none of the genes have been identified [8,21]. There are several other mutations, such as those responsible for familial hypertriglyceridemia. Another genetic and therapeutic target important for lipid metabolism is that of HDL. Its predominant role is to transport cholesterol from peripheral cells back to the liver for secretion into bile. HDL particles are 7–14 nm in diameter and consist of multiple phosphoproteins. The major protein is ApoA-I, which accounts for 70% of the protein mass, followed by ApoA-II (20%), ApoA-IV, ApoE and several others [22]. Increased plasma HDL levels are generally associated with significant protection against atherosclerosis and CAD. Tangier's disease [22], a deficiency of HDL, is due to mutations in the adenosine triphosphate (ATP) binding cassette (ABC) A1 gene (*ABCA1*), which functions in regulating cholesterol efflux from cells to lipid-poor ApoA-I. Mutations in *ABCA1* are associated with early heart disease. Overall heritability of plasma levels of cholesterol HDL (HDL-C) is approximately 60% [23,24]. While genetic disorders of HDL metabolism may account for 10–20% of premature CAD, they account for <2% of heart disease in the general population. Nevertheless, rare mutations in the *ABCA1* and *APOAI* genes strongly support the etiological importance of genes affecting cholesterol transport in atherosclerosis.

Genetic linkage analyses in families in which premature CAD segregates as a Mendelian trait have identified several chromosomal loci at 2q21, XQ23 [25], 1p34 [26], 16p13, 14qTER [27], and 15q26 [28]. The gene at 15q26 was reported by Wang *et al.* [28] to be *MEF2A*. A relationship between sequence variations in *MEF2A* and premature CAD has not been confirmed by several other investigators and the large 21 bp deletion originally reported by Wang *et al.* [28] has been observed in normal individuals; thus it remains controversial as to whether *MEF2A* contributes to atherosclerosis [29,30]. Recently, a missense mutation in LRP6 [31], located on chromosome 12p, encoding a coreceptor in the Wnt pathway has been linked to the metabolic syndrome and CAD but the pathophysiologic basis of this relationship remains to be explored.

Obstacles in the identification of genes for atherosclerosis

Efforts to map the chromosomal location of genes responsible for single-gene disorders utilizing genetic linkage analysis have been amazingly successful: over 100 single-gene disorders have been identified [32], including diseases such as familial hypercholesterolemia, atrial fibrillation [33], and familial cardiomyopathies [34]. Genetic linkage analysis is appropriate for single-gene disorders segregating in families exhibiting a Mendelian pattern of inheritance such as autosomal dominant or recessive [34]. Utilizing a panel of 300 markers spanning the genome at intervals of 10 million bp to genotype family members across two or more generations one can detect which marker(s) is coinherited with affected versus nonaffected members of the families. Knowing the chromosomal location of each marker enables one to identify the chromosomal locus responsible for the disease in the affected individuals and subsequently map and clone the gene. While these inherited disorders have helped tremendously to elucidate the etiology and pathogenesis of many diseases, including atherosclerosis, the mutations responsible for these disorders are rare, occurring in the range of only 1:500 to 1:10 000 of the general population.

However, the genetics of common disorders such as CAD and cancer has remained in its infancy. There are several major stumbling blocks (Box 10.3 and Table 10.1). First, multiple genes rather than a single gene are responsible for the genetic predisposition in these disorders, each contributing minimal or moderate effect to the resulting phenotype. In single-gene disorders, the mutation is both necessary and adequate to induce the phenotype as opposed to multigene disorders, such as atherosclerosis, in which any one mutation is neither necessary nor sufficient to induce the phenotype. Second, atherosclerosis is markedly influenced by multiple environmental and genetic risk factors, with the phenotype resulting from the interaction of many genes with internal and external environmental factors. Since multiple genes are necessary to induce the phenotype of atherosclerosis, it does not exhibit the phenotype pattern of recessive or dominant inheritance needed for the application of genetic linkage analysis [35–37]. Third, since each gene may contribute only 5% of the phenotype, detection of the locus requires DNA markers spanning the whole genome at intervals of 6000 bp or less, requiring 500 000 single nucleotide polymorphism (SNP) markers per sample [37]. This was not possible until recently and the cost would be prohibitive. Fourth, it requires a large sample size with replication in independent

Box 10.3 Obstacles to finding genes for atherosclerosis

- Atherosclerosis is due to multiple genes with each gene contributing only a modest effect to the phenotype
- Phenotype markedly influenced by multiple environmental factors
- Requires hundreds of thousands of DNA markers (≥300 000)
- Requires a large sample size with replication in independent populations

Table 10.1 Management of single gene lipid metabolism disorders predisposing to atherosclerosis

Genetic disorder	Genetic management	Dietary and drug therapy
Familial hyper-cholesterolemia	Genetic counseling Screen (full lipid profile) first-degree relatives	Lifestyle changes – Diet low in saturated fats and cholesterol – Physical activity and control other risk factors
		Drug therapy – Initiate statin therapy (high dosages often required) – Add ezetimibe as second agent as required to achieve optimal LDL-C – Bile acid sequestrants and/or niacin may be considered – Low-dose aspirin
Familial combined dyslipidemia		Lifestyle changes – Diet low in saturated fats and cholesterol – Physical activity and control other risk factors such as smoking, hypertension, hyperglycemia
		Drug therapy – Initiate statin therapy, which usually requires moderate to high dosage – Niacin may be a useful second agent to lower triglycerides and increase HDL
Familial hyper-triglyceridemia		Lifestyle changes – Weight control essential – Limit intake of alcohol, refined carbohydrates and simple sugars – increase physical activity
		Drug therapy – Consider fibric acid (e.g., fenofibrate) if triglycerides >500 mg/dl – Niacin or statin may be useful as a second agent (do not combine gemfibrozil with a statin) – Omega-3 fatty acids 3–4 mg/day may lower triglycerides by an additional 20–25%

LDL-C, low-density lipoprotein cholesterol; HDL, high-density lipoprotein.

populations. This necessitates high-throughput phenotyping and genotyping of thousands of unrelated individuals.

The candidate gene approach and its lack of success

For multigene disorders, case–control association studies (Box 10.4) in unrelated individuals are more sensitive than genetic linkage analysis [35,36]. This may be performed by the indirect approach of genome-wide genotyping, not feasible until recently, and the other is the direct approach referred to as the candidate gene approach discussed in Chapter 2. This approach consists of comparing the frequency of gene variants in cases with controls to determine whether the suspected predisposing variant is more common in the cases. The candidate gene approach, being less expensive and less time consuming, has been the predominant approach [38].

The candidate genes selected for atherosclerosis usually involve known risk factors for CAD such as hypertension [39], obesity [40], and diabetes [41,42]. Over 100 candidate genes suspected for their involvement in atherosclerosis or its sequelae [38] have been analyzed in various populations. In a recent study, 103 candidate genes shown in various genetic studies to be associated with atherosclerosis or CAD were reassessed in >1400 individuals from the Saguenay Lac St-Jean (SLSJ) region of Quebec [38]. The group tested 1536 DNA markers (SNPs). Those showing a positive association were assessed for replication in an independent sample size of 806 individuals. The investigators expressed surprise that none of the candidate genes were replicated. In another study there was an equally disturbing result, 70 genes exhibiting 85 variants previously shown to be associated with CAD were analyzed in 811 patients with acute coronary syndrome and 650 controls matched for age and sex [30]. Only one of the variants (–455 promoter variant in β-fibrinogen) replicated with statistical significance. These 70 genes included the A and B haplotypes of 5-lipoxygenase activating protein (ALOX5AP) and variants in the *ABCA1* gene. The former variant was reported to be strongly associated with myocardial infarction in the Icelandic population [43]. Several large reviews concluded none of the candidate genes for CAD had reached an association robust enough to be considered of clinical significance [35,36,44], owing to either small sample size or lack of replication in an independent population.

Box 10.4 Case–control association studies

- Direct (candidate gene approach)
- Indirect (genome-wide scan)

Genome-wide case–control association studies: an idea whose time has come

Mapping genes for common polygenic disorders such as coronary atherosclerosis requires hundreds of thousands of markers at intervals of at least every 6000 bp [37], which was not possible until recently. A new era emerged following the discovery of the SNP. These polymorphisms, although usually not in coding regions, occur randomly throughout the genome at an average frequency of 1 SNP per 1000 bp [6]. A marker set initially consisting of over 500 000 SNPs and, more recently, 1 million SNPs has been developed for genome-wide studies in large populations. This marker set is selected to detect most of the common SNPs from being either in close physical proximity or in genetic disequilibrium. Common SNPs are defined as those occurring at a frequency of ⩾5% [35–37,45]. Furthermore, common SNPs are thought to be the major genetic variants accounting for human variation and predisposition to disease [45]. The DNA sequence (3 billion base pairs) of the human genome is identical in 99.9% of all humans. Thus, all differences including predisposition or protection from disease are included in the 0.1% which represents 3 million base pairs. It is claimed that over 80% of the variation is due to SNPs and the remainder are due to insertions or deletions [46]. There are now over 11 million SNPs recognized in the general population. Commercial platforms are available to perform high-throughput genotyping, and, while still expensive, are rapidly coming into an affordable range enabling genome-wide studies with 1 million markers to be performed on large sample sizes. Thus, genome-wide association studies with adequate markers have been catapulted into plausibility. This approach makes no prior assumption as it is an unbiased search for genes associated with atherosclerosis or CAD on a genome-wide basis.

The basis of the genome-wide association analysis consists of determining the frequency of alleles in controls versus cases based on genotyping each sample with DNA markers spanning the whole genome. If one is genotyping with 500 000 markers one can expect 2500 associations by chance alone with a *P*-value of 0.05, or 500 with a *P*-valve at 0.01, or 50 at a *P*-value of 0.001. To eliminate false positives it is essential to analyze for replication in at least one independent population. It is preferable to demand more stringent statistical significance for association in the second population, which requires a larger population. In selecting both the initial and second population, one must arbitrarily decide on the numeric value of several parameters; namely the level of allelic risk expected, the minor allele frequency, the power function, and the size effect between the two populations (Box 10.5). The Ottawa Heart Genomics Study (OHGS) [5], designed to detect genes responsible for CAD, illustrates these features (Figs 10.1 and 10.2) in estimating sample size as well as the phenotyping criteria. The initial screening genome-wide association study was designed to detect genes with increased risk of atherosclerosis

Box 10.5 Perimeters for genome-wide scans

- Minor allele frequency
- Level of increased risk to be detected
- Power function
- Statistical significance for association
- Size difference to be detected between controls and cases

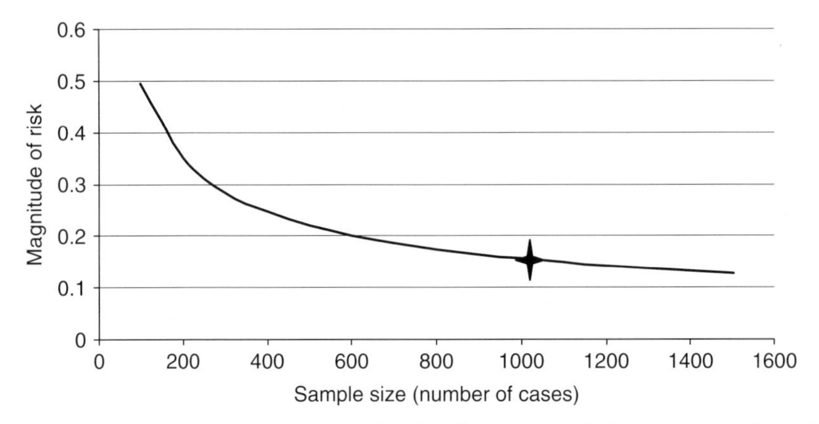

Fig. 10.1 Sample size versus magnitude of difference in risk between controls and affected ($P \leqslant 0.001$). Shown here is the estimation of the sample size required to detect genes with increased risk of atherosclerosis ≥1.3, with a minor allele frequency ≥10%, and a size difference between controls and cases of ≥0.2 at a power function of 0.90. The total sample size is 1000 cases and 1000 controls to detect an association at a $P \leqslant 0.001$.

≥1.3 [5], with a minor allele frequency ≥10% and a size difference between controls and affecteds of ≥0.2 at a power function of 0.90. In the initial population a *P*-value of ≥0.001 was required for an association and the sample size calculated to be 2000 (1000 controls and 1000 affecteds). In estimating the sample size for the second population to be used to ascertain replication, the parameters remain the same but it is very important to determine the number of positive associations carried forward from the initial screening population. We assume a maximum of 500 markers showing an association of at least 0.001 to be taken forward, and on this basis the required sample size was estimated to be 12 000 (8000 affecteds and 4000 controls) assuming a more stringent *P*-value of 10^{-6}. It would also be possible to prioritize the top 10 SNPs showing an association and ascertain replication in a smaller population of 1000. There is no agreed standard on the *P*-value for confirmation in the replication population, which varies from 0.05 to 0.000001. Genome-wide genotyping

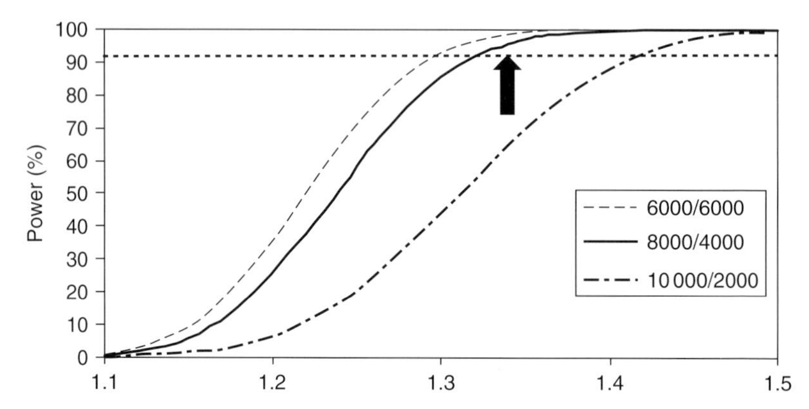

Fig. 10.2 Calculation of sample size using minor allele frequency ⩾0.05, risk ⩾1.3 at a power of 90% to map genetic loci associated with coronary artery disease ($P \leqslant 0.000001$). Shown here is the estimation of the sample size required to detect genes with increased risk of atherosclerosis ⩾1.3, with a minor allele frequency ⩾10%, and a size difference between controls and cases of ⩾0.2 at a power function of 0.90. The total sample size is 8000 cases and 4000 controls, or 6000 cases and 6000 controls, or 10000 cases and 2000 controls to detect an association at a $P \leqslant 0.000001$.

of the initial population (2 billion genotypes) has been completed and analysis showed over 384 SNPs exhibiting a significant association with CAD [5], which will be analyzed for replication in larger populations.

Genome-wide association studies: current progress

Several reviews in 2006 [35,36] concluded that no appropriately designed genome-wide scan had been performed because of inadequate sample size, too few markers, or lack of attempts to replicate in an independent population. However, genome-wide scans with a limited number of markers (50000–100000) covering only 20–30% of the genome have been performed and, despite their limitation, several loci have been identified. Loci showing genetic association with macular degeneration [47], diabetes mellitus [48], lupus [49], and prostate cancer [50] have been confirmed in independent populations. In the cardiovascular field, a major locus has been identified on chromosome 9p21. In an initial Ottawa population of 322 cases versus 312 controls utilizing 72864 SNPs, a locus on chromosome 9p21 was identified to be associated with CAD. This association with CAD [51] was confirmed in six independent white populations comprising 23000 individuals. The locus is heterozygous in 50% of whites and homozygous in 25% with an increased risk of 15–20% and 30–40% respectively. The risk of 9p21 is independent of known risk factors, implying a novel risk factor with targets for novel therapy. The mechanism is unknown and is likely to represent a major research thrust

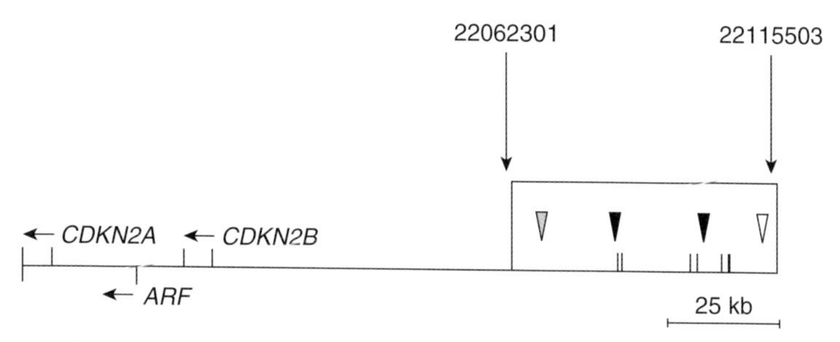

Fig. 10.3 Coronary artery disease (CAD) risk locus on chromosome 9p21. Physical map of the human 9p21 locus showing the location of the risk interval (grey box) relative to adjacent genes *CDKN2A*, *ARF*, and *CDKN2B*. Black arrowheads indicate SNPs rs10757274 and rs2383206; grey arrowhead points at SNP rs10757278 [6] and white arrowhead depicts SNP rs1333049. A total of eight SNPs in tight linkage disequilibrium in this 58 kbp region are associated with CAD independently of known risk factors. (Modified from McPherson *et al.* [52].)

for the immediate future. The 9p21 as a risk factor has now been confirmed by several independent groups worldwide [52–56], which represents a total population of over 65 000 whites. Recent studies have also confirmed that 9p21 is a risk factor in Chinese [57], Japanese, Korean [58], and East Indian [59] subjects. Furthermore, 9p21 has also been shown to be a risk factor for abdominal aortic and intracranial aneursyms [60] as well as ischemic strokes [61]. These studies strongly indicate that the defect induced by 9p21 is within the vessel wall since aneursyms are not a feature of atherosclerosis *per se*. The 9p21 locus (Fig. 10.3) does not contain any protein-coding gene but does contain ANRIL, a noncoding RNA. These studies strongly support genome-wide association studies over the candidate gene approach.

Phenotyping coronary artery disease cases and controls

A major scientific goal for the medical community over the next 10–15 years will be to identify and determine the function of thousands of SNPs as they relate to disease and therapy. The phenotyping should be a call to arms by the medical community and particularly the physician scientists to participate with vim and vigor as will be necessary to attain this goal. A major breakthrough for high-throughput phenotyping for coronary atherosclerosis recently occurred with the introduction of the multislice computed tomography (CT) scanner. This enables one to obtain a coronary angiogram noninvasively and rapidly with the imaging time being less than 1 minute. Ongoing studies have accepted <50% coronary obstruction for normal coronary arteriograms obtained by invasive cardiac catheterization and <30% for multislice CT (Box 10.6). Several populations collected in the past have used the criteria of a documented coronary event such as myocardial infarction on ECG or an

Box 10.6 Criteria for premature atherosclerosis

- Male <55 years or female <65 years
- Absence of diabetes (untreated HbA1c < 0.060)
- Absence LDL-C < 5.0 mmol/l, TC/HDL-C < 7.0 (not on lipid modifying medication)
- Untreated BP < 140/90
- Coronary artery disease confirmed by cardiac event or coronary angiography (catheterization or fast CT)

BP, blood pressure; CT, computed tomography; HDL-C, high-density lipoprotein cholesterol; LDL-C, low-density lipoprotein cholesterol; TC, total cholesterol.

Box 10.7 Criteria for controls without coronary artery disease

- Asymptomatic men >65 years or women >70 years
- Matched for sex, plasma lipids, HbA1c, and blood pressure
- Perfusion scan or coronary angiogram preferred

abnormal myoperfusion scan. Documented myocardial infarction or inadequate perfusion on myocardial imaging would appear to be adequate without coronary arteriograms.

Phenotyping the controls for diseases such as atherosclerosis or coronary artery disease is much more difficult. There is at this time no agreed criteria for controls for atherosclerosis or coronary artery disease. Since atherosclerosis or coronary artery disease onset is age dependent, it presents even greater concern (Box 10.7). It is generally accepted that individuals should be asymptomatic and ⩾65 years for men and ⩾70 years for women. For the OHGS, the criteria used have included a negative perfusion study or an arteriogram with <50% obstruction. The criteria for controls in the OHGS serves as a template but are likely to be significantly altered as we acquire more knowledge of both the phenotype and the genotype of atherosclerosis and its cardiac sequelae.

Gene to gene interactions and their interaction with the environment

It is anticipated that large samples of several populations will be genotyped with millions of markers selected to span the whole genome. This would cast a wide nonspecific and nonprejudiced search for genes predisposing to atherosclerosis in a population carefully and appropriately phenotyped. Replication in similar and different ethnic populations will ultimately identify those genes predisposing to atherosclerosis common to all populations and those unique to certain ethnic groups. Genes superimposing additional predisposition for sequelae such as ischemia or myocardial infarction will be separately determined in populations enriched for these sequeale. Results of genome-wide scans performed in populations with specific risk factors for atherosclerosis, such as hypertension, obesity, or diabetes, enable analysis for the separate effect of each risk factor and, in combinatorial arrangements, for their integrated impact. It is only after such studies that it will be possible to more precisely quantify the genetic and environmental components. This will lay the necessary infrastructure to begin to assess gene to gene interactions and how they are affected by the environment.

Personalized medicine: a new paradigm for prevention and treatment

The routine genotyping of risk alleles, while a prerequisite for personalized medicine, will require changes in society before having widespread application. There are many legal, social, and ethical issues to be resolved. Legislature to protect individual privacy will be foremost to assure one's genotype is not used inappropriately such as denial of life or medical insurance. Technology for cheap, rapid, and accurate genome-wide genotyping will probably arrive before the social, legal, and ethical issues are resolved. Sequencing of a genome for a few thousand dollars is considered feasible in the near future. Application of genetic screening will be the beginning of a new paradigm in the prevention of atherosclerosis and coronary artery disease. Genetic screening of those with a family history of heart disease or risk factors should occur in individuals who are at an age to enable early comprehensive prevention. In men it should occur in the second or third decade, if not earlier, and for women before the fifth decade. Concomitant with the discovery of CAD risk alleles, one can expect surprises which will lead to a broader understanding of the pathways leading to atherosclerosis and provide targets for novel therapy. It is to be expected that other devastating common chronic diseases will similarly succumb to the genome-wide search and hopefully with beneficial results. Identifying genes responsible for common disorders such as atherosclerosis should be a compelling reason for the physician and scientist to work together. The technology, the need, and the benefit should provide the impetus required to enable new therapies, genetic screening, prevention, and ultimate elimination of this disease.

References

1 American Heart Association. *Heart and Stroke Disease Statistics - 2008 Update.* American Heart Association, Dallas, 2007.
2 Rosamond W, Flegal K, Furie K *et al.* American Heart Association statistics Committee and stroke statistics subcommittee. Heart disease and stroke statistics - 2008 update: a report from the American Heart Association Statistics Committee and Stroke Statistics Subcommittee. *Circulation*; **117**: e25–e146, 2008. Epub 2007 Dec 17.

3 Chaer RA, Billeh R, Massad MG. Genetics and gene manipulation therapy of premature coronary artery disease. *Cardiology* 2004; **101**: 122–130.
4 Wald NJ, Law MR. A strategy to reduce cardiovascular disease by more than 80%. *BMJ* 2003; **326**: 1419–1423.
5 Roberts R., Stewart AFR. Personalized medicine: a future prerequisite for the prevention of coronary artery disease. *American Heart Journal* 2006; **4**: 222–227.
6 The International HapMap Consortium. The International HapMap Project. *Science* 2003; **426**: 789–796.
7 Chan L, Boerwinkle E. Gene-environment interactions and gene therapy in atherosclerosis. *Cardiology in Review* 1994; **2**: 130–137.
8 Genest JJ, Martin-Munley SS, McNamara JR *et al*. Familial lipoprotein disorders in patients with premature coronary artery disease. *Circulation* 1992; **85**: 2025–2033.
9 Blumenthal S, Jesse MJ, Hennekens CH *et al*. Risk factors for coronary artery disease in children of affected families. *Journal of Pediatrics* 1975; **87**: 1187–1192.
10 Rissanen A, Nikkila EA. Identification of the high-risk groups in familial coronary heart disease. *British Heart Journal* 1977; **39**: 875.
11 Allen G, Harvald B, Shields JP. Measures of twin concordance. *Acta Genetica* 1967; 1775–1781.
12 Berg K. Twin studies of coronary heart disease and its risk factors. *Acta Genetica* 2005; **33**: 349–361.
13 Slack J, Evans KA. The increased risk of death from ischaemic heart disease in first-degree relatives of 121 men and 96 women with ischaemic heart disease. *Journal of Medical Genetics* 2004; **3**: 239–257.
14 Rissanen A. Familial occurrence of coronary heart disease: effect of age at diagnosis. *American Journal of Cardiology* 1979; **44**: 60–66.
15 Hamsten A, de Faire U. Risk factors for coronary artery disease in families of young men with myocardial infarction. *American Journal of Cardiology* 1987; **59**: 14–19.
16 Hunt SC, Gwinn M, Adams TD. Family history assessment: strategies for prevention of cardiovascular disease. *American Journal of Preventive Medicine* 2003; **24**: 136–142.
17 Online Mendelian Inheritance in Man. 144250 Hyperlipidemia, familial combined (FCHL). *Nature Biotechnology* 2005.
18 Online Mendelian Inheritance in Man. 144010 Hypercholesterolemia, autosomal dominant, type B (familial defective apolipoprotein B-100). *Nature Biotechnology* 2005.
19 Austin MA, Hutter CM, Zimmern RL, Humphries SE. Familial hypercholesterolemia and coronary heart disease: a huge association review. *American Journal of Epidemiology* 2004; **160**: 421–429.
20 Goldstein JL, Schrott HG, Hazzard WR *et al*. Hyperlipidemia in coronary heart disease. Genetic analysis of lipid levels in 176 families and delineation of a new inherited disorder, combined hyperlipidemia. *Journal of Clinical Investigation* 2007; **52**: 1544–1568.
21 Shoulders CC, Jones EL, Naoumova RP. Genetics of familial combined hyperlipidemia and risk of coronary heart disease. *Human Molecular Genetics* 2004; **13**: R149–R160.
22 Genest JJ. Genetics and prevention: a new look at high-density lipoprotein cholesterol. *Cardiology Review* 2002; **10**: 61–71.
23 Rader DJ, Maugeais C. Genes influencing HDL metabolism: new perspectives and implications for atherosclerosis prevention. *Molecular Medicine Today* 2000; **6**: 170–175.
24 Cohen JC, Kiss RS, Pertsemlidis A *et al*. Multiple rare alleles contribute to low plasma levels of HDL cholesterol. *Science* 2004; **305**: 869–872.

25 Pajukanta P, Lilja HE, Sinsheimer JS *et al.* Familial combined hyperlipidemia is associated with upstream transcription factor 1 (USF1). *American Journal of Human Genetics* 2005; **67**: 1481–1493.

26 Wang Q, Rao S, Shen G-Q *et al.* Premature myocardial infarction novel susceptibility locus on chromosome 1P34–36 identified by genomewide linkage analysis. *American Journal of Human Genetics* 2004; **74**: 262–271.

27 Broeckel U, Hengstenberg C, Mayer B *et al.* A comprehensive linkage analysis for myocardial infarction and its related risk factors. *Nature Genetics* 2002; **30**: 210–214.

28 Wang L, Fan C, Topol SE. Mutation of MEF2A in an inherited disorder with features of coronary artery disease. *Science* 2003; **302**: 1578–1581.

29 Weng L, Kavaslar N, Ustaszewska A *et al.* Lack of MEF2A mutations in coronary artery disease. *Journal of Clinical Investigation* 2005; **115**: 1016–1020.

30 Morgan TM, Krumholz HM, Lifton RP, Spertus JA. Nonvalidation of reported genetic risk factors for acute coronary syndrome in a large-scale replication study. *JAMA: The Journal of the American Medical Association* 2007; **297**: 1551–1561.

31 Mani A, Radhakrishnan J, Wang H *et al.* LRP6 mutation in a family with early coronary disease and metabolic risk factors. *Science* 2007; **315**: 1278–1282.

32 Hamosh A, Scott AF, Amberger J *et al.* Online Mendelian Inheritance in Man (OMIM), a knowledgebase of human genes and genetic disorders. *Nucleic Acids Research* 2002; **30**: 52–55.

33 Brugada R, Tapscott T, Czernuszewicz GZ *et al.* Identification of a genetic locus for familial atrial fibrillation. *New England Journal of Medicine* 1997; **336**: 905–911.

34 Marian AJ, Brugada R, Roberts R. Cardiovascular diseases due to genetic abnormalities In Valentin Fuster *et al.*(eds) *Hurst's the Heart*, 11th edn. 2004; pp. 1747–1783.

35 Wang WY, Barratt B, Clayton DG, Todd JA. Genome-wide association studies: theoretical and practical concerns. *Nature Reviews Genetics* 2005; **6**: 109–118.

36 Hirshhorn JN, Daly MJ. Genome-wide association studies for common diseases and complex traits. *Nature Reviews Genetics* 2005; **6**: 95–108.

37 Kruglyak L. Prospects for whole-genome linkage disequilibrium mapping of common disease genes. *Nature Genetics* 1999; **22**: 139–144.

38 Pare G, Serre D, Brisson D *et al.* Genetic analysis of 103 candidate genes for coronary artery disease and associated phenotypes in a founder population reveals a new association between endothelin-1 and high-density lipoprotein cholesterol. *Annals of Human Genetics* 2007; **80**: 673–682.

39 Krushkal J, Xiong M, Ferrell RE *et al.* Linkage and association of adrenergic and dopamine receptor genes in the distal portion of the long arm of chromosome 5 with systolic blood pressure variation. *Human Molecular Genetics* 2005; **7**: 1379–1383.

40 Heinonen P, Koulu M, Pesonen U *et al.* Identification of a three-amino acid deletion in the alpha2B-adrenergic receptor that is associated with reduced basal metabolic rate in obese subjects. *Journal of Clinical Endocrinology and Metabolism* 1999; **84**: 2429–2433.

41 Horikawa Y, Oda N, Cox NJ *et al.* Genetic variation in the gene encoding calpain-10 is associated with type 2 diabetes mellitus. *Nature Genetics* 2000; **26**: 163–175.

42 Stone LM, Kahn SE, Fujimoto WY *et al.* A variation at position -30 of the beta-cell glucokinase gene promoter is associated with reduced beta-cell function in middle-aged Japanese-American men. *Diabetes* 2005; **45**: 422–428.

43 Helgadottir A, Manolescu A, Thorleifsson G *et al.* The gene encoding 5-lipoxygenase activating protein confers risk of myocardial infarction and stroke. *Nature Genetics* 2004; **36**: 233–239.

44 Thomas DC, Haile RW, Duggan D. Recent developments in genomewide association scans: a workshop summary and review. *American Journal of Human Genetics* 2005; **77**: 337–345.

45 Hinds DA, Stuve LL, Nilsen GB *et al*. Whole-genome patterns of common DNA variation in three human populations. *Science* 2005; **307**: 1072–1079.

46 Goncalo A, Kwong-Hang Tam P, Bustamante C *et al*. Human genome variation 2006: emerging views on structural variation and large-scale SNP analysis. *Nature Genetics* 2007; **39**: 153–155.

47 Klein RJ, Zeiss C, Chew EY *et al*. Complement factor H polymorphism in age-related macular degeneration. *Science* 2005; **308**: 385–389.

48 Sladek R, Rocheleau G, Rung J *et al*. A genome-wide association study identifies novel risk loci for type 2 diabetes. *Nature* 2007; **445**: 881–885.

49 Graham RR, Kozyrev SV, Baechler EC *et al*. A common haplotype of interferon regulatory factor 5 (IRF5) regulates splicing and expression and is associated with increased risk of systemic lupus erythematosus. *Nature Genetics* 2006; **38**: 550–555.

50 Amundadottir LT, Sulem P, Gudmundsson J *et al*. A common variant associated with prostate cancer in European and African populations. *Nature Genetics* 2006; **38**: 652–658.

51 McPherson R, Pertsemlidis A, Kavaslar N, Stewart AFR, Roberts R, Cox DR *et al*. A common allele on Chromosome 9 associated with coronary heart disease. Available from: http://www.sciencemag.org/cgi/content/full/1142447/DCI .2007. 3-11-2006.

52 McPherson R, Pertsemlidis A, Kavaslar N *et al*. A common allele on chromosome 9 associated with coronary Artery disease. *Science* 2007; **316**: 1488–1491.

53 Helgadottir A, Thorleifsson G, Manolescu A *et al*. A common variant on chromosome 9p21 affects the risk of myocardial infarction. *Science* 2007; **316**: 1491–1493.

54 Wellcome Trust Case Consortium. Genome-wide association study of 14,000 cases of seven common diseases and 3,000 shared controls. *Nature* 2007; **447**: 661–668.

55 Samani N, Erdmann J, Hall A. Genome-wide association analysis of coronary artery disease. *New England Journal of medicine* 2007; **357**: 443–453.

56 Broadbent H, Peden JF, Lorkowski S *et al*. Susceptibility to coronary artery disease and diabetes is encoded by distinct, tightly linked, SNPs in the ANRIL locus on chromosome 9p. *Human Molecular Genetics* 2008; **17**: 806–814.

57 Chen Z, Qian Q, Ma G *et al*. A common variant on chromosome 9p21 affects the risk of early-onset coronary artery disease. *Molecular Biology Reports,* 2008; pp. 1–5.

58 Hinohara K, Nakajima T, Takahashi M *et al*. Replication of the association between a chromosome 9p21 polymorphism and coronary artery disease in Japanese and Korean populations. *Journal of Human Genetics* 2008; **53**: 357–359.

59 Assimes TL, Knowles JW, Basu A *et al*. Susceptibility locus for clinical and subclinical coronary artery disease at chromosome 9p21 in the multi-ethnic ADVANCE Study. *Human Molecular Genetics* 2008; **17**: 2320–2328.

60 Helgadottir A, Thorleifsson G, Magnusson KP *et al*. The same sequence variant on 9p21 associates with myocardial infarction, abdominal aortic aneurysm and intracranial aneurysm. *Nature Genetics* 2008; **40**: 217–224.

61 Matarin M, Brown WM, Singleton A *et al*. Whole genome analyses suggest ischemic stroke and heart disease share an association with polymorphisms on chromosome 9p21. *Stroke* 2008; **39**: 1586–1589.

Chapter 11

Hypertension

Donna K. Arnett

Introduction

The American Heart Association classifies individuals as hypertensive if they satisfy one or more of the following criteria: (1) have an untreated systolic blood pressure (BP) ≥140 mmHg, (2) have an untreated diastolic BP ≥90 mmHg, (3) take antihypertensive medication, (4) have been told two or more times by a health professional that they have high BP. Clinicians categorize hypertension as "secondary" or "essential." Secondary hypertension develops as a sequela to specific diseases or conditions or in response to an underlying, identifiable, often correctable cause. For example, obstructive sleep apnea is known to raise BP; treating the apnea often reduces BP [1]. Secondary hypertension accounts for only 5–10% of all diagnosed hypertension [2,3]. Essential hypertension is that for which no specific cause can be found but likely results from the complex interaction of many physiological (including genetic) and environmental factors.

Hypertension is associated with increased morbidity and mortality [4]. For example, about 91% of individuals who develop congestive heart failure have a history of hypertension [5]; about half of all cases of nonlobar intracerebral hemorrhage are attributable to hypertension [6], and hypertension is an independent risk factor for myocardial infarction (MI) [7] and confers an increased risk for adverse outcomes after MI [8]. Hypertension is also associated with shorter overall life expectancy [9]. In recent years, prehypertension (having untreated systolic BP 120–139 mmHg and/or having untreated diastolic BP 80–89 mmHg and not having been told twice by a health professional that one has hypertension) has also been observed to increase the risk of myocardial infarction and coronary artery disease [10].

Cardiovascular Genetics and Genomics. Edited by Dan Roden. © 2009 American Heart Association, ISBN: 978-14051-7540-1.

Roughly one in three US adults is hypertensive [11]; worldwide, some 1 billion people have high BP [12]. Before age 45, more men than women are hypertensive; from age 45 to 54, the percentages of hypertensive men and women are similar; after age 55 a much higher percentage of women are hypertensive than men [13]. Race/ethnicity also modifies the risk for hypertension. For example, the prevalence of hypertension for non-Hispanic whites in the USA is about 28%, whereas the prevalence for African Americans is about 40% [14]. Environmental factors, such as diet and the use of prescription drugs, can also increase the risk for hypertension. For example, hypertension is 2–3 times more common in women who take oral contraceptives than those who do not [12]. In addition to the significant human burden of hypertension, the financial burden is considerable: the estimated direct and indirect cost of hypertension in the USA for 2008 is $69.4 billion [13].

The familial nature of hypertension has long been recognized. During the 1950s, the St. Mary's Study was the first to convincingly document that the occurrence of hypertension is more common among family members with hypertension than among the general population [15–18]. This study recruited first-degree relatives of probands with high BP (diastolic BP >100 mmHg) and normal BP (diastolic BP >85 mmHg). Familial aggregation of BP in families of high BP probands was similar to normal BP probands [15]. Subsequent studies have verified and refined these observations: Overall, first-degree relatives of a person of any age with hypertension are at a 2.3-fold greater risk of developing hypertension before age 49 than the general population. This risk increases to almost fourfold when an individual has two or more family members diagnosed with hypertension before age 55 [19,20]. Twin and adoption studies have demonstrated that familial correlation in blood pressure is influenced by both shared genes and shared environment [21,22]. The heritability (i.e., the proportion of a trait's variation in a population that has a familial basis) of BP estimated from twin studies is around 60% [23]; because twin studies integrate both genetic and environmental influences, heritability estimates of about 30% from pedigree studies are more reasonable estimates of population variability due to genetic factors [24].

The importance of hypertension as a risk factor for stroke, chronic kidney disease, and cardiovascular disease; the considerable prevalence of hypertension in many populations; and the well-documented heritable nature of hypertension have made it an important phenotype for genetic and genomic study. Although considerable progress has been made in characterizing monogenic forms of hypertension, the complex nature of essential hypertension has made it more resistant to genetic dissection. However, the combined facts that blood pressure is maintained by a complex network of physiological systems, that it is susceptible to environmental influence, and that gender, race, and ethnicity interact with other sources of variation make the phenotype a critical test case and potential source of methodological innovation for genomic science and its translation to clinical practice. This chapter traces developments in the genetics and genomics of hypertension, outlines the notable research challenges posed by the phenotype, and concludes by speculating on the potential clinical implications of blood pressure genomics.

Mendelian disorders resulting in hypertension

The contribution of Mendelian forms of hypertension (and hypotension) to blood pressure variation in populations as a whole is small; however, the study of these single-gene disorders with clear Mendelian patterns of inheritance has revealed much about the primary mechanisms of blood pressure and volume control. Fewer than a dozen forms of monogenic hypertension have been described; all tend to have large effects on blood pressure, and most act via a physiologic pathway in the kidney by altering renal salt reabsorption [25]. Mutations that increase salt reabsorption necessarily increase water reabsorption and vascular volume, and thereby increase blood pressure; conversely, mutations that decrease salt reabsorption lower blood pressure.

The cascade of events leading from a single mutation to hypertension is often complex, but for many such mutations the pathophysiologic chain is well characterized. For example, glucocorticoid remediable aldosteronism (GRA) is an autosomal dominant disorder resulting from an unequal crossing over between two closely related genes on chromosome 8 that are involved in adrenal steroid biosynthesis. The coding region of the cytochrome P450, subfamily XIB, polypeptide 2 gene (*CYP11B2*, commonly known as the aldosterone synthase gene) forms a meiotic mismatch with the promoter region of the cytochrome P450, subfamily XIB, polypeptide 1 gene (*CYP11B1*, commonly known as the 11-β-hydroxylase gene), resulting in a chimeric protein with composite properties of the two parent enzymes. Aldosterone synthase is the rate-limiting enzyme in aldosterone synthesis; aldosterone, in turn, is the steroid hormone that regulates the mineralocorticoid receptor that regulates epithelial sodium channel activity and, ultimately, salt reabsorption and blood pressure. In short, increased aldosterone normally results in increased blood pressure. The 11-β-hydroxylase enzyme is involved in the synthesis of cortisol, a corticosteroid hormone whose expression is regulated by the adrenocorticotropic hormone (ATCH). The chimeric enzyme resulting from the mismatched genes takes on the synthetic role of aldosterone synthase (i.e., it regulates aldosterone production) but, like 11-β-hydroxylase, it is regulated by ATCH. As a result, in the process of maintaining normal cortisol levels, ATCH also boosts aldosterone synthase activity with the expected commensurate increase in aldosterone, plasma volume, and blood pressure. The salt and water retention suppresses the secretion of renin, but, because aldosterone is effectively under the control of ATCH and not the normal renin–angiotensin–aldosterone pathway, the secretion of aldosterone remains unchecked [26]. GRA has a clinical expression ranging from mild blood pressure elevation to severe, early-onset hypertension, often diagnosed in childhood. Treatment with a glucocorticoid such as dexamethasone often reduces blood pressure in young patients. Adults are more variable in their response and are typically treated with additional antihypertensive medications such as thiazide diuretics.

Other Mendelian disorders are similarly documented. Luft [27] offers an excellent review of Mendelian forms of hypertension with special emphasis on clinical diagnosis.

Complex genetic forms of hypertension

Although the characterization of monogenic forms of hypertension is a bright spot in the field of clinical genetics, the predominance of essential hypertension and the development of increasingly powerful genetic and genomic methods have focused efforts on explicating essential hypertension and its polygenic nature. Both linkage and candidate gene association studies have been used to identify genes with modest effects on the BP phenotype that may contribute to essential hypertension.

Linkage studies

Linkage studies have pointed to regions on all human chromosomes that appear to contribute to hypertension and BP-related traits. Although the LOD (logarithm to the base 10 of the odds) score signals in most studies offer only statistically suggestive evidence of linkage, a number of meta-analyses have attempted to integrate findings across multiple studies, populations, and ethnic groups [28–31]. Table 11.1 summarizes regions showing suggestive or significant evidence of linkage for BP-related phenotypes in two or more meta-analyses. In most cases, further linkage follow-up work through detailed fine mapping and positional candidate gene association testing will be needed to positively identify the hypertension susceptibility gene underlying reported linkage peaks.

Association studies

Candidate gene association studies have sought to connect specific genes with high BP or hypertension. To date, at least 40 genes have been investigated for association with BP-related traits [32,33]. As has been the case with other cardiovascular phenotypes, however, almost every published positive hypertension–gene variant association result has been followed by a published negative result [34]. The reasons for these inconsistencies may include genetic heterogeneity (i.e., different genetic risks lead to hypertension); differing patterns of linkage disequilibrium in different populations (i.e., the causal variant captured by a genetic marker in one population is not captured by that same marker in another); lack of statistical power; confounding by environmental

Table 11.1 Chromosomal regions showing suggestive or significant evidence of linkage for blood pressure-related phenotypes in two or more meta-analyses.

Phenotype(s)	Race/ethnicity	Region
HT, DBP, HT+SBP*, HT+DBP	White	2p12–q22.1
HT, SBP, HT+SBP	Black+white	2p14–p13.1
HT, SBP, HT+SBP	Mixed	2p23.2–p12
HT, DBP, HT+SBP*, HT+DBP*	White	3p14.1–q12.3
HT, HT+SBP	Mixed	6q25.3–qter
DBP, HT+SBP, HT+DBP*	White	16p13–q12.2
HT*, HT+DBP	Mixed	17p12–q21.33

*Phenotypes were suggestive or significant in all meta-analyses reporting linkage in the region.

HT, hypertension; SBP, systolic blood pressure; DBP, diastolic blood pressure; +, compound phenotype.

factors; or phenotypic heterogeneity (i.e., hypertension can be caused by different processes, and some processes may be operating in some forms of hypertension but not others). Genes frequently investigated in association studies include those for α_{1b}-adrenergic receptor, β_2-adrenergic receptor, angiotensin I-converting enzyme (ACE), and endothelin 1. As with linkage studies, meta-analyses have been conducted in an effort to integrate findings from independent association studies [35–37]. For example, in a meta-analysis of 127 studies, Sethi and colleagues [35] concluded that the angiotensin I (AGT) M235T genotype was associated with an increased risk of hypertension in both white and Asian subjects. In their meta-analysis of the four networks of the NHLBI Family Blood Pressure Program, Province *et al.* [36] concluded that the AGT −6 G–A polymorphism had minimal to no effect on interindividual variation of BP levels. Although there is often considerable heterogeneity among studies, meta-analyses such as these represent one way to search for genes with modest effects on BP in populations.

Gene–gene and gene–environment interactions

Blood pressure is influenced by multiple genes interacting with each other and with the environment. Gene–gene interaction, or "epistasis," occurs when the actions of two or more genes influence a phenotype. Much of the difficulty in the genetic dissection of essential hypertension stems from the epistatic nature of the phenotype. However, recent research has begun to untangle the complex interplay of genes influencing BP. For example, using the novel method of Cheverud and Routman [38], Kardia and colleagues [39] recently found significant evidence of interaction between the ACE in/del and the AGT −6 G–A polymorphisms and systolic BP in men and women. The method used in this work is notable because it acknowledges that multiple polymorphisms can affect phenotypes in complex ways that, in the past, have not necessarily been captured by standard analytical approaches. In the era of increasingly complex genomic datasets, development of novel statistical techniques such as this will be critical to unraveling the genetic basis of hypertension.

Gene–environment interaction occurs when the same genotype produces a different phenotype under different environmental exposures, such as age, salt consumption, or a pharmacological treatment such as an ACE inhibitor or diuretic. Interventional studies, in which an environmental exposure is standardized across individuals, are excellent ways to identify gene–environment interactions and provide evidence for translation of those findings into clinical practice. For example, blood pressure response to a low-sodium diet has been shown to vary by polymorphisms of renin–angiotensin–aldosterone system genes, in particular the AGT −6 G–A polymorphism. Results from the Dietary Approaches to Stop Hypertension (DASH) study showed the AGT −6 AA genotype is associated with a significant decrease in blood pressure (−6.93 mmHg systolic and −3.68 mmHg diastolic) for individuals on the DASH diet [40]. Similarly, in the Treatment of Hypertension Prevention Trial, the incidence of hypertension was significantly lower after sodium reduction for persons with the AA genotype [relative risk 0.57 (95% confidence intervals 0.34, 0.98) versus usual care] but not for persons with the GG genotype [relative risk 1.2 (95% confidence intervals 0.79, 1.81), test for trend $P = 0.02$] [41]. Based on such results, individuals with the AGT −6 AA genotype could be placed on a low-sodium diet prior to exhibiting elevated BP, thereby avoiding hypertension and consequent organ damage. Gene–environment interaction also impels the field of antihypertensive pharmacogenetics, which seeks to find the genetic determinants of interindividual variation in response to antihypertensive drugs. For example, studies have reported interactions with respect to BP response between diuretics and variants in the nitric oxide synthase 3 gene [42]. Recent reviews of antihypertensive pharmacogenetics describe other potentially important interactions [43,44]. Given the many drugs available for treatment of hypertension and the large number of patients eligible to receive these drugs, even small sources of variation in drug efficacy and safety have important implications for clinical and public health. However, there is still a lack of research that provides the evidence necessary to justify pharmacogenetic testing in routine practice. To show that pharmacogenetic testing has clinical value, it is not enough to demonstrate gene–drug interaction; there must also be an alternative treatment that could be triggered by knowledge of genotype and proof that such measures are more clinically effective or cost-effective (or both) than traditional practice. More research is necessary before genetic testing becomes a routine precursor to managing antihypertensive therapy in essential hypertension.

Hypertension genetics and genomics: challenges, opportunities, and clinical implications

Additional research is needed to better understand genetic and genomic predictors of hypertension and the response of blood pressure to environmental (including pharmacologic) exposures. Although many of the challenges in moving hypertension genetics and genomics from bench to bedside are common to other cardiovascular disease phenotypes, hypertension researchers must overcome limitations if their work is to be translated into clinical practice. For example, Farahani *et al.* [45] examined 16 studies that focused on hypertension and genes in the renin–angiotensin–aldosterone system; they concluded that many studies had methodological limitations related to subject selection and combining different alleles, therapeutics, and end points. These factors may contribute to the often discordant results among studies. In their review of the pharmacogenomics of essential hypertension, Filigheddu and colleagues [46] also cited methodological variability as a possible source of discordant findings. However, they also argue that the complexity of the BP phenotype itself can lead to discrepancies in findings, and they suggest that, ideally, all pharmacogenetic studies should dissect the chain of intermediate phenotypes leading from gene polymorphism to final hypertensive phenotype. Given the complexity and number of pathways (and their interactions) regulating BP, the number of genes involved in these pathways [43], and the fact that the pharmacodynamics of some antihypertensives are incompletely understood, implementing this suggestion presents its own substantial challenges. The fact that the genetic basis of essential hypertension can be attributed to many common variants with individually small phenotypic effects certainly also demands that future studies must be adequately powered. However, it will be equally important for independent investigators to coordinate their efforts with respect to sample selection and characterization, phenotype selection and measurement, genotyping, interventional protocols, and analytical methods.

In terms of clinical relevance, given the incontrovertible evidence of the familial nature of hypertension, screening family members of probands with hypertension should be a top priority for all clinicians. The research measures discussed above may someday provide compelling data regarding the clinical application of genetic and genomic knowledge in the management of hypertension. In the meantime, however, there are a number of measures clinicians can take to proactively prepare for this eventuality. For example, clinicians should develop a basic genetic literacy and prepare themselves to help their patients understand the technical and negotiate the ethical aspects of genetic screening. Staying abreast of the tools being developed for genetic screening for hypertension will allow clinicians to be early adopters of new diagnostic technologies. Clinicians must also be involved in the development of appropriate treatment guidelines for particular genetic susceptibility findings. As the genetics and genomics of hypertension mature, clinicians' involvement in disciplinary discussions will ensure that their perspectives and needs will help shape clinical integration.

References

1 Stradling JR, Partlett J, Davies RJ *et al.* Effect of short term graded withdrawal of nasal continuous positive airway pressure on systemic blood pressure in patients with obstructive sleep apnoea. *Blood Pressure* 1996; **5**: 234–240.
2 Berglund G, Andersson O, Wilhelmsen L. Prevalence of primary and secondary hypertension: studies in a random population sample. *BMJ* 1976; **2**: 554–556.
3 Omura M, Saito J, Yamaguchi K *et al.* Prospective study on the prevalence of secondary hypertension among hypertensive patients visiting a general outpatient clinic in Japan. *Hypertension Research* 2004; **27**: 193–202.
4 Kannel WB. Blood pressure as a cardiovascular risk factor: prevention and treatment. *JAMA: the Journal of the American Medical Association* 1996; **275**: 1571–1576.
5 Levy D, Larson MG, Vasan RS *et al.* The progression from hypertension to congestive heart failure. *JAMA: the Journal of the American Medical Association* 1996; **275**: 1557–1562.
6 Woo D, Sauerbeck LR, Kissela BM *et al.* Genetic and environmental risk factors for intracerebral hemorrhage: preliminary results of a population-based study. *Stroke* 2002; **33**: 1190–1195.
7 Croft P, Hannaford PC. Risk factors for acute myocardial infarction in women: evidence from the Royal College of General Practitioners' oral contraception study. *BMJ* 1989; **298**: 165–168.
8 Haider AW, Chen L, Larson MG *et al.* Antecedent hypertension confers increased risk for adverse outcomes after initial myocardial infarction. *Hypertension* 1997; **30**: 1020–1024.
9 Franco OH, Peeters A, Bonneux L, de Laet C. Blood pressure in adulthood and life expectancy with cardiovascular disease in men and women: life course analysis. *Hypertension* 2005; **46**: 280–286.
10 Qureshi AI, Suri MF, Kirmani JF *et al.* Is prehypertension a risk factor for cardiovascular diseases? *Stroke* 2005; **36**: 1859–1863.
11 Fields LE, Burt VL, Cutler JA *et al.* The burden of adult hypertension in the United States 1999 to 2000: a rising tide. *Hypertension* 2004; **44**: 398–404.
12 Chobanian AV, Bakris GL, Black HR *et al.* Seventh report of the Joint National Committee on Prevention, Detection, Evaluation, and Treatment of High Blood Pressure. *Hypertension* 2003; **42**: 1206–1252.
13 Rosamond W, Flegal K, Furie K *et al.* Heart disease and stroke statistics—2008 update: a report from the American Heart Association Statistics Committee and Stroke Statistics Subcommittee. *Circulation* 2008; **117**: e25–146.

14 Hertz RP, Unger AN, Cornell JA, Saunders E. Racial disparities in hypertension prevalence, awareness, and management. *Archives of Internal Medicine* 2005; **165**: 2098–2104.

15 Hamilton M, Pickering GW, Roberts JA, Sowry GS. The aetiology of essential hypertension. 4. The role of inheritance. *Clinical Science (London)* 1954; **13**: 273–304.

16 Hamilton M, Pickering GW, Roberts JA, Sowry GS. The aetiology of essential hypertension. II. Scores for arterial blood pressures adjusted for differences in age and sex. *Clinical Science (London)* 1954; **13**: 37–49.

17 Hamilton M, Pickering GW, Roberts JA, Sowry GS. The aetiology of essential hypertension. I. The arterial pressure in the general population. *Clinical Science (London)* 1954; **13**: 11–35.

18 Ward R. Familial aggregation and genetic epidemiology of blood pressure. In: Laragh JH, Brenner BM, eds. *Hypertension: Pathophysiology, Diagnosis, and Management*, 2nd edn. Raven Press, New York, 1995: 67–88.

19 Hunt SC, Williams RR, Barlow GK. A comparison of positive family history definitions for defining risk of future disease. *Journal of Chronic Diseases* 1986; **39**: 809–821.

20 Williams RR, Hunt SC, Hasstedt SJ *et al.* Are there interactions and relations between genetic and environmental factors predisposing to high blood pressure? *Hypertension* 1991; **18** (3 Suppl): I29–37.

21 Annest JL, Sing CF, Biron P, Mongeau JG. Familial aggregation of blood pressure and weight in adoptive families. II. Estimation of the relative contributions of genetic and common environmental factors to blood pressure correlations between family members. *American Journal of Epidemiology* 1979; **110**: 492–503.

22 Feinleib M, Garrison RJ, Fabsitz R *et al.* The NHLBI twin study of cardiovascular disease risk factors: methodology and summary of results. *American Journal of Epidemiology* 1977; **106**: 284–285.

23 Hunt SC, Hasstedt SJ, Kuida H *et al.* Genetic heritability and common environmental components of resting and stressed blood pressures, lipids, and body mass index in Utah pedigrees and twins. *American Journal of Epidemiology* 1989; **129**: 625–638.

24 Longini IM, Jr., Higgins MW, Hinton PC *et al.* Environmental and genetic sources of familial aggregation of blood pressure in Tecumseh, Michigan. *American Journal of Epidemiology* 1984; **120**: 131–144.

25 Lifton RP. Molecular genetics of human blood pressure variation. *Science* 1996; **272**: 676–680.

26 Lifton RP, Dluhy RG, Powers M *et al.* A chimaeric 11 beta-hydroxylase/aldosterone synthase gene causes glucocorticoid-remediable aldosteronism and human hypertension. *Nature* 1992; **355**: 262–265.

27 Luft FC. Mendelian forms of human hypertension and mechanisms of disease. *Clinical Medicine and Research* 2003; **1**: 291–300.

28 Rice T, Cooper RS, Wu X *et al.* Meta-analysis of genome-wide scans for blood pressure in African American and Nigerian samples. The National Heart, Lung, and Blood Institute GeneLink Project. *American Journal of Hypertension* 2006; **19**: 270–274.

29 Koivukoski L, Fisher SA, Kanninen T *et al.* Meta-analysis of genome-wide scans for hypertension and blood pressure in Caucasians shows evidence of susceptibility regions on chromosomes 2 and 3. *Human Molecular Genetics* 2004; **13**: 2325–2332.

30 Liu W, Zhao W, Chase GA. Genome scan meta-analysis for hypertension. *American Journal of Hypertension* 2004; **17** (12 Pt 1): 1100–1106.

31 Wu X, Kan D, Province M *et al.* An updated meta-analysis of genome scans for hypertension and blood pressure in the NHLBI Family Blood Pressure Program (FBPP). *American Journal of Hypertension* 2006; **19**: 122–127.

32 Luft FC. Present status of genetic mechanisms in hypertension. *Medical Clinics of North America* 2004; **88**: 1–18, vii.

33 Turner ST, Boerwinkle E. Genetics of blood pressure, hypertensive complications, and antihypertensive drug responses. *Pharmacogenomics* 2003; **4**: 53–65.

34 Oparil S, Weber MA. *Hypertension: a Companion to Brenner & Rector's The Kidney.* W.B. Saunders, Philadelphia, 2000.

35 Sethi AA, Nordestgaard BG, Tybjaerg-Hansen A. Angiotensinogen gene polymorphism, plasma angiotensinogen, and risk of hypertension and ischemic heart disease: a meta-analysis. *Arteriosclerosis Thrombosis and Vascular Biology* 2003; **23**: 1269–1275.

36 Province MA, Boerwinkle E, Chakravarti A *et al.* Lack of association of the angiotensinogen-6 polymorphism with blood pressure levels in the comprehensive NHLBI Family Blood Pressure Program. National Heart, Lung and Blood Institute. *Journal of Hypertension* 2000; **18**: 867–876.

37 Kato N, Sugiyama T, Morita H *et al.* Angiotensinogen gene and essential hypertension in the Japanese: extensive association study and meta-analysis on six reported studies *Journal of Hypertension* 1999; **17**: 757–763.

38 Cheverud JM, Routman EJ. Epistasis and its contribution to genetic variance components. *Genetics* 1995; **139**: 1455–1461.

39 Kardia SL, Bielak LF, Lange LA *et al.* Epistatic effects between two genes in the renin-angiotensin system and systolic blood pressure and coronary artery calcification. *Medical Science Monitor* 2006; **12**: CR150–158.

40 Svetkey LP, Moore TJ, Simons-Morton DG *et al.* Angiotensinogen genotype and blood pressure response in the Dietary Approaches to Stop Hypertension (DASH) study. *Journal of Hypertension* 2001; **19**: 1949–1956.

41 Hunt SC, Cook NR, Oberman A *et al.* Angiotensinogen genotype, sodium reduction, weight loss, and prevention of hypertension: trials of hypertension prevention, phase II. *Hypertension* 1998; **32**: 393–401.

42 Turner ST, Chapman AB, Schwartz GL, Boerwinkle E. Effects of endothelial nitric oxide synthase, alpha-adducin, and other candidate gene polymorphisms on blood pressure response to hydrochlorothiazide. *American Journal of Hypertension* 2003; **16**: 834–839.

43 Arnett DK, Claas SA, Glasser SP. Pharmacogenetics of antihypertensive treatment. *Vascular Pharmacology* 2006; **44**: 107–118.

44 Johnson JA, Turner ST. Hypertension pharmacogenomics: current status and future directions. *Current Opinion in Molecular Therapy* 2005; **7**: 218–225.

45 Farahani P, Dolovich L, Levine M. Exploring design-related bias in clinical studies on receptor genetic polymorphism of hypertension. *Journal of Clinical Epidemiology* 2007; **60**: 1–7.

46 Filigheddu F, Troffa C, Glorioso N. Pharmacogenomics of essential hypertension: are we going the right way? *Cardiovascular and Hematological Agents in Medicinal Chemistry* 2006; **4**: 7–15.

Chapter 12

Stroke genomics

Mark J. Alberts

Introduction

The genetics of cerebrovascular disease is a complex and evolving area owing to several factors. Stroke and cerebrovascular disease are very heterogeneous disorders, ranging from ischemic strokes to intracerebral hemorrhage (ICH) to subarachnoid hemorrhage (SAH). There is even more heterogeneity within each of these categories (Table 12.1), which further complicates defining phenotypes for genetic studies. In addition, there are numerous risk factors that may contribute to each type of stroke or the development of cerebrovascular disease, and each of these risk factors (i.e., hypertension, hyperlipidemia, diabetes) can have their own complex genetic background. Considering all of these challenges, it is somewhat surprising that much progress has been made in unraveling the genetics of cerebrovascular disease [1].

The importance of understanding the genetics of cerebrovascular disease and stroke cannot be underestimated. By its very nature, most strokes occur without much warning, making identification of high-risk people an important strategy for targeting prevention and perhaps prophylactic surgical or endovascular therapies. If we could identify which people harbor a berry aneurysm at risk of rupture, or which people have a high-grade carotid stenosis before it causes a massive hemispheric stroke, this would have direct and dramatic medical and public health implications. Furthermore, the etiology and pathogenesis of some vascular malformations such as arteriovenous malformations (AVMs), aneurysms, and dissections remain unclear or unknown despite much study. A better understanding of the genetics of these various processes would be invaluable for identifying opportunities to intervene and prevent a devastating stroke perhaps by even curing the underlying genetic defect.

Cardiovascular Genetics and Genomics. Edited by Dan Roden. © 2009 American Heart Association, ISBN: 978-14051-7540-1.

Table 12.1 Classification and pathogenesis of genetic cerebrovascular diseases

Stroke type	Genetic factors
Ischemic strokes	
Atherothrombosis/atherosclerosis	Risk factors: hypertension, diabetes, hyperlipidemia, hypercoagulable states
Embolic	Cardiac diseases; cardiomyopathies; atrial fibrillation
Vasculopathy	Dissections, fibromuscular dysplasia, CADASIL, moyamoya disease, sickle cell disease, Fabry disease, CTD
Parenchymal	MELAS, migraine
Venous thrombosis	Hypercoagulable state
Hemorrhagic strokes	
Intracerebral	Amyloid angiopathy, AVMs, CCM, coagulopathy
Subarachnoid	PKD, CTD, familial aneurysms

This is a broad classification of cerebrovascular disease with a focus on common genetic etiologies. AVM, arteriovenous malformation; CADASIL, cerebral autosomal dominant arteriopathy with subcortical infarcts and leukoencephalopathy; CCM, cerebral cavernous malformations; CTD, connective tissue disease; MELAS, mitochondrial encephalomyelopathy, lactic acidosis, and stroke-like episodes; PKD, polycystic kidney disease.

This chapter will examine the genetic aspects of cerebrovascular disease by a review of (1) population, familial, and genetic epidemiology studies; (2) genetics of specific ischemic stroke types and mechanisms; and (3) genetics of hemorrhagic strokes and related vascular lesions. While there are a plethora of studies of polymorphisms associated with stroke, they will for the most part not be reviewed in this chapter since the biological and clinical significance of most of these remains unclear or unproven. Polymorphisms that are particularly important or promising based on data and clinical studies will be discussed in more detail.

Population, familial, and genetic epidemiologic studies

Several years ago, before the revolution in genetic epidemiology, linkage, and association techniques, there were several groups that investigated the familial clustering of stroke cases. Most of these studies were retrospective and hospital or clinic based; few were population based. They were limited by (in most cases) a combining of all stroke cases regardless of etiology, and in some cases limited study of patients with modern brain imaging studies. Nonetheless, most but not all did report some degree of familial clustering or association for "stroke" as a loosely defined disorder [2–7].

One of the most powerful techniques to investigate the heritability of a disorder is the use of twin studies. There have been several studies of stroke genetics using the Veterans' Administration Twin Database [8–10]. These studies do support a significant genetic component underlying the etiology of stroke, although as noted above the type of stroke was not clearly defined in some of these studies.

Polymorphism association studies and candidate gene association studies are quite common in all types of vascular disease [11]. Although these studies often appear promising, the overall approach can have significant limitations and often lacks reproducibility when applied to diverse or different populations. While a myriad of such associations have been published, most reported polymorphisms lack functional significance and many have not been confirmed on larger or diverse populations [12]. However, there have been some well-done metaanalyses for some of the more common and well-studied polymorphisms, including methylene tetrahydrofolate reductase (MTHFR), apolipoprotein E (ApoE), and the angiotensin-converting enzyme (ACE) deletion/insertion. These studies have shown significant associations between ischemic stroke and the MTHFR C677T change, as well as with the ApoE ε4 genotype. The ACE gene association is either negative or only slightly positive in most large studies [13–15].

There may be a significant association between ApoE genotype and recovery or outcome after stroke. Some studies and meta-analyses have shown that the ε4 allele is associated with a worse prognosis after hemorrhagic stroke (subarachnoid and intracerebral hemorrhage) but not ischemic stroke [16,17]. The mechanism(s) by which ApoE genotype may affect outcome remains unclear.

Genome-wide screening studies have been under way for several years. The goal of such large studies is to identify genetic variations such as single nucleotide polymorphisms (SNPs) or groups of such variations (haplotypes) that are associated with one or more types of stroke [18]. One of the best known projects is DeCode, which is based in Iceland and makes use of the extensive medical database kept on almost all citizens in Iceland. This project has reported two significant associations for ischemic stroke. One is for the phosphodiesterase 4D gene (*PDE4D*) on chromosome 5q12, and the other is for the 5-lipoxygenase activating protein (ALOX5AP) gene [19]. The linkage association for both genes is through a series of haplotypes that appear to confer differential degrees of risk among carriers. Some of the genetic association and haplotype findings have been replicated by other groups in other populations, but some have not [20–27]. It is unclear whether any of these haplotypes results in any significant functional alteration in the gene/protein or how such changes might impact stroke risk, although some theories have been advanced, including effects on the vessel wall, myeloperoxidase, and leukotrienes [28]. Other ongoing projects have genotyped several hundred subjects looking for other moderate or strong genetic factors using a high-density (400 000) SNP map [29]. Several markers and areas of interest have been identified, although the identity of any specific gene has not yet been reported.

Genetics of ischemic stroke

A small percentage of strokes are due to single-gene (monogenic) disorders or syndromes; these include sickle cell disease, CADASIL, Fabry disease, Marfan syndrome, neurofibromatosis, sickle cell disease, and some of the hemorrhagic stroke types, particularly cavernous malformations [30]. The connective tissue disorders associated with stroke are summarized in Table 12.2.

CADASIL (cerebral autosomal dominant arteriopathy with subcortical infarcts and leukoencephalopathy) is one of the prototypical monogenic ischemic stroke disorders. It was recognized and well characterized by Bousser and colleagues [31,32] in France in the early 1990s. The cluster of a positive family history, ischemic strokes and transient ischemic attacks (TIAs), cognitive decline, migraines, abnormal brain imaging, and progressive nature form a very suggestive complex (see Box 12.1 for a list of common symptoms). Classic magnetic resonance imaging (MRI) findings include bilateral lesions on T2 and FLAIR (fluid-attenuated inversion recovery) sequences involving the deep white matter, basal ganglia, anterior temporal pole, and pons [33]. CADASIL is due to mutations in the NOTCH3 gene/protein, which maps to the proximal

Table 12.2 Inherited connective tissue disorders associated with cerebrovascular disease

Disorder	Type of cerebrovascular disease
Ehlers–Danlos type IV	Dissections, aneurysms, CCF
Marfan syndrome	Dissections, aneurysms, CCF, aortic disease
Fibromuscular dysplasia	Dissections, aneurysms
Pseudoxanthoma elasticum	Vessel occlusions, aneurysms, CCF, moyamoya disease, dissections
Neurofibromatosis type I	Aneurysms, CCF, moyamoya disease, vessel occlusions

CCF, carotid-cavernous fistula.

short arm of chromosome 19 [34]. It is still unknown how the gene and protein mutations lead to the small vessel arteriopathy that leads to the CADASIL phenotype. The deposition of osmophilic granules near the basal lamina of cells is a characteristic pathologic finding of CADASIL. There is degeneration of vascular smooth muscle cells, although the precise mechanism remains elusive [35]. The burden of lacunar strokes largely correlates with the cognitive decline, suggesting that CADASIL causes a true vascular dementia [36].

The NOTCH3 mutations that cause CADASIL have been well characterized. The common mutations often involve epidermal growth factor-like repeat domains in the extracellular part of the Notch3 protein. Most mutations are missense, and most are located in exons 2–6 in some reports [37]. However, other groups have found clusters of mutations in other exons [38]. Based on these observations, a complete screen of all 33 exons is advised for the molecular diagnosis of CADASIL. This is now relatively easy since there are several companies that offer screening of the entire *NOTCH3* gene for mutations.

CADASIL often displays significant variability between and among affected family members with the same mutation as well as between families with different mutations. Testing for heritability of MRI-quantified lesions suggests that other genetic modifiers exist that affect disease burden [39]. The prognosis for patients with CADASIL is highly variable. In general men tend to have a worse prognosis than women, with men dying in their mid-sixties compared with women dying in their early seventies. Most deaths are due to pulmonary complications (pneumonia, asphyxiation) or sudden death [40].

Sickle cell disease is another common monogenic disorder that frequently causes stroke, both ischemic and hemorrhagic, as a major complication. It is due to a single base substitution in the β-hemoglobin gene on chromosome 11. Children with sickle cell disease have a 5–17% risk of stroke, which increases to 32% by age 40. About 75% of strokes are ischemic and 25% are hemorrhagic. In general, younger individuals have more ischemic strokes, while adults are

Box 12.1 Common clinical and radiologic features of CADASIL

- Positive family history
- Subcortical ischemic strokes and/or TIAs
- White-matter lesions on MRI (new and chronic strokes)
- Dementia
- Migraine headaches
- Depression
- Pseudobulbar palsy

CADASIL, cerebral autosomal dominant arteriopathy with subcortical infarcts and leukoencephalopathy; MRI, magnetic resonance imaging; TIA, transient ischemic attack.

more at risk for ICH or SAH [41,42]. Major mechanisms for ischemic stroke include a proliferative vasculopathy affecting the large vessels at the base of the brain, vessel obstruction due to sludging and clotting of sickling red cells, hemolytic anemia, and traditional factors such as hypertension and diabetes [41,43,44]. Hemorrhages may be due to rupture of intracranial vessels forming moyamoya networks as a response to proximal vessel stenosis, and rupture of intracranial aneurysms [41,42]. Screening of individuals with transcranial Doppler can identify those with high velocities who are at highest risk of subsequent strokes. These patients benefit from prophylactic blood transfusions that reduce the percentage of abnormal hemoglobin and reduce the risk of subsequent stroke [45,46].

Fabry disease is an X-linked disorder due to deficiency in the α-galactosidase A gene. It is associated with renal, cardiac, and cerebrovascular disease, particularly ischemic strokes [47,48]. In the brain it tends to affect small vessels in the vertebral–basilar territory, causing thickening of the vessel walls and elongated, tortuous vessels in some cases [49,50]. Studies of cryptogenic stroke in young adults have found mutations in the α-galactosidase A gene in about 5% of males [51]. This suggests that Fabry disease may be an underrecognized cause of stroke in young adults. It is of note since it is one of the few genetic disorders that can be treated using enzyme replacement therapy. Studies of recombinant α-galactosidase A (Fabrazyme) at doses of 1 mg/kg intravenously every 2 weeks have shown significant improvement in many of the systemic manifestations of the disease, including the cerebrovascular component [52].

Dissections of various arteries, particularly the extracranial carotid and vertebral arteries, can cause TIAs and ischemic strokes. In rare cases there appears to be a familial component [53,54]. There have been several reports of mutations in various collagen genes in patients with such dissections. However, other reports have failed to find such mutations except in very rare (i.e., $<5\%$) of cases [55–57]. In some cases such dissections are thought to indicate underlying fibromuscular dysplasia (FMD). A familial occurrence of FMD is typically seen in only about 10% of cases [58]. FMD is often seen as a beaded appearance of the extracranial carotid and vertebral arteries. It is also associated with intracranial aneurysms. Moyamoya disease is another unique vasculopathy characterized by occlusion or stenosis of the distal intracranial internal carotid arteries and proximal middle cerebral arteries. It can cause ischemic strokes or cerebral hemorrhages due to rupture of small collateral vessels that form as a response to the vascular occlusions [59,60]. Familial clustering is seen in about 10% of cases [60,61]. Studies are under way to identify causative genes for moyamoya disease, which is more common in Asian populations.

MELAS (mitochondrial encephalomyelopathy, lactic acidosis, and stroke-like episodes) is an important genetic cause of stroke. It is maternally inherited and is most commonly due to a single-base mutation of A to G in the transfer RNA for leucine in the mitochondrial DNA [62]. The stroke-like episodes typically occur in the occipital, parietal, and temporal regions and involve the cortex or the gray–white junction. They are not in typical arterial territories. Bright lesions on T2 and FLAIR MRI can be seen, which may resolve in a few days without permanent damage in some cases [63]. Magnetic resonance spectroscopy may show high levels of lactate in the abnormal region. Other symptoms of MELAS include myopathy, dementia, headaches, hearing loss, seizures, lactic acidosis, diabetes, and myoclonus [41,64].

Inherited thrombophilias are now well recognized as a cause of ischemic strokes, particularly in patients under the age of 45–50 years, those taking oral contraceptives, and those with otherwise cryptogenic strokes [65]. The association between these conditions is stronger for venous than for arterial thrombosis, but they can certainly cause ischemic strokes as well as cerebral venous thrombosis. The most common affected genes and proteins include factor V Leiden, prothrombin gene, antithrombin III, protein C, and protein S [66]. On occasion, familial associations for antiphospholipid antibodies and Sneddon syndrome have been reported [67,68].

Gene expression studies in peripheral blood are also being used to develop a genetic "signature" that might be useful for diagnosing acute stroke. Much of this work has focused on ischemic stroke phenotypes. Limitations include issues such as sensitivity and specificity, and the need for such signatures to provide some prognostic guidance, which is not yet possible [69].

Genetics of hemorrhagic strokes and malformations

Cerebral amyloid angiopathy (CAA) defines a number of disorders characterized by the deposition of one or more amyloid or amyloid-like proteins in the wall of cerebral vessels [70]. A listing of proteins that can produce amyloid angiopathy is given in Box 12.2 [70]. The clinical features include intracerebral hemorrhage, dementia, and small-vessel ischemic stroke. Many cases are sporadic, but a significant minority are familial, often with an autosomal dominant inheritance pattern. The classic genetic/familial forms are the Dutch type and the Icelandic type, which typically present with one or more ICHs and dementia in some cases [71,72]. The sporadic form of CAA is only rarely due to a mutation in one of the amyloid genes, but has been associated with specific isoforms of the apolipoprotein E gene, particularly the ε4 and ε2 alleles and lobar ICHs [73,74]. Typical changes seen in MRI are numerous cortical or subcortical dark gradient echo lesions which represent microhemorrhages. However, small-vessel ischemic lesions are also commonly seen in patients with CAA [75,76]. Clinically significant ICHs occur most often in a lobar location, and may be recurrent 20% of cases. Clinical dementia and pathologic changes consistent with Alzheimer disease is present in about 50% of all cases [75,77]. Antithrombotic agents should be avoided in patients with known or suspected CAA due to the high risk of ICH.

Box 12.2 Proteins causing cerebral amyloid angiopathy

- Aβ-amyloid
- Cystatin C
- Transthyretins
- Apolipoprotein E
- Gelsolin
- Prion protein
- ABri
- ADan

See text for details and references.

There have been some preliminary reports of mutations in the collagen type IV α_1 gene being causative for small-vessel disease, particularly microhemorrhages, larger bleeds, and leukoencephalopathy [78]. Further study is needed to determine whether these mutations are a common cause of small-vessel disease in larger populations.

Intracranial aneurysms (IAs) and their rupture lead to subarachnoid hemorrhage, which is among the most deadly of all stroke types. It is well recognized that a number of risk factors, some genetic and some modifiable, can increase the risk of having an IA and predispose to the rupture of an IA. Female gender is a major risk factor for IAs and SAH, as is hypertension and smoking [79]. Family history of an IA, especially in a sibling, is a powerful risk factor for IA [80]. However, the familial risk of an SAH appears to be somewhat less [81]. Some genetic disorders are well known to be associated with IAs and SAH, the most well known being adult polycystic kidney disease (APKD). Other genetic disorders such as Marfan syndrome, neurofibromatosis, and Ehlers–Danlos type III are also associated with IAs, although these may be fusiform aneurysms more than berry aneurysms (see Table 12.2) [82].

Despite these associations, the vast majority of IAs and SAH occur in individuals without any known genetic risk factors. There are increasing reports of IAs and SAH with a familial clustering, but this accounts for only about 5–20% of all cases [83,84]. The importance of identifying genetic markers for "sporadic" IAs and SAH cannot be understated [85]. The ability to do a blood test to identify individuals at high risk for developing an IA would be of tremendous value in terms of focusing screening and monitoring programs on high-risk individuals.

Genetic linkage studies using association paradigms as well as classic linkage models have reported various loci that are associated with IAs and SAH. A Japanese group has found linkage to chromosome 19q13.3 in several families [86]. Other groups have reported an association between a SNP in or near lysyl oxidase 2 and IAs, which may be mediated through interactions with the elastin and LIM kinase 1 gene [87]. Another study found strong evidence for linkage to the ANIB4 locus on chromosome 5p15.2–14.3; it is unclear which candidate genes are near that locus [88]. Linkage has also been reported to chromosomes 11q24–25, 14q23–31 [89] and 1p34.3–36.13 [90].

The most positive reports for genetic and IA focus on markers in the region of the elastin gene (chromosome 7q11). Linkage studies have shown convincing evidence of a major locus for IA in the area around the elastin gene, particularly the 3′ untranslated region and the *LIMK1* gene. However, subsequent studies have suggested that the gene of interest may not be elastin, but perhaps another gene or genes in that general area [91–93]. Although elastin has long been considered a strong candidate gene for some cases of IA, it appears that the underlying genetic defect may be more complex and span several genes and pathways [94]. One form of collagen, type $\alpha_{2(1)}$, has also been linked to some cases of IA [95].

Polycystic kidney disease (PKD) is a classic example of a genetic systemic disorder that can cause IAs. PKD is characterized by the formation of cysts in the kidney and liver, progressive renal failure, and the development of IAs [96]. A history of PKD increases the risk of having an IA by 4.4 times [80]. The major types of PKD are autosomal dominant (ADPKD) and autosomal recessive (ARPKD) [97]. There are two major forms of ADPKD, termed PKD1 and PKD2. PKD1 is most common, accounting for 80–85% of all cases, and is due to mutation in the polycystin 1 gene (chromosome 16q13.3). PKD2 accounts for about 10–15% of cases, is less severe, and is due to mutation in polycystin 2 (chromosome 4q21–23) [96,98]. The polycystin genes quite large, encompassing several million bases of DNA, with a large number of exons, a variety of mutations, and duplication of the part or all of the gene in some cases of PKD [99]. These factors make mutational screening problematic. Mutational analyses have shown that mutations in the 5′ end of polycystin 1 are more closely associated with IAs than other locations [100,101]. The autosomal recessive form, ARPKD, is due to a variety of mutations of the *PKHD1* gene on chromosome 6p12 [102].

Polycystin 1 and 2 are expressed in the vascular smooth muscle cells of large blood vessels [103]. The polycystin proteins are responsible for forming cell–cell desmosomal junctions as well as cell–cell adhesions [104]. If such junctions and adhesions were interrupted in the cell matrix of the intracranial vessels, this could lead to areas of weakness, thereby forming the basis for IA formation.

Cerebral cavernous malformations (CCMs) are now recognized to have a genetic basis in one-third to one-half of all cases, particularly those with multiple lesions seen on brain MRI [105]. CCMs often present with headaches, small hemorrhages, seizures, or focal neurologic symptoms. Genetic studies have shown an autosomal dominant pattern of inheritance, with three causative genes identified: CCM1 is caused by mutations in the *KRIT1* gene, CCM2 is due to *MGC4607*, and CCM3 is due to *PDCD10* [106]. In general, families with the CCM3 mutation had fewer affecteds, but those affected tended to be younger with hemorrhage being more common. In patients with the CCM1 mutations, the number of lesions increased with age more than was seen in families with CCM2 mutations [107]. Studies of sporadic cases of CCMs have shown that 29% of such cases with multiple lesions are due to mutations in the CCM1 gene, whereas no sporadic case with just one lesion was found to have a CCM1 mutation [108]. These proteins appear to function via protein kinase-mediated modulation of angiogenesis [109].

Hereditary hemorrhagic telangiectasia (HHT, also known as Rendu–Osler–Weber disease) is an autosomal dominant disorder. Patients typically have numerous small telangiectasias involving the skin, mucosa, gastrointestinal tract, and brain, as well as AVMs involving the brain, lung, and liver [110]. These lesions cause symptoms by bleeding, producing peripheral hemorrhages as well as ICHs and SAHs. Cerebral ischemic strokes and brain abscesses are also common due to pulmonary AVMs [41]. HHT type 1 is due to mutations in the endoglin gene (chromosome 9), and HHT type 2 is due to mutations in the *ALK1* gene (chromosome 12) [111,112].

There are a number of inherited bleeding disorders, typically due to deficiencies of a clotting factor (i.e., hemophilia). In general, the factor deficiencies causing hemorrhages are inherited as autosomal recessive traits, whereas the protein deficiencies (protein C and protein S) are autosomal dominant disorders [113]. Protein C and S deficiency are associated with an increased risk of thrombosis, not bleeding.

Summary

Although much progress has been made in understanding the genetics of stroke, most of the major advances have been in specific disorders and special phenotypes such as CADASIL, PKD, and CCMs. More work needs to be done to better understand the genetic risk factors underlying the common types of ischemic strokes and cerebral hemorrhage. The potential for such knowledge to lead to improved prevention, diagnosis, and treatment is almost unlimited—but the challenges remain substantial at this time. The use of new genetic technologies will be important for better identifying and dissecting the role of genetic factors in some of these disorders. The use of gene therapy to treat any of these disorders remains a niche application at present, but again holds great promise for the future.

References

1 Wang MM. Genetics of ischemic stroke: future clinical applications. *Seminars in Neurology* 2006; **26**: 523–530.

2 Alter M. Genetic factors in cerebrovascular disease. *Transactions of the American Neurological Association* 1967; **92**: 205–208.
3 Alter M, Kluznik J. Genetics of cerebrovascular accidents. *Stroke* 1972; **3**: 41–48.
4 Brass LM, Shaker LA. Family history in patients with transient ischemic attacks. *Stroke* 1991; **22**: 837–841.
5 Kubota M, Yamaura A, Ono J *et al.* Is family history an independent risk factor for stroke? *Journal of Neurology and Neurosurgery and Psychiatry* 1997; **62**: 66–70.
6 Liao D, Myers R, Hunt S *et al.* Familial history of stroke and stroke risk: The Family Heart Study. *Stroke* 1997; **28**: 1908–1912.
7 Marshall J. Familial incidence of cerebrovascular disease. *Journal of Medical Genetics* 1971; **8**: 84–89.
8 Brass LM, Merikangas KR, Robinette CDR. A twin study of stroke. *Annals of Neurology* 1990; **28**: 256.
9 Brass LM, Isaacsohn JL, Merikangas KR, Robinette CD. A study of stroke in twins. *Stroke* 1992; **23**: 221–223.
10 Brass LM, Carrano D, Hartigan PM *et al.* Genetic risk for stroke: A follow-up study of the NAS/VA twin registry. *Neurology* 1996; **46**: A212.
11 Hoppe C. From bench to bedside and back: the value of candidate gene association studies in translational research. *Stroke* 2007; **38**: 6.
12 Nikolopoulos GK, Tsantes AE, Bagos PG *et al.* Integrin, alpha 2 gene C807T polymorphism and risk of ischemic stroke: a meta-analysis. *Thrombosis Research* 2007; **119**: 501–510.
13 Banerjee I, Gupta V, Ganesh S. Association of gene polymorphism with genetic susceptibility to stroke in Asian populations: a meta-analysis. *Journal of Human Genetics* 2007; **52**: 205–19.
14 Gormley K, Bevan S, Markus HS. Polymorphisms in genes of the renin-angiotensin system and cerebral small vessel disease. *Cerebrovascular Disease* 2007; **23**: 148–155.
15 Pera J, Slowik A, Dziedzic T *et al.* ACE I/D polymorphism in different etiologies of ischemic stroke. *Acta Neurologica Scandinavica* 2006; **114**: 320–322.
16 Martinez-Gonzalez NA, Sudlow CL. Effects of apolipoprotein E genotype on outcome after ischaemic stroke, intracerebral haemorrhage and subarachnoid haemorrhage. *Journal of Neurology and Neurosurgery and Psychiatry* 2006; **77**: 1329–1335.
17 Sarzynska-Dlugosz I, Gromadzka G, Baranska-Gieruszczak M *et al.* APOE does not predict poor outcome 1 year after ischemic stroke. *Neurological Research* 2007; **29**: 64–69.
18 Nilsson-Ardnor S, Janunger T, Wiklund PG *et al.* Genome-wide linkage scan of common stroke in families from northern Sweden. *Stroke* 2007; **38**: 34–40.
19 Gretarsdottir S, Thorleifsson G, Reynisdottir ST *et al.* The gene encoding phosphodiesterase 4D confers risk of ischemic stroke. *Nature Genetics* 2003; **35**: 131–138.
20 Staton JM, Sayer MS, Hankey GJ *et al.* Association between phosphodiesterase 4D gene and ischaemic stroke. *Journal of Neurology and Neurosurgery and Psychiatry* 2006; **77**: 1067–1069.
21 Rosand J, Bayley N, Rost N, de Bakker PI. Many hypotheses but no replication for the association between PDE4D and stroke. *Nature Genetics* 2006; **38**: 1091–1092; author reply 1092–1093.
22 Zee RY, Brophy VH, Cheng S *et al.* Polymorphisms of the phosphodiesterase 4D, cAMP-specific (PDE4D) gene and risk of ischemic stroke: a prospective, nested case-control evaluation. *Stroke* 2006; **37**: 2012–2017.

23 Woo D, Kaushal R, Kissela B *et al.* Association of phosphodiesterase 4D with ischemic stroke: a population-based case-control study. *Stroke* 2006; **37**: 371–376.

24 Song Q, Cole JW, O'Connell JR *et al.* Phosphodiesterase 4D polymorphisms and the risk of cerebral infarction in a biracial population: the Stroke Prevention in Young Women Study. *Human Molecular Genetics* 2006; **15**: 2468–2478.

25 Brophy VH, Ro SK, Rhees BK *et al.* Association of phosphodiesterase 4D polymorphisms with ischemic stroke in a US population stratified by hypertension status. *Stroke* 2006; **37**: 1385–1390.

26 Meschia JF, Brott TG, Brown RD, Jr., *et al.* Phosphodiesterase 4D and 5-lipoxygenase activating protein in ischemic stroke. *Annals of Neurology* 2005; **58**: 351–361.

27 Bevan S, Porteous L, Sitzer M, Markus HS. Phosphodiesterase 4D gene, ischemic stroke, and asymptomatic carotid atherosclerosis. *Stroke* 2005; **36**: 949–953.

28 Hakonarson H. Role of FLAP and PDE4D in myocardial infarction and stroke: target discovery and future treatment options. *Current Treatment Options in Cardiovascular Medicine* 2006; **8**: 183–192.

29 Matarin M, Brown WM, Scholz S *et al.* A genome-wide genotyping study in patients with ischaemic stroke: initial analysis and data release. *Lancet Neurology* 2007; **6**: 414–420.

30 Razvi SS, Bone I. Single gene disorders causing ischaemic stroke. *Journal of Neurology* 2006; **253**: 685–700.

31 Tournier-Lasserve E, Joutel A, Melki J *et al.* Cerebral autosomal dominant arteriopathy with subcortical infarcts and leukoencephalopathy maps to chromosome 19q12. *Nature Genetics* 1993; **3**: 256–259.

32 Chabriat H, Vahedi K, Iba-Zizen MT *et al.* Clinical spectrum of CADASIL: a study of 7 families. Cerebral autosomal dominant arteriopathy with subcortical infarcts and leukoencephalopathy. *Lancet* 1995; **346**: 934–939.

33 Gladstone JP, Dodick DW. Migraine and cerebral white matter lesions: when to suspect cerebral autosomal dominant arteriopathy with subcortical infarcts and leukoencephalopathy (CADASIL). *Neurologist* 2005; **11**: 19–29.

34 Joutel A, Corpechot C, Ducros A *et al.* Notch3 mutations in CADASIL, a hereditary adult-onset condition causing stroke and dementia. *Nature* 1996; **383**: 707–710.

35 Kalaria RN, Viitanen M, Kalimo H *et al.* The pathogenesis of CADASIL: an update. *Journal of the Neurological Sciences* 2004; **226**: 35–39.

36 Liem MK, van der Grond J, Haan J *et al.* Lacunar infarcts are the main correlate with cognitive dysfunction in CADASIL. *Stroke* 2007; **38**: 923–928.

37 Peters N, Opherk C, Bergmann T *et al.* Spectrum of mutations in biopsy-proven CADASIL: implications for diagnostic strategies. *Archives of Neurology* 2005; **62**: 1091–1094.

38 Dotti MT, Federico A, Mazzei R *et al.* The spectrum of Notch3 mutations in 28 Italian CADASIL families. *Journal of Neurology and Neurosurgery and Psychiatry* 2005; **76**: 736–738.

39 Opherk C, Peters N, Holtmannspotter M *et al.* Heritability of MRI lesion volume in CADASIL: evidence for genetic modifiers. *Stroke* 2006; **37**: 2684–2689.

40 Opherk C, Peters N, Herzog J *et al.* Long-term prognosis and causes of death in CADASIL: a retrospective study in 411 patients. *Brain* 2004; **127**: 2533–2539.

41 Andrews P, Ryan M, Kandt R. Genetics causes of pediatric stroke. In: Alberts M, ed. *Genetics of Cerebrovascular Disease*. Future Publishing Co., Armonk, NY, 1999: 261–311.

42 Kirkham FJ. Therapy insight: stroke risk and its management in patients with sickle cell disease. *Nature Clinical Practice Neurology* 2007; **3**: 264–278.
43 Debaun MR, Derdeyn CP, McKinstry RC, 3rd. Etiology of strokes in children with sickle cell anemia. *Mental Retardation and Developmental Disabilities Research Reviews* 2006; **12**: 192–199.
44 Switzer JA, Hess DC, Nichols FT, Adams RJ. Pathophysiology and treatment of stroke in sickle-cell disease: present and future. *Lancet Neurology* 2006; **5**: 501–512.
45 Qureshi N, Lubin B, Walters MC. The prevention and management of stroke in sickle cell anaemia. *Expert Opinion in Biological Therapy* 2006; **6**: 1087–1098.
46 Lee MT, Piomelli S, Granger S *et al.* Stroke Prevention Trial in Sickle Cell Anemia (STOP): extended follow-up and final results. *Blood* 2006; **108**: 847–852.
47 Fellgiebel A, Muller MJ, Ginsberg L. CNS manifestations of Fabry's disease. *Lancet Neurology* 2006; **5**: 791–795.
48 Moller AT, Jensen TS. Neurological manifestations in Fabry's disease. *Nature Clinical Practice Neurology* 2007; **3**: 95–106.
49 Grewal RP. Stroke in Fabry's disease. *Journal of Neurology* 1994; **241**: 153–156.
50 Mitsias P, Levine SR. Cerebrovascular complications of Fabry's disease. *Annals of Neurology* 1996; **40**: 8–17.
51 Rolfs A, Bottcher T, Zschiesche M *et al.* Prevalence of Fabry disease in patients with cryptogenic stroke: a prospective study. *Lancet* 2005; **366**: 1794–1796.
52 Desnick RJ, Banikazemi M. Fabry disease: clinical spectrum and evidence-based enzyme replacement therapy. *Nephrologie et Therapeutique* 2006; **2** Suppl 2: S172–185.
53 Mokri B, Piepgras DG, Wiebers DO, Houser OW. Familial occurrence of spontaneous dissection of the internal carotid artery. *Stroke* 1987; **18**: 246–251.
54 Majamaa K, Portimojarvi H, Sotaniemi KA, Myllyla VV. Familial aggregation of cervical artery dissection and cerebral aneurysm. *Stroke* 1994; **25**: 1704–1705.
55 Brandt T, Orberk E, Weber R *et al.* Pathogenesis of cervical artery dissections: association with connective tissue abnormalities. *Neurology* 2001; **57**: 24–30.
56 Wiest T, Hyrenbach S, Bambul P *et al.* Genetic analysis of familial connective tissue alterations associated with cervical artery dissections suggests locus heterogeneity. *Stroke* 2006; **37**: 1697–1702.
57 Martin JJ, Hausser I, Lyrer P *et al.* Familial cervical artery dissections: clinical, morphologic, and genetic studies. *Stroke* 2006; **37**: 2924–2929.
58 Plouin PF, Perdu J, La Batide-Alanore A *et al.* Fibromuscular dysplasia. *Orphanet Journal of Rare Diseases* 2007; **2**: 28.
59 Battistella PA, Pardatscher K, Laverda AM *et al.* [Moya-moya syndrome. Progression of the angiographic picture and therapeutic prospectives]. *La Pediatria Medica e Chirurgica: Medical and Surgical Pediatrics* 1987; **9**: 41–46.
60 Chabriat H, Tournier-Lasserve E, Bousser M-G. Vasculopathies. In: Alberts M, ed. *Genetics of Cerebrovascular Disease*. Futura Publishing Co., Armonk, NY, 1999: 195–208.
61 Kitahara T, Ariga N, Yamaura A *et al.* Familial occurrence of moya-moya disease: report of three Japanese families. *Journal of Neurology and Neurosurgery and Psychiatry* 1979; **42**: 208–214.
62 Thambisetty M, Newman NJ. Diagnosis and management of MELAS. *Expert Review of Molecular Diagnostics* 2004; **4**: 631–644.
63 Clark JM, Marks MP, Adalsteinsson E *et al.* MELAS: Clinical and pathologic correlations with MRI, xenon/CT, and MR spectroscopy. *Neurology* 1996; **46**: 223–227.

64 Damian MS, Seibel P, Reichmann H *et al*. Clinical spectrum of the MELAS mutation in a large pedigree. *Acta Neurologica Scandinavica* 1995; **92**: 409–415.
65 Pezzini A, Grassi M, Iacoviello L *et al*. Inherited thrombophilia and stratification of ischaemic stroke risk among users of oral contraceptives. *Journal of Neurology and Neurosurgery and Psychiatry* 2007; **78**: 271–276.
66 de Moerloose P, Boehlen F. Inherited thrombophilia in arterial disease: a selective review. *Seminars in Hematology* 2007; **44**: 106–113.
67 Pettee AD, Wasserman BA, Adams NL *et al*. Familial Sneddon's syndrome: clinical, hematologic, and radiographic findings in two brothers. *Neurology* 1994; **44**: 399–405.
68 Ford PM, Brunet D, Lillicrap DP, Ford SE. Premature stroke in a family with lupus anticoagulant and antiphospholipid antibodies. *Stroke* 1990; **21**: 66–71.
69 Baird AE. Blood genomic profiling: novel diagnostic and therapeutic strategies for stroke? *Biochemical Society Transactions* 2006; **34**: 1313–1317.
70 Revesz T, Ghiso J, Lashley T *et al*. Cerebral amyloid angiopathies: a pathologic, biochemical, and genetic view. *Journal of Neuropathology and Experimental Neurology* 2003; **62**: 885–898.
71 Palsdottir A, Snorradottir AO, Thorsteinsson L. Hereditary cystatin C amyloid angiopathy: genetic, clinical, and pathological aspects. *Brain Pathology* 2006; **16**: 55–59.
72 Levy E, Lopez OC, Ghiso J *et al*. Stroke in Icelandic patients with hereditary amyloid angiopathy is related to a mutation in the cystatin C gene, an inhibitor of cysteine proteases. *Journal of Experimental Medicine* 1989; **169**: 1771–1778.
73 Attems J. Sporadic cerebral amyloid angiopathy: pathology, clinical implications, and possible pathomechanisms. *Acta Neuropathologica (Berlin)* 2005; **110**: 345–359.
74 Kim M, Bae HJ, Lee J *et al*. APOE epsilon2/epsilon4 polymorphism and cerebral microbleeds on gradient-echo MRI. *Neurology* 2005; **65**: 1474–1475.
75 Yip AG, McKee AC, Green RC *et al*. APOE, vascular pathology, and the AD brain. *Neurology* 2005; **65**: 259–265.
76 Roman GC, Erkinjuntti T, Wallin A *et al*. Subcortical ischaemic vascular dementia. *Lancet Neurology* 2002; **1**: 426–436.
77 Nicoll JA, Yamada M, Frackowiak J *et al*. Cerebral amyloid angiopathy plays a direct role in the pathogenesis of Alzheimer's disease. Pro-CAA position statement. *Neurobiology of Aging* 2004; **25**: 589–597; discussion 603–604.
78 Gould DB, Phalan FC, van Mil SE *et al*. Role of COL4A1 in small-vessel disease and hemorrhagic stroke. *New England Journal of Medicine* 2006; **354**: 1489–1496.
79 Nahed BV, Bydon M, Ozturk AK *et al*. Genetics of intracranial aneurysms. *Neurosurgery* 2007; **60**: 213–225; discussion 225–226.
80 Rinkel GJ. Intracranial aneurysm screening: indications and advice for practice. *Lancet Neurology* 2005; **4**: 122–128.
81 Teasdale GM, Wardlaw JM, White PM *et al*. The familial risk of subarachnoid haemorrhage. *Brain* 2005; **128**: 1677–1685.
82 Alberts M. Inherited systemic disorders that cause stroke. In: Alberts M, ed. *Genetics of Cerebrovascular Disease*. Futura Publishing Co., Armonk, NY, 1999: 313–332.
83 Kim DH, Van Ginhoven G, Milewicz DM. Incidence of familial intracranial aneurysms in 200 patients: comparison among Caucasian, African-American, and Hispanic populations. *Neurosurgery* 2003; **53**: 302–308.
84 Wang MC, Rubinstein D, Kindt GW, Breeze RE. Prevalence of intracranial aneurysms in first-degree relatives of patients with aneurysms. *Neurosurgery Focus* 2002; **13**: e2.

85 Broderick JP, Sauerbeck LR, Foroud T *et al.* The Familial Intracranial Aneurysm (FIA) study protocol. *BMC Medical Genetics* 2005; **6**: 17.
86 Mineharu Y, Inoue K, Inoue S *et al.* Model-based linkage analyses confirm chromosome 19q13.3 as a susceptibility locus for intracranial aneurysm. *Stroke* 2007; **38**: 1174–1178.
87 Akagawa H, Narita A, Yamada H *et al.* Systematic screening of lysyl oxidase-like (LOXL) family genes demonstrates that LOXL2 is a susceptibility gene to intracranial aneurysms. *Human Genetics* 2007; **121**: 377–387.
88 Verlaan DJ, Dube MP, St-Onge J *et al.* A new locus for autosomal dominant intracranial aneurysm, ANIB4, maps to chromosome 5p15.2–14.3. *Journal of Medical Genetics* 2006; **43**: e31.
89 Ozturk AK, Nahed BV, Bydon M *et al.* Molecular genetic analysis of two large kindreds with intracranial aneurysms demonstrates linkage to 11q24–25 and 14q23–31. *Stroke* 2006; **37**: 1021–1027.
90 Nahed BV, Seker A, Guclu B *et al.* Mapping a Mendelian form of intracranial aneurysm to 1p34.3-p36.13. *American Journal of Human Genetics* 2005; **76**: 172–179.
91 Akagawa H, Tajima A, Sakamoto Y *et al.* A haplotype spanning two genes, ELN and LIMK1, decreases their transcripts and confers susceptibility to intracranial aneurysms. *Human Molecular Genetics* 2006; **15**: 1722–1734.
92 Berthelemy-Okazaki N, Zhao Y, Yang Z *et al.* Examination of ELN as a candidate gene in the Utah intracranial aneurysm pedigrees. *Stroke* 2005; **36**: 1283–1284.
93 Mineharu Y, Inoue K, Inoue S *et al.* Association analysis of common variants of ELN, NOS2A, APOE and ACE2 to intracranial aneurysm. *Stroke* 2006; **37**: 1189–1194.
94 Ruigrok YM, Rinkel GJ, Wijmenga C. Genetics of intracranial aneurysms. *Lancet Neurology* 2005; **4**: 179–189.
95 Yoneyama T, Kasuya H, Onda H *et al.* Collagen type I alpha2 (COL1A2) is the susceptible gene for intracranial aneurysms. *Stroke* 2004; **35**: 443–448.
96 Ong AC, Harris PC. Molecular pathogenesis of ADPKD: the polycystin complex gets complex. *Kidney International* 2005; **67**: 1234–1247.
97 Torres VE, Harris PC. Mechanisms of disease: autosomal dominant and recessive polycystic kidney diseases. *Nature Clinical Practice Nephrology* 2006; **2**: 40–55; quiz 55.
98 Al-Bhalal L, Akhtar M. Molecular basis of autosomal dominant polycystic kidney disease. *Advances in Anatomic Pathology* 2005; **12**: 126–133.
99 Rossetti S, Consugar MB, Chapman AB et al. Comprehensive molecular diagnostics in autosomal dominant polycystic kidney disease. *Journal of the American Society of Nephrology* 2007; 18: 2143–2160.
100 Rossetti S, Chauveau D, Kubly V *et al.* Association of mutation position in polycystic kidney disease 1 (PKD1) gene and development of a vascular phenotype. *Lancet* 2003; **361**: 2196–2201.
101 Peltola P, Lumiaho A, Miettinen R *et al.* Genetics and phenotypic characteristics of autosomal dominant polycystic kidney disease in Finns. *Journal of Molecular Medicine* 2005; **83**: 638–646.
102 Bergmann C, Kupper F, Schmitt CP *et al.* Multi-exon deletions of the PKHD1 gene cause autosomal recessive polycystic kidney disease (ARPKD). *Journal of Medical Genetics* 2005; **42**: e63.
103 Torres VE, Cai Y, Chen X *et al.* Vascular expression of polycystin-2. *Journal of the American Society of Nephrology* 2001; **12**: 1–9.

104 Russo RJ, Husson H, Joly D *et al.* Impaired formation of desmosomal junctions in ADPKD epithelia. *Histochemistry and Cell Biology* 2005; **124**: 487–497.

105 Mindea SA, Yang BP, Shenkar R *et al.* Cerebral cavernous malformations: clinical insights from genetic studies. *Neurosurgery Focus* 2006; **21**: e1.

106 Revencu N, Vikkula M. Cerebral cavernous malformation: new molecular and clinical insights. *Journal of Medical Genetics* 2006; **43**: 716–721.

107 Denier C, Labauge P, Bergametti F *et al.* Genotype-phenotype correlations in cerebral cavernous malformations patients. *Annals of Neurology* 2006; **60**: 550–556.

108 Verlaan DJ, Laurent SB, Sure U *et al.* CCM1 mutation screen of sporadic cases with cerebral cavernous malformations. *Neurology* 2004; **62**: 1213–1215.

109 Plummer NW, Zawistowski JS, Marchuk DA. Genetics of cerebral cavernous malformations. *Current Neurology and Neuroscience Reports* 2005; **5**: 391–396.

110 Sabba C, Pasculli G, Lenato GM *et al.* Hereditary hemorrhagic telangiectasia: clinical features in ENG and ALK1 mutation carriers. *Journal of Thrombosis and Haemostasis* 2007; **5**: 1149–1157.

111 Sadick H, Sadick M, Gotte K *et al.* Hereditary hemorrhagic telangiectasia: an update on clinical manifestations and diagnostic measures. *Wiener Klinische Wochenschrift* 2006; **118**: 72–80.

112 Prigoda NL, Savas S, Abdalla SA *et al.* Hereditary haemorrhagic telangiectasia: mutation detection, test sensitivity and novel mutations. *Journal of Medical Genetics* 2006; **43**: 722–728.

113 Ortel T. Genetics of coagulation disorders. In: Alberts M, ed. *Genetics of Cerebrovascular Disease*. Futura Publishing Co., Armonk, NY, 1999: 129–156.

Chapter 13

Genetic determinants of arterial thrombosis

Yasmin Khan, Nauder Faraday, William Herzog, and Alan R. Shuldiner

Introduction

Cardiovascular disease (CVD) is the leading cause of mortality in men and women in the USA, accounting for 1 in every 2.8 deaths in 2005 [1]. Coronary heart disease causes 1 in 5 deaths in the USA. An estimated 770 000 Americans will have a new myocardial infarction (MI) and about 430 000 will have a recurrent MI. Each year, approximately 780 000 Americans will experience a new or recurrent stroke. The conventional risk factors that have long been associated with MI and stroke, such as hypertension, tobacco use, dyslipidemia, physical inactivity, obesity, and diabetes mellitus, account for only some of the interindividual variation observed in risk. More recently emerging CVD risk factors, such as hyper coagulability, hypertriglyceridemia, endothelial dysfunction, and inflammation have been identified and are actively being investigated [2–4]. Of those who die suddenly from MI, 50% of men and 64% of women have no previous symptoms. This clinical observation, coupled with our increased appreciation of the interdependence between atherosclerosis, inflammation, and thrombosis, suggests that platelet aggregation and arterial thrombosis is a decisive factor leading to vasculo-occlusive or atherothrombotic events.

In the nineteenth century, Rudolph Virchow described the primary features of thrombosis: injury to the vessel wall, decrease in blood flow, and hypercoagulability (Virchow's triad). The complex biochemical and cellular pathways leading to thrombosis likely evolved to pose a selective advantage by preventing excessive bleeding and death during injury. Thrombosis resulting in pathological states can occur either in the low-flow venous system (e.g., deep venous thrombosis) or the high-flow arterial system (e.g., MI and stroke). The pathogenesis

Cardiovascular Genetics and Genomics. Edited by Dan Roden. © 2009 American Heart Association, ISBN: 978-14051-7540-1.

of arterial thrombosis is heterogeneous and complex, involving chronic progressive atherosclerotic damage to blood vessels, acute platelet activation, ultimately, and clot formation. Both genetic and environmental factors play important roles in determining risk for atherosclerosis and arterial thrombosis [5].

In the past decade, there has been growing literature on the relationship between mutations and variants in specific genes that influence hemostasis and thrombotic occlusion. Mutations in single genes that have a profound impact on hemostasis, e.g., factors VIII, IX, and XI in hemophilia, are rare in the population, but have provided important insights into the molecular mechanisms and pathophysiology of the process. By contrast, very little is known about the genes that influence thrombosis in the common forms of atherothrombotic disease. Like other complex diseases and traits, it is likely that thrombosis is polygenic in which common variants in several (many) genes, each with modest effect, interacting with environmental exposures, influence risk. In addition to common gene variants, some of the genetic risk may be determined by many different rare variants in relevant genes in thrombotic pathways. Variants, both common and rare, may include single nucleotide polymorphisms, insertions/deletions, copy number variants, inversions, or other structural variations. Susceptibility gene variants for the common forms of thrombosis will be difficult to identify, but will have a greater impact on the population attributable risk and may provide new avenues for therapy and prevention of thrombotic diseases.

This chapter addresses candidate genes and their variants that predispose to arterial thrombosis through their direct effect on platelet function. Candidate genes that may indirectly affect platelet function through their effects on inflammation, oxidative damage, or metabolic derangement, e.g., homocysteine and uric acid, will not be covered in this chapter. Although variants in several genes have been identified that increase risk of venous thrombosis, e.g., factor V Leiden, prothrombin 20210 A/G, protein C and S deficiency, these will not be reviewed since the underlying physiological processes and their pathological consequences largely differ from those of arterial thrombosis. The genetic basis of venous thrombosis is the subject of several recent reviews [6–8].

Mechanisms of arterial thrombosis: insights into candidate genes

Platelets play the preeminent role in primary hemostasis and are the hemostatic element most responsible for development of arterial thrombosis. Under normal physiological conditions, circulating platelets are quiescent and do not adhere to each other or to endothelial cells, which provide a protective barrier that separates blood from the layers of the vessel wall. Arterial thrombus formation is a tightly regulated process involving cellular (platelet, endothelial cells, leukocytes) and soluble blood components (coagulation proteins, anticoagulant proteins, fibrinolytic proteins). Platelets can be rapidly activated in the high-shear arterial circulation in response to a variety of stimuli, including acute vascular injury (e.g., trauma) and plaque rupture or endothelial erosion (in the setting of atherosclerotic disease). The major steps (Fig. 13.1) include the following. (1) Platelets adhere to subendothelial matrix proteins exposed by vascular damage, primarily through interaction of GPIb-IX-V receptors with von Willebrand

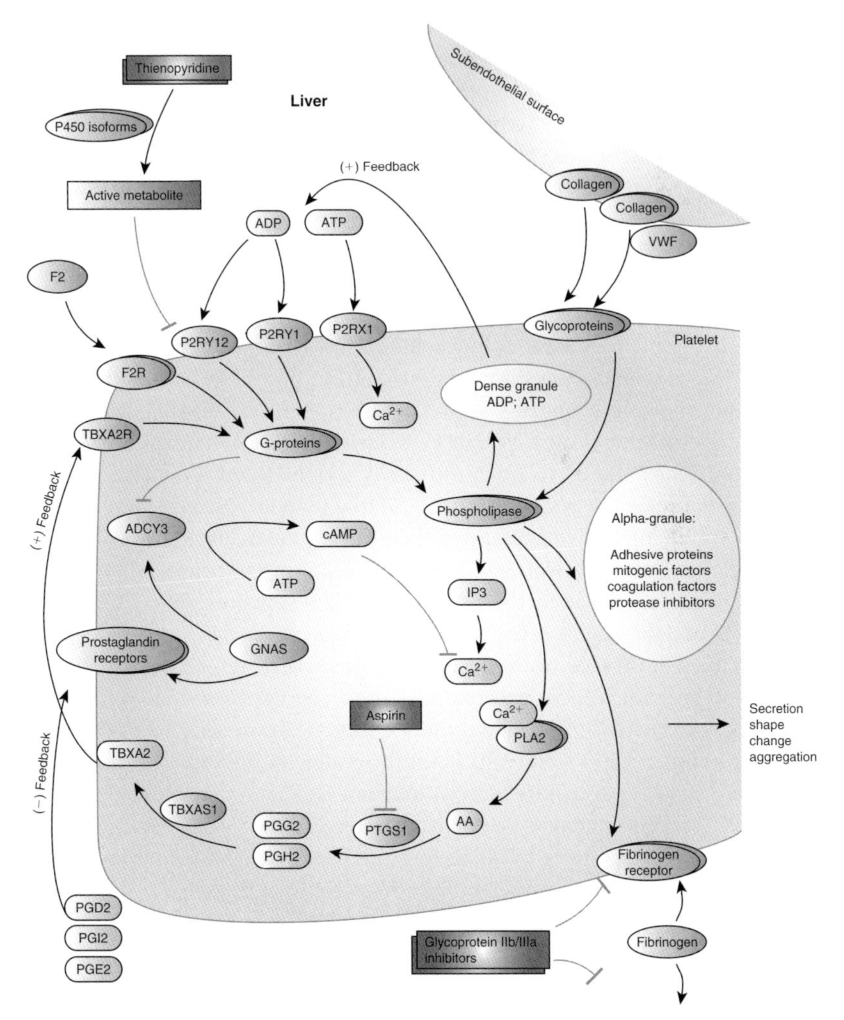

Fig. 13.1 Platelet aggregation pathway. AA, arachidonic acid; ADCY3, adenylate cyclase 3; ADP, adenosine diphosphate; ATP, adenosine triphosphate; cAMP cyclic adenosine mono-phosphate; F2, factor II; F2R, factor II (thrombin) receptor; GNAS guanine nucleotide binding protein, alpha stimulating); IP3, inositol triphosphate; PG, prostaglandin; PLA2, phospholipase A2; PTGS1, prostagladin-endoperoxide synthase 1 (COX1); P2Y purine nucleotide receptor; TBXA2, thromboxane A2, VWF, von Willebrand Factor. (Adapted from http://www.pharmgkb.org.)

factor (vWF). (2) Platelet agonists bind to specific platelet surface receptors. The most important agonist–receptor interactions include collagen binding to glycoprotein receptors GPIV, GPIaIIa, GPIV; adenosine diphosphate (ADP) binding to P2Y12 receptors; thromboxane binding to TbxA2R; and epinephrine binding to α_2-adrenergic receptors. (3) Receptor signals are transduced through a variety of intracellular second messengers including, phospholipases (PLA2) G-proteins and adenylate cyclase ADCY3, diacylglycerol, inositol-1,4,5-triphosphate (IP3), protein kinases, and calcium. (4) Platelet cyclooxygenase-1 (PTG51) converts arachidonic acid (AA) to thromboxane. (TbxA2) (5) GPIIb–IIIa receptors convert from a quiescent to activated conformation and bind fibrinogen, which mediates aggregation through intraplatelet crossbridges. (6) Platelets secrete and/or express on their surface procoagulant products including thromboxane, ADP, serotonin, and a series of adhesive proteins (e.g., fibrinogen, fibronectin) and receptors (e.g., P-selectin). In the second phase of hemostasis, fibrin formation occurs. This is primarily triggered by the tissue factor pathway (extrinsic pathway). A key event in the clotting cascade is formation of factor Xa, converting prothrombin (factor II) to thrombin (factor IIa), which cleaves fibrinogen into fibrin. The platelet phospholipid surface serves as the main site for assembly and activation of coagulation proteins and thrombin generation, which tends to limit thrombus formation to a specific location within the vascular space. The definitive arterial plug is a platelet–fibrin thrombus, which may partially or totally occlude the vascular lumen. In addition to pathways intrinsic to platelets and platelet activation, leukocytes and endothelial cells play a key role in modulating the thrombotic process (Fig. 13.1).

Hypercoagulable states arise from an imbalance between the procoagulant and anticoagulant forces of the blood. The binding of thrombin to thrombomodulin on endothelial cells neutralizes the procoagulant activities of thrombin and activates protein C. Activated protein C inhibits the generation of thrombin by inactivating factors Va and VIIIa. Antithrombin, another natural anticoagulant, is bound to heparin sulfate on endothelial cells and neutralizes thrombin, as well as the procoagulants factor XIa, factor IXa, and factor Xa. Protein S exerts anticoagulant effects by inhibiting the prothrombinase complex which converts prothrombin to thrombin. Reduced activity of protein S decreases the control of thrombin generation. The contribution of platelet hyperreactivity to a hypercoagulable state is somewhat controversial, particularly in primary prevention cohorts; however, in aspirin-treated patients with established coronary artery disease, increased platelet reactivity is associated with a fourfold increased risk of arterial thrombotic events such as MI and stroke [9,10].

Methods for quantifying platelet function

Various methods to quantify platelet function have been developed, several of which correlate with arterial thrombotic events [11,12]. The classical *in vivo* assay of platelet function is the bleeding time. The underside of the subject's forearm is cut to a standardized width and depth and the time it takes for bleeding to stop is measured. Bleeding time has the ability to detect gross abnormalities in platelet function, e.g., von Willebrand disease. It is dependent on several factors including the site of the incision, operator variability, and capillary density, and thus is not a useful measure of subtle interindividual differences in platelet function. By contrast, *in vitro* measures of platelet function can be more quantitative and can yield information about different pathways of platelet activation. Multiple assays have been devised, using a variety of methods to detect the formation of platelet aggregates in response to an agonist. The gold standard for assessing platelet function is optical aggregometry. This is a turbidometric technique, measuring the increased transmission of light as platelets aggregate, performed in platelet-rich plasma (PRP) using platelet-poor plasma (PPP) as a control. With this approach, varying concentrations of platelet agonists, e.g., collagen, ADP, epinephrine, and arachidonic acid, are added to a cuvette containing PRP. In a commonly used variant of this type of aggregometry, whole blood is used and platelet aggregation is determined by change in impedance across an electrode. Platelet function has also been monitored using flow cytometry to assess the expression of cell surface activation markers. In this methodology, whole blood or isolated platelets are incubated with fluorescently labeled antibodies specific for platelet activation markers (e.g., PAC1, P-selectin) and platelet reactivity is measured, with or without agonist stimulation, by the amount of fluorescence emitted from each cell.

While platelet aggregometry and flow cytometry have primarily been used as research tools, the platelet function analyzer 100 (PFA-100) is a shear-based technique that uses a more automated process. This cartridge-based system offers a limited choice of agonists and is often available in the hematology laboratory of large hospitals. Recently, the VerifyNow (Accumetrics; San Diego, CA) assay, which measures platelet function in unprocessed whole blood, has been promulgated as a bedside or point-of-care test to diagnose clinical platelet abnormalities, including aspirin and clopidogrel resistance. Another type of *in vitro* assay of platelet function is thromboelastography (TEG). This test measures the kinetics of clot formation and also provides information about the strength and stability of the clot.

Evidence for a heritable component to platelet function and arterial thrombosis

Many studies have demonstrated that genes can affect platelet function. Heritable factors accounted for 20–30% of the variance in platelet aggregation from epinephrine, ADP, and collagen agonists in siblings from the Framingham Heart Study, and this was greater than the variability attributed to measured environmental factors [13]. Gaxiola and Friedl [14] showed the heritability of epinephrine-induced platelet aggregation in a twin study with a correlation of 0.61 for monozygotic twin males and 0.43 for dizygotic twin males. Bray and coworkers [15] reported similar heritability of baseline *in vitro* platelet aggregation phenotypes in more outbred US white and African American populations.

Approaches to genetic analysis of arterial thrombosis and platelet function

As described above, observations that diseases caused by arterial thrombosis such as MI and stroke cluster in families and that platelet reactivity is heritable suggest a genetic component. However, the common form of arterial thrombosis causing MI and stroke is not inherited in a predictable Mendelian fashion characteristic of a highly penetrant monogenic disease, suggesting a more complex genetic architecture. It is likely that common variations in many genes, each with modest effect, acting through different pathways affect risk of arterial thrombosis. Defining the genetic underpinnings of susceptibility to arterial thrombosis is further complicated by interactions of these gene variants with each other and with nongenetic factors (e.g., age, diet, lifestyle).

Studies performed to date involve investigation of single genes thought to play a role in platelet aggregation and thrombosis. Many candidate genes have been investigated, but few (if any) have been reproducibly found to be associated with arterial thrombosis or platelet function. In most cases, just one or a few variants in these candidate genes have been investigated, rather than a more complete survey of common and rare variation, which is now possible using high-throughput genotyping and sequence analysis. The following sections review a few of the more intensively studied candidate genes for arterial thrombosis and platelet function. These genes include those expressed by platelets, soluble factors involved in the coagulation cascade, and products of endothelial cells that modulate platelet function (Fig. 13.1). Although some gene variants affecting lipids [e.g., apolipoprotein E (*APOE*)] and inflammation [e.g., tumor necrosis factor-α (*TNFA*), C-reactive protein (*CRP*), interleukins 1 and 6 (*IL1*, *IL6*)] have been implicated to be associated with platelet function and thrombosis, their effects are likely indirect and thus not covered in this chapter.

Platelet glycoproteins

Normal platelet function is dependent on the presence of platelet-membrane glycoproteins that regulate platelet adhesion and aggregation. Gp1b-IX-V binds to the vWF molecule on the subendothelial surface to promote adhesion. This process activates the platelet and alters the conformation of the GpIIb/IIIa receptor, leading to platelet aggregation. Genetic variation that results in altered expression or changes in the primary structure of these membrane glycoproteins could alter platelet function and thus risk of arterial thrombosis.

Platelet glycoprotein IIIa (GpIIIa)

GpIIIa is encoded by *ITGB3* (OMIM +173470), which has 15 exons spanning 60 kb on chromosome 17q21.32. Absence of GpIIIa causes Glanzmann thrombasthenia, a rare autosomal recessive bleeding disorder characterized by decreased platelet aggregation and absent or diminished clot retraction. The variant in *ITGB3* that has been studied most intensely to date with respect to typical arterial thrombotic disease is a common missense mutation in which leucine is changed to proline at codon position 59 (rs5918). The Pro59 allele (also noted in the literature as PLA2 and Leu33Pro) is found in approximately 15% of whites, 5–8% of African Americans, and is much less common in Asian populations. Maternofetal incompatibility at this codon can cause alloimmune thrombocytopenia in neonates, and post-transfusion thrombocytopenia in women who have acquired sensitization during pregnancy.

The PLA2 allele has been associated with incrementally greater aggregability *in vitro* [16,17], suggesting that this allele is prothrombotic. Weiss *et al.* [18] was the first to describe an association between the PLA2 allele and risk for MI. The allele was associated with a 2.8-fold increase in risk for coronary artery disease. The risk was especially high for those aged <60 years at the time of infarction. Subsequently, many association studies of PLA2 were reported in diverse populations and study designs, examining its role in coronary disease [19–29]. Some studies support a role of PLA2 in coronary disease while others do not. Two of the early larger studies, the ECTIM study [23] of 620 patients with MI and 700 controls, and the US Physicians Health Study [26] of 374 patients with MI and 704 controls, failed to show an association between the PLA2 allele and MI. Mamotte and coworkers [25] investigated the risk for coronary restenosis following angioplasty and found no association with the PLA2 allele. More recently, Knowles and coworkers [28] examined 1375 patients and found the PLA2 allele to be modestly more common in patients with acute MI (14.5%) than in patients with stable exertional angina (12.0%) ($P = 0.083$). Studies of cerebrovascular disease have also been equivocal. The role of the PLA2 allele of *ITBG3* in aspirin resistance has also been investigated, with some studies providing evidence for a role [30–32] and others not [33,34].

In summary, *in vitro* data support a functional consequence for the PLA2 allele with respect to platelet function. Numerous association studies with coronary disease and related phenotypes have been equivocal. The lack of consistency across studies may be due to differences in the populations studied and study design, with a true positive effect being present only in some subgroups or populations. In addition, most studies to date have been underpowered to detect alleles of modest (or even moderate) effect size, which could result in false-negative findings. Alternatively, negative results from several large studies could suggest little or no role for this allele in arterial thrombosis, with the smaller and earlier studies representing false-positive results. Additional studies of the PLA2 allele in much larger sample sizes as well as investigation of other variants in *ITBG3* will be necessary for more definitive conclusions to be made.

Other platelet glycoproteins

The GpIb-IX-V receptor complex is composed of four gene products. The two gene products that have been examined most extensively with regard to arterial thrombosis are the α and β subunits of the Gp1b gene, *ITGA2* and *GP1BA*, respectively.

ITGA2 contains 30 exons spanning 105.5 kb on chromosome 5q23–q31. A common variant 807C/T has been associated with higher expression on the surface of platelets and increased aggregatability to collagen [35–37]. It has been associated with MI and stroke in a number of studies [38–40], but not in others [41–43]. For example, Santoso and coworkers [38] studied the 807C/T variant in 2237 male patients and found strong association of the T allele with nonfatal MI in younger individuals. By contrast, in a large Italian study of 1210 young MI cases and 1210 controls, there was no evidence of association with 807C/T [42].

GP1BA contains two exons spanning 2.7 kb on chromosome 17pter–p12. Rare loss of function mutations in *GP1BA* causes Bernard–Soulier syndrome, which is characterized by thrombocytopenia and bleeding abnormalities [44,45]. The three common variants that have been studied most intensively in this gene are a threonine to methionine substitution at codon 161 (rs6065) (also known as Thr145Met and Ko) [46], a T/C variant located 5 bp upstream of the ATG initiation codon (also known as −5T/C and Kozak), and a 39 bp variable number of tandem repeat (VNTR) polymorphism in the coding region (encoding 13 amino acids) which results in four isoforms, designated D, C, B, and A. There are a few reports of association between Thr145Met *GP1BA* and acute MI [47,48]. However, other small studies examining the relationship between these polymorphisms and MI and stroke have been inconsistent. A recent study suggests that the Thr145Met *GP1BA* polymorphism may be associated with MI in subjects with dyslipidemia, but not in those without dyslipidemia [49], suggesting a possible interaction that could explain inconsistencies among studies.

In summary, a large number of association analyses have been performed on specific polymorphisms in platelet glycoprotein genes. Some have clear effects on expression of the protein and/or platelet function. However, no definitive conclusions can be made with regard to their role in arterial thrombosis events. It is intriguing that, for both the 807C/T *ITBG2* and Thr145Met *GP1BA* variants, larger more consistent associations with thrombotic disease appear in those with younger onset and in smokers, suggesting an effect in those more predisposed to thrombosis. Additional large population-based and prospective studies will be necessary to define further the possible role of common platelet glycoprotein genes in atherosclerosis.

Soluble factors

Fibrinogen

Human fibrinogen is a 340 kDa glycoprotein consisting of three nonidentical polypeptides (α, β, γ) linked by disulfide bonds. There is a linear relationship between fibrinogen levels and traditional risk factors such as tobacco use, age, diabetes, total cholesterol, physical inactivity, and hypertension. Elevated fibrinogen levels have been consistently associated with arterial thrombosis, especially in smokers [50–53]. Prospective studies have shown an 84% increase in the 5 year risk of ischemic heart events for each standard deviation increase in serum fibrinogen above the mean [50]. In the PROCAM study, the incidence of coronary events in the upper tertile of the plasma fibrinogen distribution was twofold higher than in the lower tertile. Maresca and coworkers [54] performed a meta-analysis of 22 studies and found that the risk of cardiovascular events in subjects with plasma fibrinogen levels in the highest tertile was twice as high as that of subjects in the lower one (odds ratio 1.99). What remains to be determined is whether fibrinogen levels are a causal risk factor or the result of inflammation associated with atherosclerosis.

High concentrations of fibrinogen lead to formation of a tightly packed fibrin clot and increased blood viscosity. Mechanisms that may explain the association of increased fibrinogen with arterial thrombosis include increased platelet aggregation, increased fibrin formation, and smooth muscle proliferation. Fibrinogen contributes to atherosclerosis by migrating into injured vessel walls where it forms crosslinked fibrin. This process leads to release of inflammatory mediators, platelet aggregation, and smooth muscle proliferation. Fibrinogen is also an acute phase reactant, in part due to IL-6 responsive elements in the promoter regions of all three fibrinogen chains.

The three fibrinogen polypeptides are encoded by three genes (*FGA*, *FGB*, *FGG*) located on chromosome 4q28. A large number of rare mutations in the fibrinogen genes have been identified as causes of familial dysfibrinogenemia and afibrinogenemia syndromes [55,56]. Typically encoding missense or frameshift mutations, individuals carrying such mutations are often asymptomatic, but also may have bleeding diathesis and/or thrombotic tendencies typically associated with trauma. Amyloidosis with renal complications have also been reported.

Several common polymorphisms have been identified in the three fibrinogen subunit genes. Those most intensively studied are summarized in Table 13.1. Despite being located in all three genes, these variants are in linkage

Table 13.1 Common variants in the three fibrinogen gene subunits

β-Chain	G854A	Elevated plasma fibrinogen
β-Chain	−455G/A	Elevated plasma fibrinogen
β-Chain	BclI	Elevated plasma fibrinogen
α-Chain	Thr312Ala	Increased α/α-crosslinking
γ-Chain	T9340C	Elevated plasma fibrinogen

disequilibrium, thus making it difficult to dissect genetically which (if any) is responsible for association with fibrinogen levels or related traits. These variants have been associated with altered levels of fibrinogen; however their relationship with thrombotic events is less well established [57]. β-Chain polymorphisms have been the most intensely studied because β-chain synthesis is the rate-limiting step in the production of fibrinogen. The two most studied polymorphisms are a BclI polymorphism in the 3′ untranslated region and −455G/A, the latter of which is in close proximity to the IL-6 responsive element in the regulatory region. Early studies investigated these single-gene variants with equivocal results with regard to association with arterial thrombosis [58–60]. Recently, Jood and coworkers [61] used a haplotype tagging approach in 600 Scandinavian stroke cases and an equal number of controls and found two distinct haplotype blocks, one encompassing *FGG* and *FGA* and the other encompassing *FGB*, that were associated with ischemic stroke. In the Rotterdam Study, similar associations between haplotypes and small-vessel ischemic disease were found [62], but there was no evidence for association with coronary disease in this same population [63]. Similarly, lack of association of fibrinogen locus haplotypes with MI were reported in a large study of German subjects [64]. By contrast, Mannila and coworkers [65] identified certain fibrinogen locus haplotypes that were associated with MI. Consistent associations of fibrinogen genotypes with fibrinogen levels but less consistent associations with arterial thrombosis may be because the effect of these genotypes on fibrinogen levels are too modest to be of major clinical significance.

Plasminogen activator inhibitor 1

Plasminogen activator inhibitor 1 (PAI1) is a key component of the fibrinolytic system. Genetic deficiency of PAI1 due to a homozygous frameshift mutation results in abnormal bleeding after trauma or surgery in affected individuals [66,67]. Elevated levels of PAI1 are associated with increased arterial thrombotic disease [68].

The gene encoding PAI1 is located on chromosome 7q21.3–q22 and contains nine exons spanning 11.9 kb. Many studies have examined common variants in this gene. The most often studied variant is a single G insertion in the regulatory region (−675 4G/5G). *In vitro* studies indicate a functional consequence, with the 4G variant resulting in increased transcription compared with the 5G variant [69]. However, studies of association of this variant with thrombotic events have been inconsistent, with some studies showing modest evidence for association with MI and atherosclerotic disease and others not [70–72]. Meta-analysis supports a modest role for this variant in MI risk [73] and stroke [74]; however such analyses are subject to publication bias since some negative studies are never published. Thus, in general, meta-analyses must be interpreted with caution.

Other soluble factors that have been investigated, but without definitive results, include tissue plasminogen activator (TPA), von Willebrand factor (vWF), factors V, VII, XII, and XIII, and prothrombin. As with other soluble factor candidate genes described above, association between common variants and arterial thrombosis phenotypes have been inconclusive.

The endothelium, nitric oxide, and nitric oxide synthase

To a large extent, nitric oxide (NO) modulates the interaction between platelets and the endothelium. In the critical microenvironment where circulating platelets come into contact with the endothelium, nitric oxide affects platelet functions in at least two ways. It is a direct platelet inhibitor via a cyclic guanosine monophosphate (GMP)-mediated mechanism. NO also reduces oxidative stress via a free radical scavenging mechanism and this, in turn, leads to a relative suppression of transcriptional activation of genes which code for adhesion molecules [75]. As platelets encounter normally functioning endothelium, nitric oxide acts to prevent the initiation of platelet activation. Decreased nitric oxide production by endothelium damaged by trauma or rendered dysfunctional by disease creates a prothrombotic state. This is one of the molecular mechanisms underlying Virchow's original observation that injury to the vessel wall predisposes to thrombosis.

Polymorphisms of the endothelium nitric oxide synthase gene (*NOS3*) that cause deficiency of nitric oxide production have long been postulated to contribute to an arterial prothrombotic state. *NOS3* is encoded by 27 exons spanning 23.5 kb on chromosome 7q36. Several polymorphisms of *NOS3* have been described, the most commonly studied include a nonsynonymous variant Glu298Asp, −786T/C in the promoter region, and a VNTR in intron 4. As early as 1999, small studies suggested that the Glu298Asp variant was associated with coronary artery disease [76]. Subsequent studies in different populations made this original observation controversial [77]. Casas and coworkers [78] performed a meta-analysis of 26 case–control studies evaluating the association between the NOS3 polymorphisms and ischemic heart disease (MI or angiographic coronary artery occlusion), involving 9867 cases and 13 161 controls. They found that homozygosity for Asp298 or the intron 4 A allele was associated with an increased risk of ischemic heart disease (odds ratios 1.31 and

1.34, respectively), but no significant association was found with the −786C allele. A few recent studies in a variety of populations support the concept that certain polymorphisms of the eNOS gene increase risk for atherothrombotic disease [79–85]. Additional work in larger populations will be required to better understand the role of this endothelium-expressed gene in arterial thrombosis.

Summary and future directions

To date, candidate gene studies seeking association of common variants with arterial thrombosis have been equivocal. These studies suffer from a number of limitations. The genetic architecture of the candidate genes investigated to date has not been studied in sufficient detail. Now with much greater knowledge of common variation across the genome coupled with less expensive and higher throughput genotyping and sequencing technologies, it is now possible to study multiple variants in candidate genes to capture most or all of the common variation in the candidate gene under study. A more comprehensive investigation of candidate genes is now possible with a commercially available chip in which 50 000 single nucleotide polymorphisms in more than 2000 cardiovascular candidate genes can be studied [86]. Second, candidate gene approaches are limited by our incomplete knowledge of the pathways and mechanisms responsible for arterial thrombosis. Moving toward genome-wide approaches in which common variation throughout the genome, agnostic to specific candidate genes, will be an important next step in expanding the search for genetic variation responsible for arterial thrombosis. For example, a recent genome-wide association analysis for myocardial infarction identified a locus on chromosome 9p21 [87,88]. This locus, near the CDK2NA/B genes, has been robustly replicated by several groups. Our work suggests that this increased risk may be mediated, in part, through alternations in platelet function [89].

Both genome-wide analyses and comprehensive candidate gene analyses enhance the likelihood of false-positive findings owing to the fact that many gene variants are being analyzed. Thus, much larger sample sizes and similarly powered replication sample sets will be necessary to confirm putative associations. Another limitation is that arterial thrombosis is very heterogeneous in which multiple factors and pathways contribute risk. Defining a more homogeneous group of individuals through more detailed phenotyping may afford better opportunities for success. Finally, finding true positive and well-replicated associations between a gene variant (or chromosomal region) and arterial thrombosis is the first step toward understanding its biology. Follow-up *in vitro* and *in vivo* animal and human studies to better understand molecular mechanisms by which specific genetic variants increase risk will be critical to the application of such knowledge to develop new strategies for prevention and treatment of diseases caused by arterial thrombosis.

References

1 Rosamond W, Flegal K, Furie K *et al.* American Heart Association Statistics Committee and Stroke Statistics Subcommittee. Heart disease and stroke statistics—2008 update: a report from the American Heart Association Statistics Committee and Stroke Statistics Subcommittee. *Circulation* 2008; 117: e25–146.

2 Ross R. Atherosclerosis is an inflammatory disease. *American Heart Journal* 1999; **138**: S418–S420.

3 Wagner DD, Burger PC. Platelets in inflammation and thrombosis. *Arteriosclerosis Thrombosis and Vascular Biology* 2003; **23**: 2131–2137.

4 Hokanson JE. Hypertriglyceridemia and risk of coronary heart disease. *Current Cardiology Reports* 2002; **4**: 488–493.

5 Rader DJ, Daugherty A. Translating molecular discoveries into new therapies for atherosclerosis. *Nature* 2008; **451**: 904–913.

6 Marchiori A, Mosena L, Prins MH, Prandoni P. The risk of recurrent venous thromboembolism among heterozygous carriers of factor V Leiden or prothrombin G20210A mutation. A systematic review of prospective studies. *Haematologica* 2007; **92**: 1107–1114.

7 Rosendorff A, Dorfman DM. Activated protein C resistance and factor V Leiden: a review. *Archives of Pathology and Laboratory Medicine* 2007; **131**: 866–871.

8 Feero WG. Genetic thrombophilia. *Primary Care* 2004; **31**: 685–709.

9 Snoep JD, Hovens MMC, Eikenboom JCJ *et al.* Association of laboratory-defined aspirin resistance with a higher risk of recurrent cardiovascular events: a systematic review and meta-analysis. *Archives of Internal Medicine* 2007; **167**: 1593–1599.

10 Krasopoulos G, Brister SJ, Beattie WS, Buchanan MR. Aspirin "resistance" and risk of cardiovascular morbidity: systematic review and meta-analysis. *BMJ* 2008; **336**: 195–198.

11 Shah U, Ma AD. Tests of platelet function. *Current Opinion in Hematology* 2007; **14**: 432–437.

12 Zeidan AM, Kouides PA, Tara MA, Fricke WA. Platelet function testing: state of the art. *Expert Reviews of Cardiovascular Therapy* 2007; **5**: 955–967.

13 O'Donnell CJ, Larson MG, Feng D *et al.* Genetic and environmental contributions to platelet aggregation: the Framingham heart study. *Circulation* 2001: **103**; 3051–3056.

14 Gaxiola B, Friedl W, Propping P. Epinephrine-induced platelet aggregation. A twin study. *Clinical Genetics* 1984; **26**: 543–548.

15 Bray PF, Mathias RA, Faraday N *et al.* Heritability of platelet function in families with premature coronary artery disease. *Journal of Thrombosis and Haemostasis* 2007; **5**: 1617–1623.

16 Feng D, Lindpaintner K, Larson MG *et al.* Increased platelet aggregability associated with platelet GPIIIa PlA2 polymorphism: the Framingham Offspring Study. *Arteriosclerosis Thrombosis and Vascular Biology* 1999; **19**: 1142–1147.

17 Michelson AD, Furman MI, Goldschmidt-Clermont P *et al.* Platelet GP IIIa Pl(A) polymorphisms display different sensitivities to agonists. *Circulation* 2000; **101**: 1013–1018.

18 Weiss EJ, Bray PF, Tayback M *et al.* A polymorphism of a platelet glycoprotein receptor as an inherited risk factor for coronary thrombosis. *New England Journal of Medicine* 1996; **334**: 1090–1094.

19 Carter AM, Ossei-Gerning N, Wilson IJ, Grant PJ. Association of the platelet Pl(A) polymorphism of glycoprotein IIb/IIIa and the fibrinogen Bbeta 448 polymorphism with myocardial infarction and extent of coronary artery disease. *Circulation* 1997; **96**: 1424–1431.
20 Ardissino D, Mannucci PM, Merlini PA *et al.* Prothrombotic genetic risk factors in young survivors of myocardial infarction. *Blood* 1999; **94**: 46–51.
21 Anderson JL, King GJ, Bair TL *et al.* Associations between a polymorphism in the gene encoding glycoprotein IIIa and myocardial infarction or coronary artery disease. *Journal of the American College of Cardiology* 1999; **33**: 727–733.
22 Garcia-Ribes M, Gonzalez-Lamuño D, Hernandez-Estefania R *et al.* Polymorphism of the platelet glycoprotein IIIa gene in patients with coronary stenosis. *Thrombosis and Haemostasis* 1998; **79**: 1126–1129.
23 Herrmann SM, Poirier O, Marques-Vidal P *et al.* The Leu33/Pro polymorphism (PlA1/PlA2) of the glycoprotein IIIa (GPIIIa) receptor is not related to myocardial infarction in the ECTIM Study. Etude Cas-Temoins de l'Infarctus du Myocarde. *Thrombosis and Haemostasis* 1997; **77**: 1179–1181.
24 Scaglione L, Bergerone S, Gaschino G *et al.* Lack of relationship between the P1A1/P1A2 polymorphism of platelet glycoprotein IIIa and premature myocardial infarction. *European Journal of Clinical Investigation* 1998; **28**: 385–388.
25 Mamotte CD, van Bockxmeer FM, Taylor RR Pla1/a2 polymorphism of glycoprotein IIIa and risk of coronary arter disease and restenosis following coronary angioplasty. *American Journal of Cardiology* 1998; **82**: 13–16.
26 Ridker PM, Hennekens CH, Schmitz C *et al.* PIA1/A2 polymorphism of platelet glycoprotein IIIa and risks of myocardial infarction, stroke, and venous thrombosis. *Lancet* 1997; **349**: 385–388.
27 Williams MS, Bray PF. Genetics of arterial prothrombotic risk states. *Experimental Biology and Medicine (Maywood, NJ)* 2001; **226**: 409–419.
28 Knowles JW, Wang H, Itakura H *et al.* Association of polymorphisms in platelet and hemostasis system genes with acute myocardial infarction. *American Heart Journal* 2007; **154**: 1052–1058.
29 Di Castelnuovo A, de Gaetano G, Donati MB, Iacoviello L. Platelet glycoprotein receptor IIIa polymorphism PLA1/PLA2 and coronary risk: a meta-analysis. *Thrombosis and Haemostasis* 2001; **85**: 626–633.
30 Cooke GE, Bray PF, Hamlington JD *et al.* PlA2 polymorphism and efficacy of aspirin. *Lancet* 1998; **351**: 1253.
31 Dropinski J, Musial J, Sanak M *et al.* Antithrombotic effects of aspirin based on PLA1/A2 glycoprotein IIIa polymorphism in patients with coronary artery disease. *Thrombosis Research* 2007; **119**: 301–303.
32 Cooke GE, Liu-Stratton Y, Ferketich AK *et al.* Effect of platelet antigen polymorphism on platelet inhibition by aspirin, clopidogrel, or their combination. *Journal of the American College of Cardiology* 2006; **47**: 541–546.
33 Kranzhofer R, Ruef J. Aspirin resistance in coronary artery disease is correlated to elevated markers for oxidative stress but not to the expression of cyclooxygenase (COX) 1/2, a novel COX-1 polymorphism or the PlA(1/2) polymorphism. *Platelets* 2006; **17**: 163–169.

34 Lev EI, Patel RT, Guthikonda S *et al.* Genetic polymorphisms of the platelet receptors P2Y(12), P2Y(1) and GP IIIa and response to aspirin and clopidogrel. *Thrombosis Research* 2007; **119**: 355–360.

35 Kunicki TJ, Kritzik M, Annis DS, Nugent DJ. Hereditary variation in platelet integrin alpha-2-beta-1 density is associated with two silent polymorphisms in the alpha-2 gene coding sequence. *Blood* 1997; **89**: 1939–1943.

36 Kritzik M, Savage B, Nugent DJ *et al.* Nucleotide polymorphisms in the alpha-2 gene define multiple alleles that are associated with differences in platelet alpha-2/beta-1 density. *Blood* 1998; **92**: 2382–2388

37 Cadroy Y, Sakariassen KS, Charlet JP *et al.* Role of 4 platelet membrane glycoprotein polymorphisms on experimental arterial thrombus formation in men. *Blood* 2001; **98**: 3159–3161.

38 Santoso S, Kunicki TJ, Kroll H *et al.* Association of the platelet glycoprotein Ia C807T gene polymorphism with nonfatal myocardial infarction in younger patients. *Blood* 1999; **93**: 2449–2453.

39 Carlsson LE, Santoso S, Spitzer C *et al.* The alpha-2 gene coding sequence T807/A873 of the platelet collagen receptor integrin alpha-2/beta-1 might be a genetic risk factor for the development of stroke in younger patients. *Blood* 1999; **93**: 3583–3586.

40 Antoniades C, Tousoulis D, Vasiliadou C *et al.* Genetic polymorphisms of platelet glycoprotein Ia and the risk for premature myocardial infarction: effects on the release of sCD40L during the acute phase of premature myocardial infarction. *Journal of the American College of Cardiology* 2006; **47**: 1959–1966.

41 Mikkelsson J, Perola M, Penttilä A, Karhunen PJ. Platelet collagen receptor GPIa (C807T/HPA-5) haplotype is not associated with an increased risk of fatal coronary events in middle-aged men. *Atherosclerosis* 2002; **165**: 111–118.

42 Atherosclerosis, Thrombosis and Vascular Biology Italian Study Group. No evidence of association between prothrombotic gene polymorphisms and the development of acute myocardial infarction at a young age. *Circulation* 2003; **107**: 1117–1122.

43 Nikolopoulos GK, Tsantes AE, Bagos P *et al.* Integrin, alpha 2 gene C807T polymorphism and risk of ischemic stroke: a meta-analysis. *Thrombosis Research* 2007; 119: 501–10.

44 Holmberg, L, Karpman D, Nilsson I, Olofsson T. Bernard-Soulier syndrome Karlstad: trp498-to-stop mutation resulting in a truncated glycoprotein Ib-alpha that contains part of the transmembranous domain. *British Journal of Haematology* 1997; **98**: 57–63.

45 Noda M, Fujimura K, Takafuta T *et al.* Heterogeneous expression of glycoprotein Ib, IX and V in platelets from two patients with Bernard-Soulier syndrome caused by different genetic abnormalities. *Thrombosis and Haemostasis* 1995; **74**: 1411–1415.

46 Murata M, Furihata K, Ishida F *et al.* Genetic and structural characterization of an amino acid dimorphism in glycoprotein Ib-alpha involved in platelet transfusion refractoriness. *Blood* 1992; **79**: 3086–3090.

47 Gonzalez-Conejero R, Lozano ML, Rivera J *et al.* Polymorphisms of platelet membrane glycoprotein Ib associated with arterial thrombotic disease. *Blood* 1998; **92**: 2771–2776.

48 Murata M, Matsubara Y, Kawano K *et al.* Coronary artery disease and polymorphisms in a receptor mediating shear stress-dependent platelet activation. *Circulation* 1997; **96**: 3281–3286.

49 Yoshida T, Yajima K, Hibino T *et al*. Association of gene polymorphisms with myocardial infarction in individuals with different lipid profiles. *International Journal of Molecular Medicine* 2007; **20**: 581–590.
50 Heinrich J, Balleisen L, Schulte H, Assmann G. Fibrinogen and factor VII in the prediction of coronary risk. Results from the PROCAM study in healthy men. *Arteriosclerosis and Thrombosis* 1994; **14**: 54–59.
51 Eriksson M, Egberg N, Wamala S *et al*. Relationship between plasma fibrinogen and coronary heart disease in women. *Arteriosclerosis Thrombosis and Vascular Biology* 1999; **19**: 67–72.
52 Kannel WB, Wolf PA, Castelli WP, D'Agostino RB. Fibrinogen and risk of cardiovascular disease. The Framingham Study. *JAMA: the Journal of the American Medical Association* 1987; **258**: 1183–1186.
53 Green D, Foiles N, Chan C *et al*. Elevated fibrinogen levels and subsequent subclinical atherosclerosis: The CARDIA Study. *Atherosclerosis* 2008. Epub ahead of print.
54 Maresca G, Di Blasio A, Marchioli R, Di Minno G. Measuring plasma fibrinogen to predict stroke and myocardial infarction: an update. *Arteriosclerosis Thrombosis and Vascular Biology* 1999; **19**: 1368–1377.
55 Asselta R, Duga S, Tenchini ML. The molecular basis of quantitative fibrinogen disorders. *Journal of Thrombosis and Haemostasis* 2006; **4**: 2115–2129.
56 Neerman-Arbez M. Molecular basis of fibrinogen deficiency. *Pathophysiology of Haemostasis and Thrombosis* 2006; **35**: 187–198.
57 Lane DA, Grant PJ. Role of hemostatic gene polymorphisms in venous and arterial thrombotic disease. *Blood* 2000; **95**: 1517–1532.
58 Tybjaerg-Hansen A, Agerholm-Larsen B, Humphries SE *et al*. A common mutation (G-455→A) in the beta-fibrinogen promoter is an independent predictor of plasma fibrinogen, but not of ischemic heart disease. A study of 9,127 individuals based on the Copenhagen City Heart Study. *Journal of Clinical Investigation* 1997; **99**: 3034–3039.
59 Zito F, Di Castelnuovo A, Amore C *et al*. Bcl I polymorphism in the fibrinogen beta-chain gene is associated with the risk of familial myocardial infarction by increasing plasma fibrinogen levels. A case-control study in a sample of GISSI-2 patients. *Arteriosclerosis Thrombosis and Vascular Biology* 1997; **17**: 3489–3494.
60 Doggen CJ, Bertina RM, Cats VM, Rosendaal FR. Fibrinogen polymorphisms are not associated with the risk of myocardial infarction. *British Journal of Haematology* 2000; **110**: 935–938.
61 Jood K, Danielson J, Ladenvall C *et al*. Fibrinogen gene variation and ischemic stroke. *Thrombosis and Haemostasis* 2008; **6**: 897–904.
62 van Oijen M, Cheung EY, Geluk CE *et al*. Haplotypes of the fibrinogen gene and cerebral small vessel disease: the Rotterdam scan study. *Journal of Neurology Neurosurgery and Psychiatry* 2008; **79**: 799–803.
63 Kardys I, Uitterlinden AG, Hofman A *et al*. Fibrinogen gene haplotypes in relation to risk of coronary events and coronary and extracoronary atherosclerosis: the Rotterdam Study. *Thrombosis and Haemostasis* 2007; **97**: 288–295.
64 Koch W, Hoppmann P, Biele J *et al*. Fibrinogen genes and myocardial infarction: a haplotype analysis. *Arteriosclerosis Thrombosis and Vascular Biology* 2008; **28**: 758–763.
65 Mannila MN, Eriksson P, Lundman P *et al*. Contribution of haplotypes across the fibrinogen gene cluster to variation in risk of myocardial infarction. *Thrombosis and Haemostasis* 2005; **93**: 570–577.

66 Fay WP, Shapiro AD, Shih JL *et al.* Complete deficiency of plasminogen-activator inhibitor type I due to a frameshift mutation. *New England Journal of Medicine* 1992; **327**: 1729–1733.
67 Hamsten A, de Faire U, Walldius G *et al.* Plasminogen activator inhibitor in plasma: risk factor for recurrent myocardial infarction. *Lancet* 1987; **2**: 3–9.
68 Scarabin PY, Aillaud MF, Amouyel P *et al.* Associations of fibrinogen, factor VII and PAI-1 with baseline findings among 10,500 male participants in a prospective study of myocardial infarction: the PRIME Study. Prospective Epidemiological Study of Myocardial Infarction. *Thrombosis and Haemostasis* 1998; **80**: 749–756.
69 Dawson SJ, Wiman B, Hamsten A *et al.* The two allele sequences of a common polymorphism in the promoter of the plasminogen activator inhibitor-1 (PAI-1) gene respond differently to interleukin-1 in HepG2 cells. *Journal of Biological Chemistry* 1993; **268**: 10739–10745.
70 Simmonds RE, Hermida J, Rezende SM, Lane DA. Haemostatic genetic risk factors in arterial thrombosis. *Thrombosis and Haemostasis* 2001; **86**: 374–385.
71 Ye S, Green FR, Scarabin PY *et al.* The 4G/5G genetic polymorphism in the promoter of the plasminogen activator inhibitor-1 (PAI-1) gene is associated with differences in plasma PAI-1 activity but not with risk of myocardial infarction in the ECTIM study. Etude Cas Temoins d'Infarctus du Mycocarde. *Thrombosis and Haemostasis* 1995; **74**: 837–841.
72 Anderson JL, Muhlestein JB, Habashi J *et al.* Lack of association of a common polymorphism of the plasminogen activator inhibitor-1 gene with coronary artery disease and myocardial infarction. *Journal of the American College of Cardiology* 1999; **34**: 1778–1783.
73 Iacoviello L, Burzotta F, Di Castelnuovo A, *et al.* The 4G/5G polymorphism of PAI-1 promoter gene and the risk of myocardial infarction: a meta-analysis. *Thrombosis and Haemostasis* 1998; **80**: 1029–1030.
74 Attia J, Thakkinstian A, Wang Y *et al.* The PAI-1 4G/5G gene polymorphism and ischemic stroke: an association study and meta-analysis. *Journal of Stroke and Cerebrovascular Diseases* 2007; **16**: 173–179.
75 Loscalzo J. Functional polymorphisms in a candidate gene for atherothrombosis. *Journal of the American College of Cardiology* 2003; **41**: 946–948.
76 Hingorani AD, Liang CF, Fatibene J *et al.* A common variant of the endothelial nitric oxide synthase (Glu→Asp) is a major risk factor for coronary artery disease in the UK. *Circulation* 1999; **100**: 1515–1520.
77 Casas JP, Cavalleri GL, Bautista LE *et al.* Endothelial nitric oxide synthase gene polymorphisms and cardiovascular disease: a HuGE review. *American Journal of Epidemiology* 2006; **164**: 921–935.
78 Casas JP, Bautista LE, Humphries SE, Hingorani AD. Endothelial nitric oxide synthase genotype and ischemic heart disease: meta-analysis of 26 studies involving 23028 subjects. *Circulation* 2004; **109**: 1359–1365.
79 Rossi GP, Cesari M, Zanchetta M *et al.* The T-786C endothelial nitric oxide synthase genotype is a novel risk factor for coronary artery disease in Caucasian patients of the GENICA study. *Journal of the American College of Cardiology* 2003; **41**: 930–937.
80 Rossi GP, Maiolino G, Zanchetta M *et al.* The $T^{-786}C$ endothelial nitric oxide synthase genotype predicts cardiovascular mortality in high-risk patients. *Journal of the American College of Cardiology* 2006; **48**: 1166–1174.

81 Rao S, Austin H, Davidoff MN, Zafari AM. Endothelial nitric oxide synthase intron 4 polymorphism is a marker for coronary artery disease in African-American and Caucasian men. *Ethnicity and Disease* 2005; **15**: 191–197.
82 Rios DL, D'Onofrio LO, Souza JK *et al.* Smoking-dependent and haplotype-specific effects of endothelial nitric oxide synthase gene polymorphisms on angiographically assessed coronary artery disease in Caucasian- and African-Brazilians. *Atherosclerosis* 2007; **193**: 135–141.
83 Kim IJ, Bae J, Lim SW *et al.* Influence of endothelial nitric oxide synthase gene polymorphisms (-786T>C, 4a4b, 894G>T) in Korean patients with coronary artery disease. *Thrombosis Research* 2007; **119**: 579–585.
84 Morray B, Goldenberg I, Moss AJ *et al.* Polymorphisms in the paraoxonase and endothelial nitric oxide synthase genes and the risk of early onset myocardial infarction. *American Journal of Cardiology* 2007; **99**: 1100–1105.
85 Tamemoto H, Ishikawa S, Kawakami M. Association of the Glu298Asp polymorphism of the eNOS gene with ischemic heart disease in Japanese diabetic subjects. *Diabetes Research and Clinical Practice* 2008; **80**; 275–279.
86 Keating BJ, Tischfield S, Murray SS *et al.* Concept, design and implementation of a cardiovascular gene-centric 50 k SNP array for large-scale genomic association studies. *PLoS One* 2008; **3**: e3583.
87 Helgadottir A, Thorleifsson G, Manolescu A *et al.* A common variant on chromosome 9p21 affects the risk of myocardial infarction. *Science* 2007; **316**: 1491–1493.
88 Samani NJ, Erdmann J, Hall AS *et al.* Genomewide association analysis of coronary artery disease. *New England Journal of Medicine* 2007; **357**: 443–453.

Pharmacogenetics and pharmacogenomics

Julie A. Johnson, Issam Zineh, and Michael A. Pacanowski

Introduction

The goal of pharmacogenetics and pharmacogenomics is to unravel the genetic underpinnings of variable drug response, with the translational potential to utilize genetic information in drug therapy decision-making (Fig. 14.1) [1]. Pharmacogenetics is often used to describe the influence of single genes on drug response, while pharmacogenomics often refers to approaches that study large numbers of genes (up to the whole genome) for associating genetic polymorphisms with drug response variability. There are several potential areas in which genetic information might be used to optimize drug therapy. First, response rates across a variety of therapeutic drug classes average about 50% [2]. Thus, if it would be possible to identify those who will not benefit from therapy based on their genetic make-up, alternative therapeutic approaches could be pursued. Similarly, drugs are associated with certain risks, some of which are serious, and identification of those at risk would also be beneficial. Finally, understanding the relationship between drug efficacy and/or toxicity and genotype might help expedite drug discovery and drug development. In the case of drug discovery, knowledge of the genetic determinants of disease can help identify potential drug targets. Such an approach is being widely utilized in development of cancer chemotherapies, but as yet is minimally utilized in cardiovascular drug discovery. Drug development might also be advanced through pharmacogenetics or pharmacogenomics, whereby a genetic group that is responsive to therapy or likely to experience an endpoint of interest might be identified in early-phase clinical trials, with later trials enriching enrollment with that group, making an

Cardiovascular Genetics and Genomics. Edited by Dan Roden. © 2009 American Heart Association, ISBN: 978-14051-7540-1.

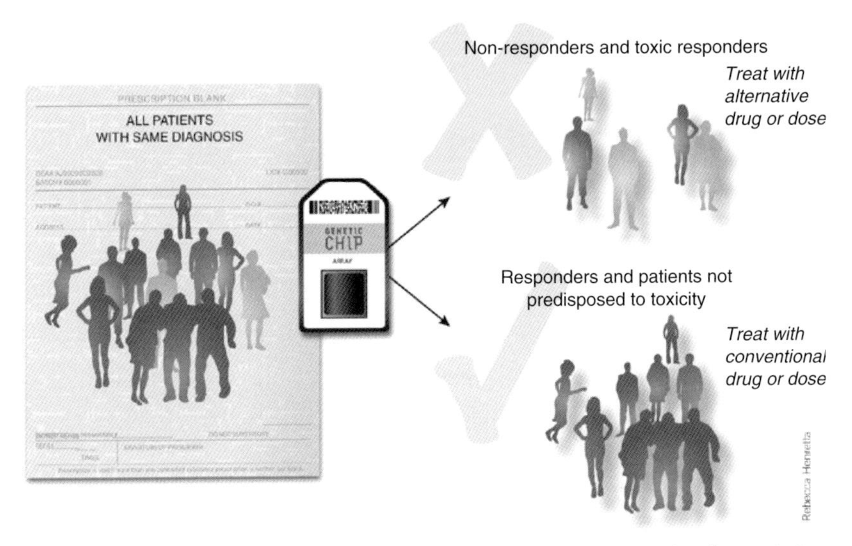

Fig. 14.1 Paradigmatic approach to pharmacogenetic medicine. (Reprinted with permission from Piquette-Miller and Grant [1].)

efficacy endpoint easier to achieve. An indirect example of this in cardiovascular disease is BiDil, the combination of isosorbide dinitrate and hydralazine. Data from earlier clinical trials with this drug combination suggested that African Americans derived more benefit from this therapy than whites. Thus, a study was conducted that enrolled only African Americans in an event-driven heart failure clinical trial, and was able to show significant clinical benefit in this targeted population [3]. Many believe that, in this study, African ancestry simply is a surrogate for a gene (or genes) that influences response to this combination, and for which the responsive allele is more common in those of African ancestry. Such a targeted approach to drug development potentially increases the likelihood for a drug to reach its efficacy endpoint in phase III clinical trials.

Herein we will discuss ongoing pharmacogenetics and pharmacogenomics research and potential clinical implications for cardiovascular drugs. While there are a large number of published cardiovascular pharmacogenetic studies, we will focus on those that have been best replicated, and thus have, at present, the best potential for translation into practice. We will also attempt to provide insight into how pharmacogenetics and pharmacogenomics might be utilized in the practice of cardiovascular medicine in the future.

Research approaches in pharmacogenetics and pharmacogenomics

There are different approaches that can be taken in identifying the genetic variants associated with variable drug response. Historically, the primary approach was to focus on a candidate gene, meaning the gene for a protein that might be reasonably expected to be associated with response variability (e.g., the protein target or metabolizing enzyme of the drug). Initially, this approach focused on only one or two genes, and a few single nucleotide polymorphisms (SNPs) within those genes. With advances in genotyping technologies, the candidate gene approaches have expanded to include tens to hundreds of genes. Additionally, based on findings from the International HapMap project [4], these studies no longer focus on a few SNPs, but often utilize an approach that selects SNPs to explain variability across the entire gene (called tag SNPs) [5]. In general the candidate gene approach has been fruitful in pharmacogenetics, owing in part to the fact that the pharmacology and pharmacokinetic properties of the drugs are typically well defined and thus genes that influence response may be easier to identify than in situations where the goal is to define the genetic basis of disease.

More recently, genome-wide association approaches have become more common. In this approach, 300 000 to 1 million SNPs across the genome are genotyped and then tested for association with the relevant drug response. The goal here is to identify additional genes that might contribute to drug response variability, particularly those that would not have been intuitive a priori in the candidate gene approach.

Most of the published literature is from candidate gene studies, and to date there have been no publications of genome-wide associations with cardiovascular drug response. However, there are numerous such studies ongoing and thus the fruits of these studies will be forthcoming. Throughout this chapter the official gene abbreviations will be utilized but the corresponding names for these genes can be found in Table 14.1.

Hypertension pharmacogenetics

Hypertension is the most common chronic disease in Westernized societies, with an estimated 72 million Americans affected [6]. There are five antihypertensive drug classes recommended as first-line therapy [7], although data suggest that, despite the plethora of agents available to treat the disease, blood pressure (BP) control is far from optimal. Specifically, estimates suggest that 42% of treated hypertensives do not have their BP controlled (i.e., <140/90 mmHg), with another 16% who know they have hypertension but are untreated [7]. These sobering statistics may be influenced in part by the fact that any given antihypertensive will produce only a reasonable antihypertensive response in about 50% of the population when used as monotherapy [8], but there are few mechanisms for identifying which patients will respond to which medications. In the case of treated but uncontrolled hypertensives, it may be possible to improve BP control if those genetically predisposed to respond to a given therapy could be identified prior to therapy. Additionally,

Table 14.1 Gene symbols and names

Gene symbol	Gene name
ABCB1	ATP-binding cassette, subfamily B, member 1
ABCG5	ATP-binding cassette, subfamily G, member 5
ABCG8	ATP-binding cassette, subfamily G, member 8
ACE	Angiotensin-converting enzyme
ADD1	α-Adducin
ADRA2C	α_{2C}-Adrenergic receptor
ADRB1	β_1-Adrenergic receptor
AGT	Angiotensinogen
AGTR1	Angiotensin II receptor, type 1
APOA1	Apolipoprotein A1
APOB	Apolipoprotein B
APOE	Apolipoprotein E
CETP	Cholesteryl ester transfer protein
CYP2C19	Cytochrome P450, subfamily 2C, polypeptide 19
CYP2C9	Cytochrome P450, subfamily 2C, polypeptide 9
CYP2D6	Cytochrome P450, subfamily 2D, polypeptide 6
CYP3A4	Cytochrome P450, subfamily 3A, polypeptide 4
CYP3A5	Cytochrome P450, subfamily 3A, polypeptide 5
CYP7A1	Cytochrome P450, subfamily 7A, polypeptide 1
FDFT1	Squalene synthase
HMGCR	3-α-3-Hydroxy-3-methylglutaryl coenzyme A reductase
KCNA5	Potassium voltage-gated channel, shaker-related subfamily, member 5
KCNH2	Potassium voltage-gated channel, subfamily H (eag-related), member 2; HERG
KCNQ1	Potassium voltage-gated channel, KQT-like subfamily, member 1
LDLR	Low-density lipoprotein receptor
LIPC	Hepatic lipase
LPL	Lipoprotein lipase
NOS3	Endothelial nitric oxide synthase
P2Y12	Purinergic receptor P2Y, G-protein coupled, 12; ADP receptor
PTGS1	Cyclooxygenase 1 or prostaglandin-endoperoxide synthase 1
SCN5A	Sodium channel, voltage-gated, type V, alpha subunit
VKORC1	Vitamin K epoxide reductase complex, subunit 1

data suggest that failure to persist with antihypertensive therapy is high among newly diagnosed hypertensives, and a potential cause of poor persistence is that the prescribed therapy either caused adverse effects or failed to reduce their blood pressure. Additionally, hypertension is treated to reduce the incidence of the long-term adverse cardiovascular outcomes [namely myocardial infarction (MI), stroke, heart failure (HF), renal failure], and, while it is possible to measure the BP response to a drug in an individual patient, it is not possible to measure prevention of these adverse outcomes in an individual patient. Thus, there are numerous potential benefits associated with identification of the genetic variants associated with blood pressure and event reduction with antihypertensive drugs.

Among the first-line antihypertensive agents, the beta-blockers have the most compelling pharmacogenetic data to date. Numerous (although not all) studies that have investigated the influence of common SNPs in the β_1-adrenergic receptor gene (*ADRB1*) have shown that the Arg389 homozygous genotype is associated with significantly better BP lowering than those who carry a Gly389 allele [9–13]. An example of differences in response by genotype is shown in Fig. 14.2, in which the influence of polymorphisms at codons 49 and 389 are depicted. These data are consistent with functional studies that suggest that the Arg389 form of the receptor couples more efficiently to G-protein, resulting in enhanced signal transduction [14]. Taken together these data suggest that the polymorphisms in *ADRB1* may have future clinical utility in identifying those hypertensives who are the best candidates for beta-blocker therapy.

Despite many studies on the genetic associations with angiotensin-converting enzyme (ACE) inhibitor or angiotensin receptor blocker (ARB) response, there have been few consistent findings across pharmacogenetic studies evaluating the

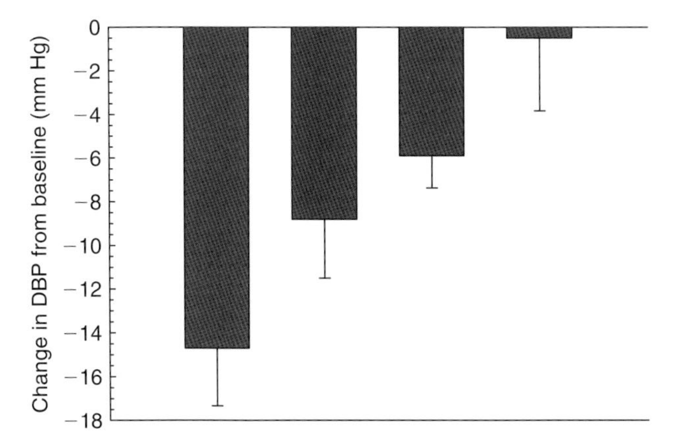

Fig. 14.2 Blood pressure response to metoprolol by *ADRB1* diplotype. SR, Ser49Arg389; SG, Ser49Gly389; GR, Gly49Arg389. (Reprinted with permission from Johnson *et al.* [13].)

drug targets, ACE, and the angiotensin II receptor [15]. There have been some recent papers suggesting that the angiotensinogen gene (*AGT*) may represent an interesting marker for BP response and outcomes in hypertension, although further work is needed because the directions of the associations are not always consistent [16–19].

Regarding the diuretics, there have been several studies (but not all) suggesting an association with the α-adducin gene (*ADD1*) and BP response [15,20–22], along with one suggesting different outcomes based on genotype among diuretic-treated hypertensives [23]. However, the latter finding was not replicated in genetic substudies from the very large ALLHAT [24] and INVEST [25] studies. Thus, the role of this polymorphism remains to be defined. There have been numerous other genes associated with the BP response to diuretics, but most have been shown in only a single study and contribute minimally to the response phenotype [15].

Clinical implications for pharmacogenetics in hypertension

Pharmacogenetics has a high potential clinical value in hypertension, through helping to identify the drug that either would lead to the best BP lowering or would be associated with the greatest event reduction. At present *ADRB1* polymorphisms (notably Arg389Gly) represent the only example with potential for near-term translation to practice. For this gene, there have been numerous genetic association studies suggesting the Arg389 homozygous genotype has the greatest blood pressure lowering, with more recent data suggesting that beta-blockers provide superior reduction in adverse cardiovascular events for those with this genotype [26]. If the latter findings can be replicated in independent cohorts, this would suggest that those with the target genotype/haplotype should receive beta-blockers to reduce adverse cardiovascular outcomes. For *ADD1* and the diuretic response, several studies suggest an association with blood pressure response, but this does not appear to translate into differences in outcomes. The other potentially interesting gene at present is *AGT*, which may influence response to ACE inhibitors (and presumably ARBs), but further work is required before such information could be translated to practice.

Dyslipidemia pharmacogenetics

Dyslipidemia is an important worldwide modifiable risk factor for first MI, and is amenable to drug therapy with such agents as HMG-CoA reductase inhibitors (statins), PPAR-α agonists (fibrates), niacin, bile acid resins, and cholesterol absorption inhibitors (ezetimibe) [27,28]. Despite widespread use of drugs to correct lipoprotein abnormalities, there is tremendous variability in drug response in terms of both lipoprotein and inflammatory protein changes and cardiovascular risk reduction [12,29–31]. Because of the healthcare resources expended on dyslipidemia management and uncertainty in drug responses, pharmacogenetics-enhanced treatment algorithms may prove to be important in streamlining primary and secondary disease prevention.

While pharmacogenetics studies have been performed for nonstatin agents, the majority of evaluations have been conducted in cohorts of statin-treated individuals [32]. Furthermore, the clear majority of statin pharmacogenetic studies has been performed using a candidate gene approach. Candidate genes in statin pharmacogenetic studies include those involved in drug metabolism (e.g., CYP enzyme genes), drug transport (e.g., organic anion transporters), cholesterol biosynthesis, and lipoprotein metabolism [33]. Furthermore, because of growing interest in the low-density lipoprotein (LDL)-independent effect of statins, candidate genes have grown to include related enzyme targets such as the gene which encodes endothelial nitric oxide synthase (*NOS*).

While relatively small published studies are increasing in number, two large studies remain the hallmarks of statin pharmacogenetics to date. The first is a 10-candidate-gene association study of the prospectively executed Pravastatin Inflammation/CRP Evaluation (PRINCE) study [34]. In this retrospective analysis, investigators explored whether any of 148 SNPs in the *ABCG5, ABCG8, APOB, APOE, CETP, CYP3A4, CYP3A5, FDFT1, HMGCR*, and *LDLR* genes were associated with variable lipoprotein responses to pravastatin 40 mg/day among the 1536 individuals treated for 24 weeks. It was found that two highly linked SNPs in the *HMGCR* gene (whose encoded protein is the target of statin therapy) were associated with variable lipid responses such that variant carriers had roughly 20% smaller reductions in total cholesterol and LDL than individuals with two common copies of the gene. This association remained robust even after rigorously controlling for multiple comparisons.

In an even larger study, Thompson *et al.* [35] investigated whether SNPs in 16 candidate genes were associated with lipoprotein responses to a variety of statins studied in the Atorvastatin Comparative Cholesterol Efficacy and Safety Study (ACCESS) program. In addition to many of the genes studied in PRINCE, the investigators also explored *ABCB1, ACE, APOA1, CYP7A1, LIPC*, and *LPL*. Analysis of this 2735-patient database revealed that the well-studied triallelic polymorphism in *APOE* (ε2/ε3/ε4) was associated with variable LDL responses to statins. This finding replicated previous studies that demonstrated variable lipoprotein responses to statins by *APOE* genotype [36].

In addition to these and other fairly large analyses, novel modeling approaches to exploring genetic determinants of statin efficacy (and myotoxicity) are being employed [37,38]. For example, Ruano *et al.* [36] conducted an analysis of 10 vascular function genes and found that creatine kinase activity (a surrogate for myopathy) in patients taking statins was associated with variation in *NOS3* and the angiotensin II type 1 receptor gene (*AGTR1*). These evolving methods highlight increasing activity in the area of statin pharmacogenetic research.

Clinical implications for pharmacogenetics in dyslipidemia

As with pharmacogenetics in general, there are limitations to the currently published statin pharmacogenetic studies. For example, there is a paucity of whole genome studies in this area, the impact of variable lipoprotein responses on clinical outcomes is uncertain, pharmacogenetic studies of statin pleiotropic effects are limited, and replication of significant genetic associations is inconsistent. However, integrative research programs that include clinicians, basic and translational scientists, statistical geneticists, and bioinformaticians are increasingly being developed. Consequently, it is conceivable that, for such widely used drugs as the statins, future policy interventions (e.g., at the health system or managed care levels) would include genotype-enhanced therapeutic decisions. Particularly relevant to clinicians, there are ongoing efforts to identify the genetic risks for statin-mediated myalgia and myopathy. Regardless of whether genotyping will be routinely performed to predict statin side-effects, studies like the above-mentioned analyses by Ruano *et al.* [37] and the Marshfield Clinic investigators will likely serve as paradigms for the conduct of pharmacogenetic evaluations of severe, rare adverse drug events. Furthermore, it is clear that LDL lowering is not the sole predictor of statin cardioprotection. Ongoing pharmacogenetic evaluations of statin antiinflammatory effects may identify an at-risk genotype group that requires clinical intervention with a statin regardless of baseline LDL or lipoprotein treatment response.

Coronary artery disease and stroke pharmacogenetics

Coronary artery disease (CAD) is the leading cause of death in the USA, followed closely by stroke [6]. Antiplatelet, anticoagulant, and thrombolytic drugs are essential to preventing and treating CAD and stroke. Whereas the potential for gene-guided warfarin therapy is fairly far advanced (see Chapter 15), pharmacogenetic studies are just now emerging for aspirin and clopidogrel, and a handful have investigated genetic predictors of response to heparin and glycoprotein IIB/IIIA inhibitors. Pharmacogenetics could also allow for personalized dosing and monitoring of antiplatelet and anticoagulant drugs, and identify potential nonresponders in whom alternative agents or combination therapy might be beneficial.

Approximately 5–60% of patients taking aspirin and about 4–30% of patients taking clopidogrel will have cardiovascular events or fail to exhibit adequate inhibition of platelet function *ex vivo*, a phenomenon referred to as antiplatelet "resistance" [39,40]. The glycoprotein IIIA PlA polymorphism (Leu33Pro) is the most commonly studied candidate for aspirin or clopidogrel resistance, although the data are conflicting [10,41–43]. Genetic variations in the target of aspirin (*PTGS1*) have been associated with aspirin response [44,45], although polymorphisms in the target of clopidogrel (*P2Y12*) [42,46,47] and other platelet surface glycoproteins [43,47,48] have generally not proven to be informative markers of antiplatelet response. Interestingly, since clopidogrel is metabolically activated *in vivo*, CYP isoenzyme polymorphisms that confer reduced activity have been linked to diminished clopidogrel response, resulting in higher cardiovascular event rates after coronary stenting [47,49,50].

Warfarin will likely be the first cardiovascular drug with genotype-guided dosing to reach the clinic. Numerous studies have documented that the *VKORC1* and *CYP2C9* variants are important determinants of warfarin dose variability, bleeding risk, and time to stable warfarin therapy (see Chapter 15). Indeed, in mid-2007, the US Food and Drug Administration (FDA) changed the warfarin label to indicate that physicians should consider lower initial doses in certain genetically defined populations. A number of other strong biological candidates have been studied, but no others have been consistently associated with warfarin dose [51]. Early studies focused on the drug metabolizing enzyme CYP2C9, but the subsequent characterization of the target protein's gene, vitamin K epoxide reductase (*VKORC1*). Along with consideration of other clinical and demographic factors it possible to explain 50–60% of warfarin dosing variability [52]. Based on these findings, the National Institutes of Health has funded a clinical trial of genotype-guided warfarin dosing, compared against dosing via a clinical algorithm. The trial is expected to begin in 2009, and, if the results are favorable for the genotype-guided approach, then genotype-guided warfarin dosing may become the preferred approach for warfarin dosing in clinical practice. Warfarin pharmacogenetics and the potential clinical implications are discussed in greater detail in Chapter 15.

Clinical implications for pharmacogenetics in coronary artery disease and stroke

In general, the pharmacogenetics of drugs acting on platelets and coagulation are very much a work in progress. A practical barrier is that most studies have evaluated biochemical resistance rather than clinical resistance. It is not entirely clear that pharmacogenetic associations with *in vitro* or *ex vivo* resistance translate to clinical resistance, or vice versa. Additionally, clinical monitoring of platelet aggregation may eventually obviate the need for genotyping. Moving forward, laboratory standards and consensus definitions for what constitutes "resistance" need to be developed. Likewise, future studies should probe for gene–gene as well as gene–drug interactions. Overall, many associations have been documented, which certainly provides the impetus for further research. Warfarin, on the other hand, has the potential to be one of the early entries in translation to practice of genotype-guided cardiovascular therapy.

Heart failure pharmacogenetics

HF consumes tremendous healthcare resources in the USA, with the economic burden alone totaling approximately $33 billion each year [6]. Polypharmacy is the cornerstone of HF therapy, and patients routinely receive a minimum of three or four drugs, including an ACE inhibitor, a beta-blocker, a diuretic, and digoxin. Vasodilators and spironolactone are added if the syndrome progresses [53]. As treatment regimens grow in complexity, genetic testing may help to streamline the battery of medications, or identify patients who might benefit from earlier intervention with additional drugs. Furthermore, given that beta-blockers vary in their receptor specificity (e.g., metoprolol vs carvedilol) and that ACE inhibitors and ARBs differ in the mechanism by which they target the renin–angiotensin–aldosterone system (RAAS), genetic tests may guide selection of the most effective drug.

A logical candidate for ACE inhibitor responsiveness is the *ACE* gene, which has an extensively studied insertion/deletion (I/D) polymorphism. In HF patients, the D allele is associated with higher levels of RAAS activity [54]. Consistent with these findings, the D allele has been associated with increased mortality, which high-dose, but not low-dose, ACE inhibitor therapy ameliorated [54]. This dose effect might be attributable to differences in the degree of ACE suppression or susceptibility to RAAS "escape," although mechanistic studies are not conclusive [54,56]. Interestingly, beta-blockers also diminished D allele risk (Fig. 14.3) [57], while another study suggested that spironolactone did not improve ventricular remodeling in patients with the D allele. These examples represent potential cases for use of genetic information to optimize heart failure pharmacotherapies [58].

Compelling evidence is now available to suggest that the genetic polymorphisms in the β_1-adrenergic receptor gene (*ADRB1*), particularly the Arg389Gly polymorphism, modifies beta-blocker responses in HF. Patients with the Arg389 allele consistently responded more favorably to beta-blockade in terms of tolerability, and echocardiographic changes [12]. Most notably, a pharmacogenetic analysis of outcomes in a large clinical trial demonstrated that bucindolol significantly lowered death and hospitalization rates among Arg389 homozygotes but not Gly389 carriers, who had similar event rates as all placebo-treated patients (Fig. 14.4) [59]. Complementary *in vitro*, *ex vivo*, and physiological studies further substantiated the genotype-dependent benefits of bucindolol [59]. Based on these findings, and additional associations with an I/D polymorphism in *ADRA2C* relative to the sympatholytic effects of bucindolol [58], a small pharmaceutical company has submitted a new drug application to the FDA for bucindolol, whereby the drug would be indicated in specific *ADRB1* and *ADRA2C* genotypes. It is also interesting to note that, while the *ADRA2C* D allele was associated with poorer outcomes with bucindolol, it was associated with better improvement in ejection fraction with metoprolol [25], a finding that is easily explained by differences in ancillary properties between metoprolol and bucindolol. Further work is needed in this area, but these data highlight that *ADRB1* and *ADRA2C* genotype might be utilized to select the most appropriate beta-blocker for an individual patient.

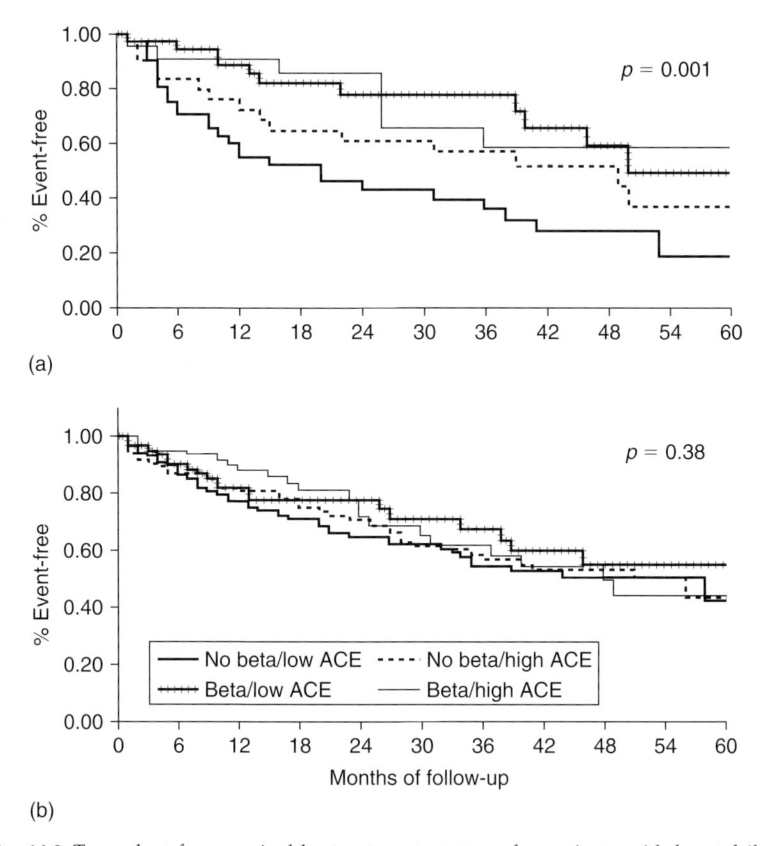

Fig. 14.3 Transplant-free survival by treatment strategy for patients with heart failure with the *ACE* DD genotype (a) and the ID or DD genotypes (b). ACE, angiotensin-converting enzyme inhibitors; Beta, beta-blockers. (Reprinted with permission from McNamara *et al.* [55].)

Another potential role for pharmacogenetics in HF is in identifying genetic subgroups of patients who do not optimally respond to current therapy and thus may benefit from additional therapy. Such therapy might be other existing heart failure drugs (e.g., isosorbide dinitrate) that are not universally indicated, or new drugs under development. Drug development in heart failure in the twenty-first century has had a dismal record, with a clinical trial failure rate exceeding 75% [20]. Thus, the approach of enrolling a broad heart failure population appears inefficient, and so some means of identifying those with the greatest potential to respond to additional therapy is needed. Use of genetic information is one potential approach to identifying such a population.

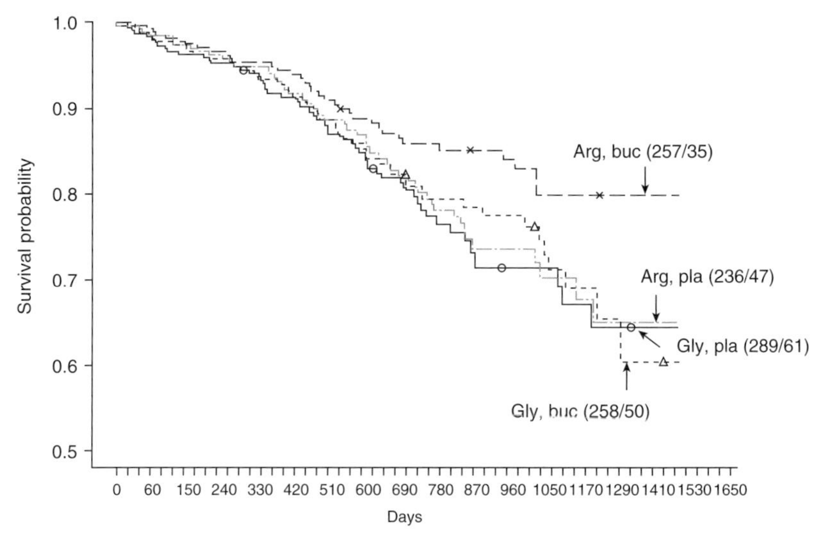

Fig. 14.4 Survival for bucindolol versus placebo by *ADRB1* Arg389Gly carrier status. Pla, placebo; Buc, bucindolol; Arg, Arg389 homozyogtes; Gly, Gly389 carriers. (Reprinted with permission from Liggett *et al.* [59].)

Clinical implications for pharmacogenetics in heart failure

Personalized medicine in HF is evolving rapidly, from biomarker-guided therapy to race to SNP genotyping. It is also becoming clear that multiple polymorphisms within a physiological system contribute to clinical outcomes. Coupled with the complex etiology of HF, comprehensive genetic studies in well-phenotyped populations are still needed. Faced with such challenges, perhaps the greater impact of pharmacogenetics in HF will be realized in drug development, especially considering that several HF drugs have failed in the late stages owing to lack of efficacy or toxicity [60]. As discussed in the introduction, BiDil highlights the potential for developing drugs in genetically defined patient subgroups, and suggests that this is an approach that should be more aggressively pursued in heart failure. Additionally, in the near future, the *ADRB1* and *ADRA2C* genotypes may help guide therapy with bucindolol, if not beta-blocker therapy in general.

Dysrhythmia pharmacogenetics

Ventricular and atrial dysrhythmias account for a significant portion of death and disability in the USA [61,62]. Consequently, treatment modalities exist to either restore patients to normal sinus rhythm or control the pulse rates and prevent thromboembolic complications of dysrhythmia. Aside from the pharmacogenetics of drugs used to treat chronic rhythm disturbances, an area of active translational research is QT interval pharmacogenetics, owing to the fact that many "antiarrhythmic," cardiovascular, and noncardiovascular drugs can prolong the QT interval, increasing the likelihood for life-threatening ventricular dysrhythmia [63].

Drug-induced QT prolongation and subsequent arrhythmia have been described for antihistamines, fluoroquinolone antibiotics, antipsychotic agents, antihypertensives, antiarrhythmics, and others. In fact, QT prolongation and its associated dysrhythmia, torsades de pointes, have been a major reason for withdrawal of drugs from the worldwide markets over the past decade [64].

In general, genes associated with congenital long QT syndromes have also been associated with drug-induced QT prolongation. For instance, variants in genes that regulate potassium and sodium channels (*KCNQ1/KvLQT1; KCNH2/HERG; SCN5A*) have been identified to occur in a subset of patients who experience drug-induced QT prolongation [63,65]. In a study by Drolet *et al.* [66], it was found that a nonsynonymous polymorphism in the *KCNA5* gene (P532L) was associated with a similar baseline potassium current (I_{Kur}) as wild type, but was resistant to the blocking effects of quinidine [66]. These genetic epidemiological and *in vitro* studies suggest that polymorphisms in genes important in cardiac conduction may be relevant in assessing a person's risk for developing drug-mediated dysrhythmia [67–70]. In addition to cardiac conduction genes, drug metabolism enzyme polymorphisms (e.g., *CYP2D6, CYP2C9, CYP2C19, CYP3A*) as well as clinical variables (e.g., sex, renal function, serum electrolytes, and drug interactions) may be considered when stratifying patient risk [71].

Clinical implications for pharmacogenetics in dysrhythmia

Exploration of genetic variants as they relate to congenital and drug-induced QT prolongation or dysrhythmia is already helping to uncover the molecular basis of cardiac rhythm disturbances. However, there is greater promise for genetics and genomics of dysrhythmia in new drug development [72]. Drugs that fail in late-phase clinical trials because of proarrhythmic properties can cost hundreds of millions of dollars. Preclinical expression profiling (e.g., DNA microarray) of new compounds may identify genomic signatures similar to existing compounds with arrhythmogenic effects. If this were the case, the novel compound can be abandoned before introduction into humans, thereby minimizing the public burden of exposure to a potentially toxic agent.

Conclusion

There is great potential for pharmacogenetics and pharmacogenomics to aid in optimizing cardiovascular drug therapies. It is evident from the previous discussion that certain examples are closer to the clinical realization of this potential than others. Figure 14.5 depicts a knowledge pyramid for moving pharmacogenetic information from research to practice.

Those examples that would appear to have great potential for translation to clinical practice in the next few years include warfarin, beta-blockers in heart failure, and beta-blockers in hypertension clopidogrel and statins (for statin induced myopathy). In each of these cases, the accrued evidence is near the top of the pyramid. At the top of the knowledge pyramid are clinical trials to document the superiority of a genotype-guided approach. As discussed, such a trial is planned for warfarin. In the case of the beta-blockers in hypertension and heart failure, that final step may not be required, given the consistency of the associations across multiple studies, and that adverse cardiovascular outcomes (e.g., death) are the outcomes of interest, making undertaking a genotype-guided clinical trial somewhat less realistic.

Others are likely to follow, but will require additional research to move the knowledge base around them to higher steps on the pyramid. There is also great potential for pharmacogenetics to aid in drug development, particularly in heart failure. While there are numerous challenges ahead, it appears that the use of genetic information to improve drug or dose selection and outcomes with cardiovascular drugs is realistic in the next decade. Once

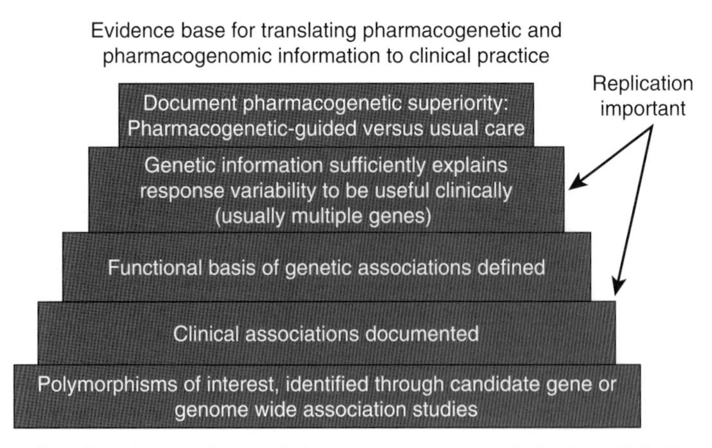

Fig. 14.5 Paradigm for translation of pharmacogenetics knowledge into clinical practice. Genetic variability that influences drug response is first identified through genetic association studies (through either a candidate gene or genome-wide approach) and the importance of the single nucleotide polymorphism/gene will typically be documented in several studies. At some point it is optimal if there is an understanding of the functional basis for the genetic polymorphism and its clinical association. Next, there must be an ability to sufficiently explain clinical response variability (likely with both genetic and nongenetic factors), and this will often require knowledge of the contribution of multiple genes to the variable response. Finally, in many cases it will be necessary to document in a controlled clinical trial that a genotype-guided approach is superior in order for there to be broad uptake in practice.

sufficient evidence is available for translation to practice, it will be incumbent on the healthcare system to find a mechanism for disseminating this information, so that it might be adopted into clinical practice.

Several significant advances in cardiovascular pharmacogenetics since the chapter was written deserve comment. Clopidogrel is a pro-drug that requires bioactivation to an active metabolite, a process for which cytochrome P450 2C19 plays a major role. *CYP2C19* contains several reduced function polymorphisms, the most common of which is the *2 allele, which leads to a loss of enzymatic activity. Three papers, published simultaneously, reported that carriers of reduced function variant *CYP2C19* alleles had increased risk for adverse cardiovascular outcomes [73–75]. Data for these papers arose from both controlled clinical trials and population cohorts, providing insight into the external validity of the findings. These consistent and compelling data suggest *CYP2C19* genotyping could quickly become a standard of care for patients being initiated on clopidogrel therapy. Additionally, certain drugs that inhibit *CYP2C19* (e.g. proton pump inhibitors) can, in essence, convert patients to the same phenotype as the genetic polymorphisms. Thus, careful attention to drugs interacting with clopidogrel's metabolism via *CYP2C19* are probably also warranted.

The chapter also noted that there was promise for genome-wide association studies, but no such studies had been completed in cardiovascular pharmacogenetics. This is no longer the case, and published studies now include evaluation of the LDL response to statins, the blood pressure lowering with a thiazide, and statin-induced myopathy. It is the latter for which the findings are most striking. The investigators discovered a common polymorphism in an organic anion transporter gene (*SLCO1B1)* was associated with statin-induced myopathy, with the data suggesting a 4.5-fold increased risk for myopathy per copy of variant allele [76]. This gene is one for which there was mounting evidence from smaller pharmacokinetic studies of a potential role in the disposition of certain statins. Thus, an understanding of the functional underpinnings of the association, along with replication of the association with myopathy in a separate clinical trial, add confidence that the finding is real. Further population-based cohorts will likely need tested to provide greater insight into the clinical utility of testing for this polymorphism prior to statin therapy. But the literature in hand suggests use of this information in the clinic may be around the corner.

In summary, in the short period between submission to proof stage, there were two major cardiovascular pharmacogenetic findings reported. This highlights the speed with which additional advances in this field might come in the future.

References

1 Piquette-Miller M, Grant DM. The art and science of personalized medicine. *Clinical Pharmacology and Therapeutics* 2007; **81**: 311–315.

2 Spear BB, Heath-Chiozzi M, Huff J. Clinical application of pharmacogenetics. *Trends in Molecular Medicine* 2001; **7**: 201–204.

3 Taylor AL, Ziesche S, Yancy C *et al.* Combination of isosorbide dinitrate and hydralazine in blacks with heart failure. *New England Journal of Medicine* 2004; **351**: 2049–2057.

4 The International HapMap Consortium. A haplotype map of the human genome. *Nature* 2005; **437**: 1299–320.

5 de Bakker PI, Burtt NP, Graham RR *et al.* Transferability of tag SNPs in genetic association studies in multiple populations. *Nature Genetics* 2006; **38**: 1298–1303.

6 Rosamond W, Flegal K, Friday G *et al.* Heart disease and stroke statistics—2007 update: a report from the American Heart Association Statistics Committee and Stroke Statistics Subcommittee. *Circulation* 2007; **115**: e69–171.

7 Chobanian AV, Bakris GL, Black HR *et al.* The Seventh Report of the Joint National Committee on Prevention, Detection, Evaluation, and Treatment of High Blood Pressure: The JNC 7 Report. *JAMA: the Journal of the American Medical Association* 2003; **289**: 2560–2571.

8 Materson BJ, Reda DJ, Cushman WC *et al.* Single-drug therapy for hypertension in men. A comparison of six antihypertensive agents with placebo. The Department of Veterans Affairs Cooperative Study Group on Antihypertensive Agents [see comments] [published erratum appears in *New England Journal of Medicine* 1994; **330**: 1689]. *New England Journal of Medicine* 1993; **328**: 914–921.

9 Liu J, Liu ZQ, Tan ZR *et al.* Gly389Arg polymorphism of beta1-adrenergic receptor is associated with the cardiovascular response to metoprolol. *Clinical Pharmacology and Therapeutics* 2003; **74**: 372–379.

10 Cooke GE, Liu-Stratton Y, Ferketich AK *et al.* Effect of platelet antigen polymorphism on platelet inhibition by aspirin, clopidogrel, or their combination. *Journal of the American College of Cardiology* 2006; **47**: 541–546.

11 Sofowora GG, Dishy V, Muszkat M *et al.* A common beta1-adrenergic receptor polymorphism (Arg389Gly) affects blood pressure response to beta-blockade. *Clinical Pharmacology and Therapeutics* 2003; **73**: 366–371.

12 Zineh I, Johnson JA. Pharmacogenetics of chronic cardiovascular drugs: applications and implications. *Expert Opinion in Pharmacotherapy* 2006; **7**: 1417–1427.

13 Johnson JA, Zineh I, Puckett BJ *et al.* Beta 1-adrenergic receptor polymorphisms and antihypertensive response to metoprolol. *Clinical Pharmacology and Therapeutics* 2003; **74**: 44–52.

14 Mason DA, Moore JD, Green SA, Liggett SB. A gain-of-function polymorphism in a G-protein coupling domain of the human beta1-adrenergic receptor. *Journal of Biological Chemistry* 1999; 274: 12670–4.

15 Johnson JA, Turner ST. *Hypertension* pharmacogenomics: current status and future directions. *Current Opinion in Molecular Therapeutics* 2005; **7**: 218–225.

16 Bis JC, Smith NL, Psaty BM *et al.* Angiotensinogen Met235Thr polymorphism, angiotensin-converting enzyme inhibitor therapy, and the risk of nonfatal stroke or myocardial infarction in hypertensive patients. *American Journal of Hypertension* 2003; **16**: 1011–1017.

17 Goldenberg I, Moss AJ, Ryan D *et al.* Polymorphism in the angiotensinogen gene, hypertension, and ethnic differences in the risk of recurrent coronary events. *Hypertension* 2006; **48**: 693–699.

18 Schelleman H, Klungel OH, Witteman JC *et al*. Angiotensinogen M235T polymorphism and the risk of myocardial infarction and stroke among hypertensive patients on ACE-inhibitors or beta-blockers. *European Journal of Human Genetics* 2007; **15**: 478–484.
19 Su X, Lee L, Li X *et al*. Association between angiotensinogen, angiotensin II receptor genes, and blood pressure response to an angiotensin-converting enzyme inhibitor. *Circulation* 2007; **115**: 725–732.
20 Cusi D, Barlassina C, Azzani T *et al*. Polymorphisms of alpha-adducin and salt sensitivity in patients with essential hypertension. *Lancet* 1997; **349**: 1353–1357.
21 Glorioso N, Manunta P, Filigheddu F *et al*. The role of alpha-adducin polymorphism in blood pressure and sodium handling regulation may not be excluded by a negative association study. *Hypertension* 1999; **34** (4 Pt 1): 649–654.
22 Sciarrone MT, Stella P, Barlassina C *et al*. ACE and alpha-adducin polymorphism as markers of individual response to diuretic therapy. *Hypertension* 2003; **41**: 398–403.
23 Psaty BM, Smith NL, Heckbert SR *et al*. Diuretic therapy, the alpha-adducin gene variant, and the risk of myocardial infarction or stroke in persons with treated hypertension. *JAMA: the Journal of the American Medical Association* 2002; **287**: 1680–1689.
24 Davis BR, Arnett DK, Boerwinkle E *et al*. Antihypertensive therapy, the alpha-adducin polymorphism, and cardiovascular disease in high-risk hypertensive persons: the Genetics of Hypertension-Associated Treatment Study. *Pharmacogenomics Journal* 2007; **7**: 112–122.
25 Gerhard T, Gong Y, Beitelshees AL *et al*. Cardiovascular outcomes, diuretic therapy and the alpha-adducin polymorphism: results for the International Verapamil SR-Trandolapril Study Genetic Substudy (INVEST-GENES). *Circulation* 2005; **112**: II-608.
26 Pacanowski MA, Gong Y, Cooper–Dehoff RM *et al*. *Clin Pharmacol Ther* 2008; **84**: 715–721.
27 Grundy SM, Cleeman JI, Merz CN *et al*. Implications of recent clinical trials for the National Cholesterol Education Program Adult Treatment Panel III guidelines. *Circulation* 2004; **110**: 227–239.
28 Yusuf S, Hawken S, Ounpuu S *et al*. Effect of potentially modifiable risk factors associated with myocardial infarction in 52 countries (the INTERHEART study): case-control study. *Lancet* 2004; **364**: 937–952.
29 Libby P. The forgotten majority: unfinished business in cardiovascular risk reduction. *Journal of the American College of Cardiology* 2005; **46**: 1225–1228.
30 Pazzucconi F, Dorigotti F, Gianfranceschi G *et al*. Therapy with HMG CoA reductase inhibitors: characteristics of the long-term permanence of hypocholesterolemic activity. *Atherosclerosis* 1995; **117**: 189–198.
31 Pedro-Botet J, Schaefer EJ, Bakker-Arkema RG *et al*. Apolipoprotein E genotype affects plasma lipid response to atorvastatin in a gender specific manner. *Atherosclerosis* 2001; **158**: 183–193.
32 Johnson JA, Zineh I. Pharmacogenetics and personalized medicine. In: Dzau VJ, Liew CC, ed. *Cardiovascular Genetics and Genomics for the Cardiologist*. Blackwell Publishing; Oxford, England 2007: 250–276.
33 Zineh I. HMG-CoA reductase inhibitor pharmacogenomics: overview and implications for practice. *Clinical Cardiology* 2005; **1**: 191–206.
34 Chasman DI, Posada D, Subrahmanyan L *et al*. Pharmacogenetic study of statin therapy and cholesterol reduction. *JAMA: the Journal of the American Medical Association* 2004; **291**: 2821–2827.

35 Thompson JF, Man M, Johnson KJ *et al.* An association study of 43 SNPs in 16 candidate genes with atorvastatin response. *Pharmacogenomics Journal* 2005; **5**: 352–358.
36 Zineh I. Pharmacogenetics of response to statins. *Current Atherosclerosis Reports* 2007; 9.
37 Ruano G, Thompson PD, Windemuth A *et al.* Physiogenomic analysis links serum creatine kinase activities during statin therapy to vascular smooth muscle homeostasis. *Pharmacogenomics* 2005; **6**: 865–872.
38 McCarty C, Wilke R, Giampietro P *et al.* The Marshfield Clinic Personalized Medicine Research Project (PMRP): design, methods and initial recruitment results for a population-based DNA Biobank. *Personal Medicine* 2005; **2**: 49–79.
39 Sanderson S, Emery J, Baglin T, Kinmonth AL. Narrative review: aspirin resistance and its clinical implications. *Annals of Internal Medicine* 2005; 142: 370–80.
40 Geisler TMD, Gawaz MMD. Variable response to clopidogrel in patients with coronary artery disease. *Seminars in Thrombosis and Hemostasis* 2007; **33**: 196–202.
41 Szczeklik A, Sanak M, Undas A. Platelet glycoprotein IIIa pl(a) polymorphism and effects of aspirin on thrombin generation. *Circulation* 2001; **103**: E33–34.
42 Lev EI, Patel RT, Guthikonda S *et al.* Genetic polymorphisms of the platelet receptors P2Y(12), P2Y(1) and GP IIIa and response to aspirin and clopidogrel. *Thrombosis Research* 2007; **119**: 355–360.
43 Macchi L, Christiaens L, Brabant S *et al.* Resistance in vitro to low-dose aspirin is associated with platelet PlA1 (GP IIIa) polymorphism but not with C807T(GP Ia/IIa) and C-5T Kozak (GP Ibalpha) polymorphisms. *Journal of the American College of Cardiology* 2003; **42**: 1115–1119.
44 Lepantalo A, Mikkelsson J, Resendiz JC *et al.* Polymorphisms of COX-1 and GPVI associate with the antiplatelet effect of aspirin in coronary artery disease patients. *Thrombosis and Haemostasis* 2006; **95**: 253–259.
45 Maree AO, Curtin RJ, Chubb A *et al.* Cyclooxygenase-1 haplotype modulates platelet response to aspirin. *Journal of Thrombosis and Haemostasis* 2005; **3**: 2340–2345.
46 Ziegler S, Schillinger M, Funk M *et al.* Association of a functional polymorphism in the clopidogrel target receptor gene, P2Y12, and the risk for ischemic cerebrovascular events in patients with peripheral artery disease. *Stroke* 2005; **36**: 1394–1399.
47 Angiolillo DJ, Fernandez-Ortiz A, Bernardo E *et al.* Contribution of gene sequence variations of the hepatic cytochrome P450 3A4 enzyme to variability in individual responsiveness to clopidogrel. *Arteriosclerosis Thrombosis and Vascular Biology* 2006; **26**: 1895–1900.
48 Jefferson BK, Foster JH, McCarthy JJ *et al.* Aspirin resistance and a single gene. *American Journal of Cardiology* 2005; **95**: 805–808.
49 Suh JW, Koo BK, Zhang SY *et al.* Increased risk of atherothrombotic events associated with cytochrome P450 3A5 polymorphism in patients taking clopidogrel. *CMAJ: Canadian Medical Association Journal* 2006; **174**: 1715–1722.
50 Hulot JS, Bura A, Villard E *et al.* Cytochrome P450 2C19 loss-of-function polymorphism is a major determinant of clopidogrel responsiveness in healthy subjects. *Blood* 2006; **108**: 2244–2247.
51 Wadelius M, Chen LY, Eriksson N *et al.* Association of warfarin dose with genes involved in its action and metabolism. *Human Genetics* 2007; **121**: 23–34.
52 Schwarz UI, Stein CM. Genetic determinants of dose and clinical outcomes in patients receiving oral anticoagulants. *Clinical Pharmacology and Therapeutics* 2006; **80**: 7–12.

53 Hunt SA. ACC/AHA 2005 guideline update for the diagnosis and management of chronic heart failure in the adult: a report of the American College of Cardiology/American Heart Association Task Force on Practice Guidelines (Writing Committee to Update the 2001 Guidelines for the Evaluation and Management of Heart Failure). *Journal of the American College of Cardiology* 2005; **46**: e1–82.
54 Tang WH, Vagelos RH, Yee YG, Fowler MB. Impact of angiotensin-converting enzyme gene polymorphism on neurohormonal responses to high- versus low-dose enalapril in advanced heart failure. *American Heart Journal* 2004; **148**: 889–894.
55 McNamara DM, Holubkov R, Postava L *et al.* Pharmacogenetic interactions between angiotensin-converting enzyme inhibitor therapy and the angiotensin-converting enzyme deletion polymorphism in patients with congestive heart failure. *Journal of the American College of Cardiology* 2004; **44**: 2019–2026.
56 Cicoira M, Zanolla L, Rossi A *et al.* Failure of aldosterone suppression despite angiotensin-converting enzyme (ACE) inhibitor administration in chronic heart failure is associated with ACE DD genotype. *Journal of the American College of Cardiology* 2001; **37**: 1808–1812.
57 McNamara DM, Holubkov R, Janosko K *et al.* Pharmacogenetic interactions between beta-blocker therapy and the angiotensin-converting enzyme deletion polymorphism in patients with congestive heart failure. *Circulation* 2001; **103**: 1644–1648.
58 Cicoira M, Rossi A, Bonapace S *et al.* Effects of ACE gene insertion/deletion polymorphism on response to spironolactone in patients with chronic heart failure. *American Journal of Medicine* 2004; **116**: 657–661.
59 Liggett SB, Mialet-Perez J, Thaneemit-Chen S *et al.* A polymorphism within a conserved beta(1)-adrenergic receptor motif alters cardiac function and beta-blocker response in human heart failure. *Proceedings of the National Academy of Sciences of the USA* 2006; **103**: 11288–11293.
60 Kaye DM, Krum H. Drug discovery for heart failure: a new era or the end of the pipeline? *Nature Reviews Drug Discovery* 2007; **6**: 127–139.
61 Zheng ZJ, Croft JB, Giles WH, Mensah GA. Sudden cardiac death in the United States, 1989 to 1998. *Circulation* 2001; **104**: 2158–2163.
62 Wattigney WA, Mensah GA, Croft JB. Increased atrial fibrillation mortality: United States, 1980–1998. *American Journal of Epidemiology* 2002; **155**: 819–826.
63 Giacomini KM, Brett CM, Altman RB *et al.* The pharmacogenetics research network: from SNP discovery to clinical drug response. *Clinical Pharmacology and Therapeutics* 2007; **81**: 328–345.
64 Giacomini KM, Krauss RM, Roden DM *et al.* When good drugs go bad. *Nature* 2007; **446**: 975–977.
65 Yang P, Kanki H, Drolet B *et al.* Allelic variants in long-QT disease genes in patients with drug- associated torsades de pointes. *Circulation* 2002; **105**: 1943–1948.
66 Drolet B, Simard C, Mizoue L, Roden DM. Human cardiac potassium channel DNA polymorphism modulates access to drug-binding site and causes drug resistance. *Journal of Clinical Investigation* 2005; **115**: 2209–2213.
67 Roden DM. Pharmacogenetics and drug-induced arrhythmias. *Cardiovascular Research* 2001; **50**: 224–231.
68 Donger C, Denjoy I, Berthet M *et al.* KVLQT1 C-terminal missense mutation causes a forme fruste long-QT syndrome. *Circulation* 1997; **96**: 2778–2781.

69 Napolitano C, Schwartz PJ, Brown AM *et al.* Evidence for a cardiac ion channel mutation underlying drug-induced QT prolongation and life-threatening arrhythmias. *Journal of Cardiovascular Electrophysiology* 2000; **11**: 691–696.
70 Sesti F, Abbott GW, Wei J *et al.* A common polymorphism associated with antibiotic-induced cardiac arrhythmia. *Proceedings of the National Academy of Sciences of the USA* 2000; **97**: 10613–10618.
71 Roden DM. Genetic polymorphisms, drugs, and proarrhythmia. *Journal of Interventional Cardiac Electrophysiology* 2003; **9**: 131–135.
72 Roden DM. Human genomics and its impact on arrhythmias. *Trends in Cardiovascular Medicine* 2004; **14**: 112–116.
73 Collet JP, Hulot JS, Pena A, *et al.* Cytochrome P450 2C19 polymorphism in young patients treated with clopidogrel after myocardial infarction: a cohort study. Lancet 2008.
74 Mega JL, Close SL, Wiviott SD, *et al.* Cytochrome P-450 Polymorphisms and Response to Clopidogrel. *N Engl J Med* 2008.
75 Simon T, Verstuyft C, Mary-Krause M, *et al.* Genetic Determinants of Response to Clopidogrel and Cardiovascular Events. *N Engl J Med* 2008.
76 Link E, Parish S, Armitage J, *et al.* SLCO1B1 variants and statin-induced myopathy–a genomewide study. *N Engl J Med* 2008; **359**: 789–799.

Case study: warfarin pharmacogenetics from single to multiple genes

Michael D. Caldwell and Richard Berg

Introduction

Warfarin is the most frequently prescribed oral anticoagulant, the fourth most prescribed cardiovascular agent, and, overall, the eleventh most commonly prescribed drug in the USA, with annual sales of approximately $500 million [1]. Despite the extensive use of the drug, in 1995 the Agency for Healthcare Policy and Research (presently the Agency for Healthcare Quality and Research) reported that warfarin was underutilized for stroke prevention, notwithstanding the evidence that warfarin therapy prevented 20 strokes for every bleeding episode that it caused. The underutilization of warfarin anticoagulation persists because physicians remain reluctant to prescribe the drug, owing to their concerns regarding hemorrhagic complications associated with warfarin utilization [2].

The extent of hemorrhagic adverse events related to warfarin therapy was investigated by Fihn *et al.* [3]. Using data on 928 patients collected across five anticoagulation clinics with 1950 patient-years of follow-up, these investigators demonstrated that the cumulative incidence of a fatal bleed with warfarin therapy reached 2% by the third year of therapy. Further, following 8 years of therapy, 9% of patients had experienced an episode of a life-threatening hemorrhage and an episode of serious bleeding was documented in an additional 40% of patients. Outcomes in randomized clinical trials of patients with deep venous thrombosis, tissue heart valves, mechanical heart valves, ischemic stroke, or atrial fibrillation have shown the frequency of major bleeding episodes was strongly related to the intensity of anticoagulant therapy [4]. The risk assessment

Cardiovascular Genetics and Genomics. Edited by Dan Roden. © 2009 American Heart Association, ISBN: 978-14051-7540-1.

model of Hylek and Singer [5] for intracerebral hemorrhage in patients receiving warfarin anticoagulation therapy predicted that risk doubled for each numerical increase of approximately 1.0 in the international normalized ratio (INR). Other studies demonstrated that variability in an individual patient's INR was associated with an increased frequency of hemorrhagic complications independent of the mean INR [3,6,7]. The clinical use of warfarin has been troublesome because both a means for estimating the stable therapeutic dose and a means to reduce variation in therapeutic response are lacking and must be established empirically. As substantiated by the recent Food and Drug Administration (FDA) black label warning, initiation of warfarin therapy and an INR of >4.0 during therapy remain predictors of serious or life-threatening hemorrhage.

Given that warfarin has been the only effective oral anticoagulant in clinical use over the last 50 years, there have been substantial efforts to improve the safety of warfarin therapy. Despite reduced hemorrhagic complications due to broader access to managed care by anticoagulation clinics with an increased focus on warfarin safety, the median annual rate of major bleeding continues to range from 0.9% to 2.7%, and the median annual rate of fatal bleeding ranges from 0.07% to 0.7% [4,8–10]. Much of the initial progress in reducing complications was related to an improved understanding of the relative impact of intensity of anticoagulation, age, body size, comorbidities, and concomitant medications on response to warfarin therapy. Little additional progress occurred, however, until the recent age of pharmacogenetics.

Pharmacodynamics of warfarin

The pharmacological action of warfarin lies in its ability to act as an antagonist to the function of vitamin K as a cofactor for γ-carboxylation of glutamic acid residues in proteins. The clotting factors II, VII, IX, and X and the naturally occurring endogenous anticoagulant proteins C, S, and Z all have γ-carboxylated glutamic acid residues [11,12].

The vitamin K-dependent (VKD) γ-carboxylase is located in the endoplasmic reticulum, allowing VKD proteins to be carboxylated during their secretion. Multiple glutamic acid residues in the of VKD proteins are converted to γ-carboxylated glutamic acid residues. Full γ-carboxylation of the proteins is required for optimal VKD protein function which results in calcium binding either to phospholipids exposed on the surfaces of cells, thus accelerating blood coagulation, or to hydroxyapatite molecules in the extracellular matrix. Expression of the γ-glutamyl carboxylase is detectable in virtually all human tissues and a single carboxylase (the product of an autosomal gene) appears to be responsible for modifying all VKD proteins [13].

Although many VKD proteins have now been described, this chapter will focus on the role of vitamin K in the production of the VKD proteins which serve as clotting factors [factors II (prothrombin), VII, IX, and X, and natural anticoagulant proteins C, S, and Z]. These factors are synthesized primarily by the hepatic carboxylase from precursor proteins containing a carboxylase recognition signal region, which is cleaved subsequent to carboxylation of the glutamic acid residues [12].

Vitamin K quinone in its reduced state is the required cofactor for γ-glutamyl carboxylase activity. This carboxylase oxidizes the vitamin K hydroquinone to a 2,3-epoxide (vitamin K epoxide). Given its structural similarity to vitamin K, it is not surprising that warfarin (Fig. 15.1) was shown to produce an anticoagulant effect by interfering with the cyclical interconversion of the reduced form of vitamin K and its 2,3-epoxide. This interconversion requires the action of an enzyme known as vitamin K 2,3-epoxide reductase (VKOR) as well as the γ-glutamyl carboxylase [14]. By inhibiting the action of VKOR and thereby inhibiting the formation of vitamin K hydroquinone, warfarin causes hepatic production of partially γ-carboxylated proteins with reduced activity [15,16] (Fig. 15.2).

Inhibition of VKOR is reversible; therefore the anticoagulant effect of even large doses of coumarin derivatives can be overcome by withdrawing the

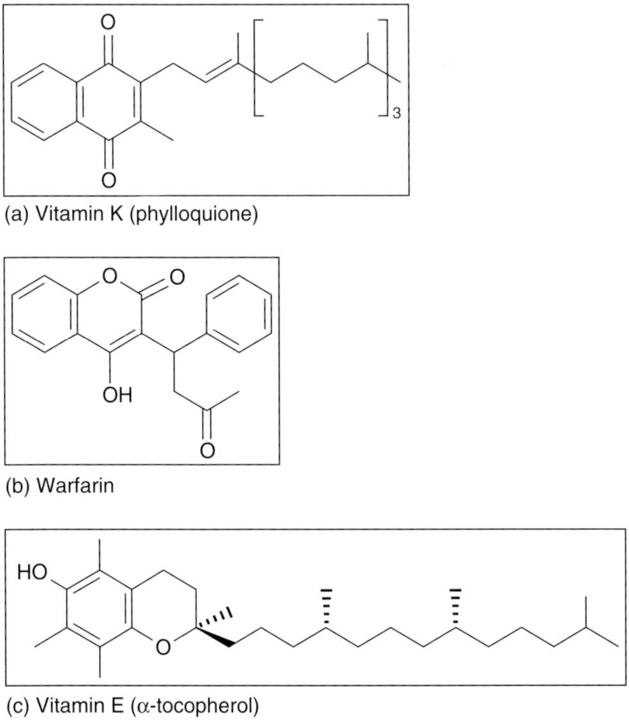

(a) Vitamin K (phylloquione)

(b) Warfarin

(c) Vitamin E (α-tocopherol)

Fig. 15.1 Structural overview of vitamins K (a), warfarin (b), and vitamin E (c). Vitamin K is the end target of inhibition by warfarin vitamin E is a known substrate of CYP4F2. Because of structural similarities between the side-chains and side-chain oxidation products of vitamins E and K [53,54], it is proposed that CYP4F2 is involved in the metabolism of vitamin K.

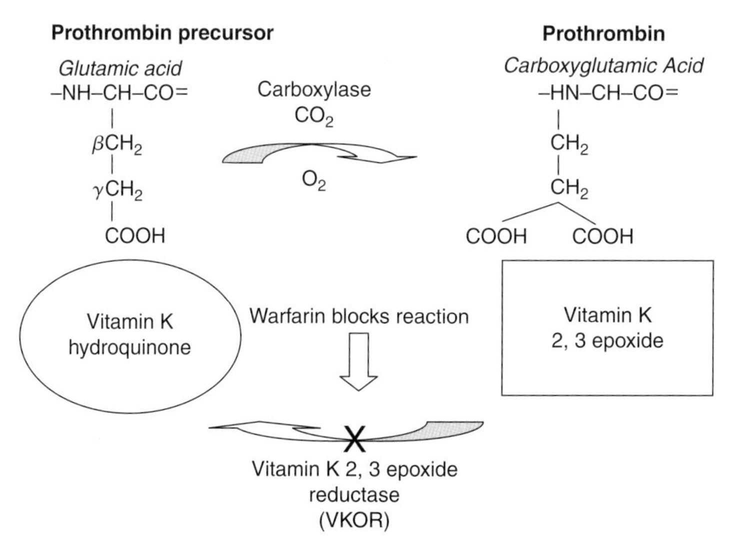

Fig. 15.2 The mechanism of action of warfarin is depicted in the diagram above. Vitamin K-hydroquinone acts as a cofactor in the generation of prothrombin during which it is oxidized to 2,3 vitamin K epoxide. Regeneration of vitamin K into its reduced state is essentially blocked by action of warfarin on VKOR, the enzyme which catalyzes conversion of vitamin K from its oxidized to its reduced state.

drug and by administering doses of vitamin K_1 (phylloquinone). The exogenous vitamin K is subsequently reduced by hepatic quinone reductases NQO1 and CBR1 (each encoded by polymorphic genes) particularly in an environment of large hepatic vitamin K stores to provide a cofactor for the γ-carboxylase [11].

Warfarin pharmacokinetics

In therapeutic form, warfarin is a racemic mixture of the *R* and *S* enantiomers. The *S* enantiomer is 3–5 times more potent an inhibitor of the vitamin K epoxide reductase complex than is *R*-warfarin [17]. Warfarin is absorbed from the upper gastrointestinal tract and is hematogenously transported bound to albumin and the acid glycoproteins orosomucoid-1 and orosomucoid-2 [18,19]. The enantiomers are metabolized by different enzymes. The *S* isomer is predominantly metabolized via cytochrome P450 (CYP) 2C9. This enzyme converts *S*-warfarin into the inactive *S*-7-hydroxy-warfarin metabolite. *R*-warfarin is metabolized mainly via CYP3A4 with involvement of CYP1A1, CYP1A2, CYP2C8, CYP2C9, CYP2C18 and CYP2C19. Phase 2 metabolism of warfarin has not been well studied, although sulfated and glucuronyl conjugates have been described [20]. Final elimination of warfarin metabolic products is primarily renal. However, interaction of warfarin with the hepatic ABCB1 transporter has been demonstrated [21].

Several drugs are known to interact with warfarin [22,23]. The list of clinically significant potentiators of warfarin action include eight antibiotics (ciprofloxacin, cotrimoxazole, erythromycin, fluconazole, isoniazid, metronidazole, miconazole, and voriconazole), seven cardiovascular drugs (amiodarone, clofibrate, diltiazem, fenofibrate, propafenone, propranolol, and sulfinpyrazone), two antiinflammatory drugs (phenylbutazone and piroxicam), four central nervous system active drugs [alcohol (only in the presence of concomitant liver disease), citalopram, entacapone, and sertraline], two gastrointestinal drugs (cimetidine and omeprazole), and other agents including herbal supplements, anabolic steroids, and zileuton. Many of these medications appear to competitively inhibit enzymatic degradation of the *S*- and *R*-warfarin enantiomers (Table 15.1). The clinically significant inhibitors of warfarin action include four antibiotics (griseofulvin, ribavirin, rifampin, and nafcillin), two drugs active on the central nervous system (barbiturates and carbamazepine), and cholestyramine, mesalamine, mercaptopurine, and foods high in vitamin K content. These last agents appear to alter warfarin metabolism by inducing warfarin metabolic enzymes (Table 15.2).

Current knowledge in warfarin pharmacogenetics: the multigenetic regulation of warfarin action

The high incidence of warfarin-related adverse events correlates strongly with the marked interindividual variability in therapeutic dose. Physicians have known that age, some comorbid conditions, and, to a lesser extent, gender affect the patient's stable therapeutic dose. As previously noted, some concomitant medications are known to alter warfarin metabolism, thereby influencing dose requirements. However, modeling the effects of all these factors and their potential interactions explained only approximately 20% of the interindividual variation in warfarin dose requirements [24].

In 1995, Furuya *et al.* [25] reported the first known association of polymorphisms in CYP2C9 and warfarin dose. This cytochrome, a part of the hepatic microsomal enzyme system known to be important in xenobiotic metabolism, was sequenced in 1980 and subsequently shown by Rettie *et al.* [26] in 1992 to actively degrade warfarin to an inactive metabolite (*S*-7-hydroxy-warfarin).

In 1999, Aithal *et al.* [27] showed a strong association between the CYP2C9 genotype of polymorphic alleles and warfarin sensitivity and postulated that hemorrhagic complications observed in warfarin-sensitive patients were associated with their CYP2C9 genotype. Over the next 5 years, many investigators confirmed the association between CYP2C9 genotype and warfarin dose and explored the effects of racial and ethnically associated polymorphisms in this gene. By 2005 a meta-analysis by Sanderson *et al.* [28] reported that the

Table 15.1 Clinically significant potentiators of warfarin

Drug potentiators	Drug classification	Putative mechanism for effect on warfarin	Primary drug metabolizing enzyme
Ciprofloxacin	Antiinfectives	Inhibits 1A2, 3A4	3A4
Cotrimoxazole			
Erythromycin		Inhibits 1A2, 3A4	3A4
Fluconazole		Inhibits 2C9, 2C19, 3A4	
Isoniazid		Inhibits 2C9, 1A2	
Metronidazole		Inhibits 2C9, 3A4	
Miconazole		Inhibits 3A4	
Voriconazole		Inhibits 3A4, 2C9	
Amiodarone	Cardiovascular	Inhibits 2C9, 1A2, 3A4	3A4, 2D6
Clofibrate			
Diltiazem		Inhibits 1A2, 3A4	3A4
Fenofibrate			
Propafenone			2D6
Propranolol			1A2, 2D6, 3A4
Sulfinpyrazone		Inhibits 2C9, induces 3A4	
Phenylbutazone	Antiinflammatory	Inhibits 2C9, induces 3A4	2C9
Piroxicam			2C9
Alcohol + liver disease	CNS drugs		
Citalopram			2C19
Entacapone			
Sertraline		Inhibits 2C9, 3A4	3A4
Cimetidine	Gastrointestinal drugs	Inhibits 2C9, 2C19, 3A4, 1A2	
Omeprazole		Induces 1A2, inhibits 2C19	2C19
Boldo-fenugreek	Herbal supplements		
Quilinggao			
Anabolic steroids	Other drugs		3A4 (testosterone)
Zileuton			1A2

Table 15.2 Inducers of warfarin metabolic enzymes

Drug inhibitors	Drug classification	Putative mechanism for effect on warfarin	Primary drug metabolizing enzyme
Griseofulvin	Antiinfective	Induces 3A4	
Nafcillin		Induces 1A2	
Ribavirin			
Rifampin		Induces 2C9, 1A2, 3A4, 2C19	
Cholestyramine	Cardiovascular		
Mesalamine	Antiinflammatory		
Barbiturates	Central nervous system drug	Induce 3A4, 2C19	
Carbamazepine		Induces 2C9, 2C19, 3A4	3A4
Mercaptopurine	Other drugs		
High content foods	Vitamin K	Bypasses VKOR	

association between CYP2C9 and warfarin dose was so compelling in the Caucasian populations that no further association studies were necessary.

Patients with variant CYP2C9 alleles exhibit decreased *S*-warfarin clearance [29,30] leading to a decrease in warfarin maintenance dose requirements [29,31–36]. Patients encoding the 2C9*2 or 2C9*3 variant alleles also required lower mean daily warfarin doses and more frequently exceeded the target therapeutic INR range during the induction phase of therapy than did patients carrying only wild-type alleles [37]. Higashi *et al.* [35] showed that the mean warfarin maintenance doses were 87% of wild type in 2C9*1/*2, 72% in 2C9*2/*2, 59% in 2C9*1/*3, 42% in 2C9*2/*3, and 28% in 2C9*3/*3. Patients with variant alleles further required longer intervals to achieve stable dose and had a significantly increased risk of serious or life-threatening hemorrhagic events than patients with the wild-type genotype [27]. Patients titrated to a consistent target INR demonstrated similar plasma *S*-warfarin concentrations independent of CYP2C9 genotype and its inherent metabolic capacity [29]. Once stabilized on warfarin therapy, patients with variant CYP2C9 alleles showed no difference in risk for over-anticoagulation compared with patients with the wild-type genotype during long-term therapy [34].

In 2004, Rost *et al.* [38] cloned the vitamin K 2,3-epoxide reductase complex subunit 1 (*VKORC1*) gene and demonstrated its relationship to warfarin resistance. The *VKORC1* gene encodes vitamin K epoxide reductase complex subunit 1, a small transmembrane protein of the endoplasmic reticulum. These investigators showed that overexpression of wild-type *VKORC1* resulted in a marked stimulation of VKOR activity with a 14- to 21-fold increase in production of vitamin K hydroquinone. They also described four different heterozygous mutations in the *VKORC1* gene in individuals with warfarin resistance.

Rieder *et al.* [39] further investigated the genetic basis of the widely variable response among patients receiving warfarin therapy. They examined *VKORC1* haplotype frequencies in African American, European American, and Asian American populations. The investigators identified 10 common *VKORC1* single nucleotide polymorphisms (SNPs) and inferred five major haplotypes. They identified a low-dose haplotype group (A) and a high-dose haplotype group (B). The *VKORC1* haplotype groups A and B explained approximately 25% of the variance in individual stable therapeutic warfarin dose. Asian Americans had a higher proportion of group A haplotypes and African Americans a higher proportion of group B haplotypes. The investigators also showed that VKORC1 mRNA levels varied according to the haplotype combination. Thus, the association of warfarin dose with VKORC1 genotype appears to be regulated at the transcriptional level [39,40].

D'Andrea *et al.* [41] showed that the combined effect of polymorphisms in CYP2C9 and VKORC1 on warfarin metabolism could explain up to 35% of the variability in stable therapeutic warfarin dose. Thus, by 2005, it was clear that approximately 55% of the variability in warfarin dosing could be explained by age, gender, comorbidities, and CYP2C9 and VKORC1 genotypes (see, for example, Sconce *et al.* [42]).

Following the successful association of polymorphisms in CYP2C9 and VKORC1 with warfarin dose requirements, investigations focused on identification of other polymorphic candidate genes involved in warfarin pharmacodynamics and pharmacokinetics that might affect stable therapeutic warfarin dose. Table 15.3 lists the genes encoding for proteins thought to be involved in warfarin pharmacokinetics and pharmacodynamics. This table was constructed based on recent comprehensive discussions by Wadelius and Pirmohamed [43], Wadelius *et al.* [44], and Krynetskiy and McDonnell [45].

Wadelius *et al.* [44] recently reported an investigation of 29 candidate genes involved in what they referred to as the "warfarin interactive pathways" in 201 patients. They evaluated approximately 800 SNPs within those candidate genes that comprehensively captured common variations based on measures of LD ($r^2 \geqslant 0.8$). This analysis identified 348 SNPs that were in Hardy–Weinberg equilibrium, exhibiting minimal allele frequencies of at least 4% in their population with call rates above 70%. Their analysis showed that 32 polymorphisms within or flanking the following genes were nominally associated with warfarin dose ($P < 0.05$): *VKORC1, CYP2C9, CYP2C18, CYP2C19, PROC,*

Table 15.3 Genes involved in warfarin pharmacokinetics and pharmacodynamics Modified from Wadelius *et al.* [44]

Abbreviation	Name	Function of encoded protein
ABCB1	ATP-binding cassette transporter B1 gene	Xenobiotic efflux pump
APOE	Apolipoprotein E gene	Ligand for receptors mediating vitamin K uptake
CALU	Calumenin gene	Binds VKOR; inhibits warfarin effect
CYP1A1	Cytochrome P450 1A1 gene	Metabolizes *R*-warfarin
CYP1A2	Cytochrome P450 1A2 gene	Metabolizes *R*-warfarin
CYP2A6	Cytochrome P450 2A6 gene	Metabolizes *S*-warfarin
CYP2C8	Cytochrome P450 2C8 gene	Minor metabolism *R*,*S*-warfarin
CYP2C9	Cytochrome P450 2C9 gene	Major metabolism *S*-warfarin
CYP2C18	Cytochrome P450 2C18 gene	Minor metabolism *R*,*S*-warfarin
CYP2C19	Cytochrome P450 2C19 gene	Minor metabolism *R*,*S*-warfarin
CYP3A4	Cytochrome P450 3A4 gene	Metabolism *R*-warfarin
CYP3A5	Cytochrome P450 3A5 gene	Metabolism *R*-warfarin
EPHX1	Epoxide hydrolase 1, microsomal gene	? Part of VKORC complex
F2	Coagulation factor II (prothrombin) gene	Converts fibrinogen to fibrin, activates V, VII, XI, XIII, protein C
F5	Coagulation factor V gene	Activates II along with Xa
F7	Coagulation factor VII gene	As VIIa converts IX to IXa and X to Xa
F9	Coagulation factor IX gene	Along with VIIIa converts X to Xa
F10	Coagulation factor X gene	Activates II along with Va
GAS6	Growth-arrest specific 6	Sequence homology with protein S protects against clotting
GGCX	γ-Glutamyl carboxylase gene	Carboxylates vitamin K-dependent clotting factors
NQO1	NADPH dehydrogenase, quinone 1 gene	Forms vitamin K hydroquinone
NR1I2	Pregnane X receptor gene	Mediates induction of 2C9, 3A4
NR1I3	Constitutive androstane receptor gene	Transcriptional regulation of 2C9 and 3A4
ORM1	Orosomucoid 1 gene	Warfarin transport in blood

Abbreviation	Name	Function of encoded protein
ORM2	Orosomucoid 2 gene	Warfarin transport in blood
PROC	Protein C gene	With protein S inactivates Va and VIIIa
PROS1	Protein S gene	With protein C degrades Va and VIIIa
PROZ	Protein Z gene	Cofactor for inactivation of Xa
SERPINC1	Antithrombin III gene	Inhibits IIa, IXa, Xa, XIa, XIIa
VKORC1	Vitamin K epoxide reductase complex C1 gene	Reduces vitamin K to form cofactor for γ-glutamyl carboxylase
CYP4F2	Cytochrome P450 4F2 gene	? Oxidative degradation of vitamin K

APOE, EPHX1, CALU, GGCX, and *ORM1-ORM2* (Table 15.3) along with haplotypes of *VKORC1, CYP2C9, CYP2C8, CYP2C19, PROC, F7, GGCX, PROZ, F9, NR112* and *ORM1-ORM2*. After correction for multiple testing, *VKORC1, CYP2C9, CYP2C18,* and *CYP2C19* were associated with dose while *PROC* and *APOE* were significant only after within-gene correction. The association of *CYP2C18* and *CYP2C19* was completely explained by linkage disequilibrium with *CYP2C9**2 and/or *CYP2C9**3. Three linked *VKORC1* SNPs and the *CYP2C9* allele *3 were the strongest genetic factors determining warfarin dose requirements. Apart from *VKORC1* and *CYP2C9*, the most significant finding was the association of SNPs in *PROC*. Applying a multiple regression model to *VKORC1, CYP2C9**2/*3, *PROC*, and nongenetic factors, these authors were able to explain 62% of the variance in warfarin dose in Swedish patients. The addition of *EPHX1, GGCX* and *ORM1-ORM2* to the model predicted approximately 10% more of the variance. In the same year Caldwell *et al.* validated the prominence of CYP2C9 and VKORC-1 polymorphisms among candidate genes involved in warfarin metabolism and function. [46].

In early 2008 another candidate gene approach designed to identify genetic polymorphisms associated with warfarin dose was reported. Using the Affymetrix drug-metabolizing enzymes and transporters (DMET) panel to identify candidate associations, Caldwell *et al.* [47] screened 1228 SNP positions within 169 genes encoding proteins involved in drug metabolism and transport. The purpose of this study was to identify a small number of individual SNPs that might explain clinically meaningful proportions of the previously unexplained variability in stable warfarin dosing requirements. In order

Table 15.4 Analysis of residuals from the CYP/VKORC1 model by CYP4F2

Genotype	N	Mean (mg/week)	Standard deviation	Lower 95%	Upper 95%
CC	213	0.9	9.7	2.2	0.4
CT	175	2.3	8.9	1.0	3.6
TT	36	6.1	8.4	3.3	9.0

Kruskal–Wallis *P*-value <0.0001.

to identify potentially informative SNPs, the Affymetrix genotyping results were merged with the residuals from the best model the authors had developed to that point and which contained *CYP2C9* and *VKORC1* genotypic and clinical data. The existing model, without inclusion of *CYP4F2*, explained 56% of the interpatient variability in stable warfarin dose requirements. Each SNP was tested for association with the residual variability and evaluated in terms of the proportion of the residual variability explained by the SNP (i.e., the R^2 from a model with the residuals as the response and the SNP grouping as a predictor).

Following this screening protocol, the association of one SNP (rs2108622) emerged clearly. This SNP represents a polymorphism in the gene encoding the CYP drug-metabolizing enzyme, CYP4F2, and results in an amino acid change at position 433 in the protein (V433M). The results showed a highly significant difference (even after correction for multiple comparisons) with homozygous (CC) patients requiring less warfarin than otherwise predicted and those with T alleles requiring more warfarin than predicted (Table 15.4). Patients having two TT alleles require about 1 mg/day more warfarin than patients having two CC alleles. Figure 15.3 illustrates the impact of the C allele on dosing requirements in the updated model and shows the additive effect of CYP4F2 to those of CYP2C9 and VKORC1. These data were replicated in two separate white patient populations from regionally distinct locations in the USA.

The physiological role of CYP4F2 in the vitamin K/warfarin pathway was unknown prior to the discovery of this association. The enzyme is known to have a role in the omega-hydroxylation of products of leukotriene B_4 and the formation of 20-hydroxyeicosatetraenoic acid from arachidonic acid [48–50]. However, it is also known that CYP4F2 omega-hydroxylates the phytyl side-chain of tocopherol molecules as the first step leading to the formation of the γ-oxidation-truncated side- chain of tocopherol urinary metabolites [51,52]. In light of the similarities between the side-chains and side-chain oxidation products of vitamins E and K [53,54] (Fig. 15.1), the authors postulated that CYP4F2 is involved in the metabolism of vitamin K. The authors have further proposed

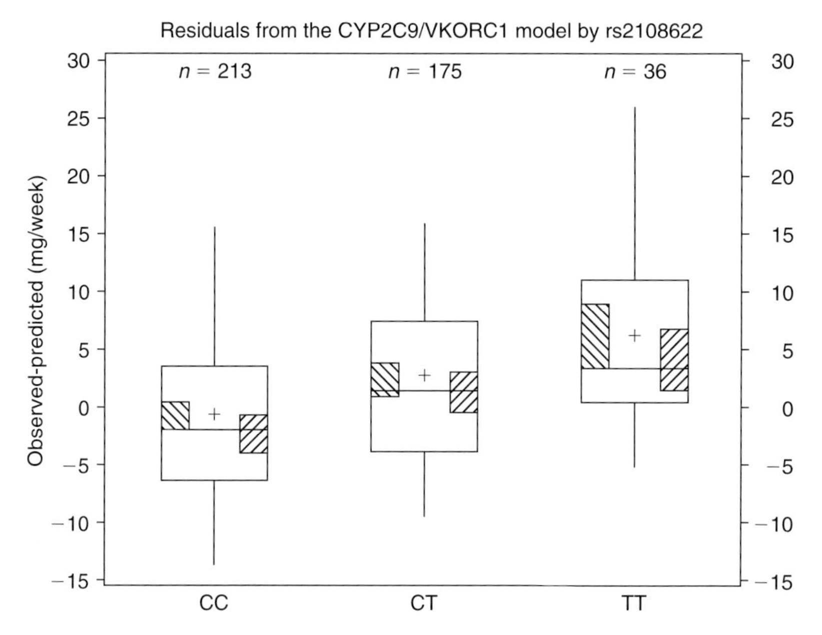

Fig. 15.3 Incrementally higher warfarin stable dose requirements were noted in patients whose CYP4F2 genotype included one and two T alleles, respectively.

that individuals with T alleles have a decreased function of the enzyme resulting in less degradation of vitamin K, thereby increasing the requirement for warfarin of individuals encoding the T allele.

Notably, the V433M polymorphism in CYP4F2 was recently shown to affect enzymatic activity. This polymorphism decreased 20-HETE production in a reconstituted recombinant protein system to about 50% of that of the wild-type enzyme [48].

Predictive models for warfarin therapy

Models have been developed for estimating the risk for major bleeding during warfarin therapy. Shireman *et al.* [55] recently examined combined data abstracted from the National Registry of Atrial Fibrillation and Medicare part A claims to identify major bleeding events requiring hospitalization. Using a split-sample technique, candidate variables that provided statistically stable relationships with major bleeding events were subsequently selected for model development. Model development and validation were conducted on 26345 patients with atrial fibrillation who were >65 years of age and had been discharged from hospital while receiving warfarin therapy. Eight variables were included in the final risk score model: age ⩾70 years, gender, remote bleeding, recent bleeding (index hospitalization), alcohol/drug abuse, diabetes, anemia, and antiplatelet use. Bleeding rates were 0.9%, 2.0%, and 5.4%, respectively, for the groups with low, moderate, and high risk, compared with the bleeding rates for groups with moderate risk (1.5% and 1.0%) and high risk (1.8% and 2.5%) from other models. The authors noted that the large size of the registry afforded the opportunity to incorporate additional risk factors [55].

Models have also been developed which may be used to estimate therapeutic dose in patients prior to initiating warfarin. These models have been able to explain over one-half of the dosing variability among patients based upon clinical and genetic (primarily *CYP2C9* and *VKORC1*) factors [39,42,44,46]. The addition of new genetic factors to these models in the future may provide substantial improvements. However, there are many challenges that remain in developing accurate dosing models for general clinical practice.

Models to date were derived from data collected in select clinical populations, generally at a single study site, so their general predictive accuracy is uncertain. Furthermore, while the size of these studies may appear large (several hundred patients), the number of important factors requires high-dimensional analysis in which the data are really quite sparse. This is particularly true because of the importance of genetic factors with low allele frequencies. A case in point is the *CYP2C9* variant *3/*3; the variant occurs in just 0.5% of white patients, but those patients may require only one-fifth the warfarin dose of patients with the most common genotype.

Assessment of interactions among the factors associated with warfarin dosing has been very limited. Interactions would be important, for example, if the magnitude of the effect of a clinical factor such as age differed substantially by gender or by genotype. In essence, modeling interactions among two or more factors poses an even higher dimensional analysis problem, further partitioning the data and increasing the likelihood that certain subgroups will be poorly represented by any model developed.

Initial data sharing has suggested that models developed at one site may demonstrate substantially reduced accuracy elsewhere. For example Sconce *et al.* [42] published the following regression equation based on data collected among patients in the Newcastle region in the UK:

$$V_{\text{dose}} = 0.628 - 0.0135\,(\text{age}) - 0.240\,(\text{CYP*2}) - 0.370\,(CYP\text{*3}) - 0.241\,(VKORC) + 0.0162\,(\text{height})$$

where dose is measured in mg/day, age is in years, CYP*2 and *3 are the respective numbers of *CYP2C9* alleles, *VKORC* is coded 1 for GG, 2 for GA, and 3 for AA, and height is measured in centimeters.

When the model was applied to appropriate historical cases from the Marshfield Clinic cohort ($n = 366$ observations), a systematic lack of fit was observed. Figure 15.2 shows the predicted values from the model on the vertical axis and the actual values on the horizontal axis, with a line of identity for reference. The R^2 was only 23% for the Marshfield Clinic cohort, compared with 54% as reported for the cohort used to develop the model.

This has provided impetus for a large collaboration known as the International Warfarin Pharmacogenetic Consortium (IWPC). The IWPC is an *ad hoc* organization of 21 participating research teams that formed in the fall of 2006 with the goal of pooling genotype and phenotype data from multiple studies (with an average size of around 300) to find the best possible dosing algorithm for warfarin, potentially including genotypes, medications, and comorbidities, as well as demographic data. The IWPC dataset included approximately 6000 patients. The dataset is diverse with respect to age, gender, and racial distribution. Data are available for *CYP2C9* and *VKORC1* in most of the study subjects.

Acknowledgments

The authors thank the Marshfield Clinic Research Foundation for its support and provision of editorial assistance in the preparation of this manuscript by Ingrid Glurich PhD and Alice Stargardt in the Office of Scientific Writing and Publication.

References

1 IMS America. *National Prescription Audit: Physician Specialty Report, Dispensed Data.* IMS America, Plymouth Meeting, PA, 1998.
2 Evans A, Davis S, Kilpatrick C *et al.* The morbidity related to atrial fibrillation at a tertiary centre in one year: 9.0% of all strokes are potentially preventable. *Journal of Clinical Neuroscience* 2002; **9**: 268–272.
3 Fihn SD, McDonell M, Martin D *et al.* Risk factors for complications of chronic anticoagulation. A multicenter study. Warfarin Optimized Outpatient Follow-up Study Group. *Annals of Internal Medicine* 1993; **118**: 511–520.
4 Levine MN, Raskob G, Beyth RJ *et al.* Hemorrhagic complications of anticoagulant treatment: the Seventh ACCP Conference on Antithrombotic and Thrombolytic Therapy. *Chest* 2004; **126** (3 suppl): 287S–310S.
5 Hylek EM, Singer DE. Risk factors for intracranial hemorrhage in outpatients taking warfarin. *Annals of Internal Medicine* 1994; **120**: 897–902.
6 Adjusted-dose warfarin versus low-intensity, fixed-dose warfarin plus aspirin for high-risk patients with atrial fibrillation: Stroke Prevention in Atrial Fibrillation III randomised clinical trial. *Lancet* 1996; **348**: 633–638.
7 Casais P, Luceros AS, Meschengieser S *et al.* Bleeding risk factors in chronic oral anticoagulation with acenocoumarol. *American Journal of Hematology* 2000; **63**: 192–196.
8 Van der Meer F, Rosendaal F, Vandenbroucke J, Briët E. Bleeding complications in oral anticoagulant therapy. An analysis of risk factors. *Archives of Internal Medicine* 1993; **153**: 1557–1562.

9 Cannegieter SC, Rosendaal FR, Wintzen AR *et al.* Optimal oral anticoagulant therapy in patients with mechanical heart valves. *New England Journal of Medicine* 1995; **333**: 11–17.
10 Palareti G, Leali N, Coccheri S *et al.* Bleeding complications of oral anticoagulant treatment: an inception-cohort, prospective collaborative study (ISCOAT). Italian Study on Complications of Oral Anticoagulant Therapy. *Lancet* 1996; **348**: 423–428.
11 Suttie JW. Vitamin K-dependent carboxylase. *Annual Review of Biochemistry* 1985; **54**: 459–477.
12 Berkner KL. The vitamin K-dependent carboxylase. *Annual Review of Nutrition* 2005; **25**: 127–149.
13 Kuo WL, Stafford DW, Cruces J *et al.* Chromosomal localization of the gamma-glutamyl carboxylase gene at 2p12. *Genomics* 1995; **25**: 746–748.
14 Hirsh J, Fuster V, Ansell J, Halperin JL; American Heart Association; American College of Cardiology Foundation. American Heart Association/American College of Cardiology Foundation guide to warfarin therapy. *Circulation* 2003; **107**: 1692–1711.
15 Friedman PA, Rosenberg RD, Hauschka PV, Fitz-James A. A spectrum of partially carboxylated prothrombins in the plasmas of coumarin-treated patients. *Biochimica et Biophysica Acta* 1977; **494**: 271–276.
16 Malhotra OP, Nesheim ME, Mann KG. The kinetics of activation of normal and gamma-carboxyglutamic acid-deficient prothrombins. *Journal of Biological Chemistry* 1985; **260**: 279–287.
17 Choonara IA, Haynes BP, Cholerton S *et al.* Enantiomers of warfarin and vitamin K1 metabolism. *British Journal of Clinical Pharmacology* 1986; **22**: 729–732.
18 Palareti G, Legnani C. Warfarin withdrawal. Pharmacokinetic-pharmacodynamic considerations. *Clinical Pharmacokinetics* 1996; **30**: 300–313.
19 Otagiri M, Maruyama T, Imai T *et al.* A comparative study of the interaction of warfarin with human alpha 1-acid glycoprotein and human albumin. *Journal of Pharmacy and Pharmacology* 1987; **39**: 416–420.
20 Jansing RL, Chao ES, Kaminsky LS. Phase II metabolism of warfarin in primary culture of adult rat hepatocytes. *Molecular Pharmacology* 1992; **41**: 209–215.
21 Sussman N, Waltershied M, Butler T *et al.* The predictive nature of high throughput toxicity screening using a human hepatocyte cell line. *Cell Notes* 2002; **3**: 7–10.
22 Holbrook AM, Pereira JA, Labiris R *et al.* Systematic overview of warfarin and its drug and food interactions. *Archives of Internal Medicine* 2005; **165**: 1095–1106.
23 Desta Z, Soukhova NV, Flockhart DA. Inhibition of cytochrome P450 (CYP450) isoforms by isoniazid: potent inhibition of CYP2C19 and CYP3A. *Antimicrobial Agents and Chemotherapy* 2001; **45**: 382–392.
24 Hirsh J, Dalen JE, Anderson DR *et al.* Oral anticoagulants: mechanism of action, clinical effectiveness, and optimal therapeutic range. *Chest* 1998; **114** (5 Suppl): 445S–469S.
25 Furuya H, Fernandez-Salguero P, Gregory W *et al.* Genetic polymorphism of CYP2C9 and its effect on warfarin maintenance dose requirement in patients undergoing anticoagulation therapy. *Pharmacogenetics* 1995; **5**: 389–392.
26 Rettie AE, Korzekwa KR, Kunze KL *et al.* Hydroxylation of warfarin by human cDNA-expressed cytochrome P-450: a role for P-4502C9 in the etiology of (S)-warfarin-drug interactions. *Chemical Research in Toxicology* 1992; **5**: 54–59.
27 Aithal GP, Day CP, Kesteven PJ, Daly AK. Association of polymorphisms in the cytochrome P450 CYP2C9 with warfarin dose requirement and risk of bleeding complications. *Lancet* 1999; **353**: 717–719.

28 Sanderson S, Emery J, Higgins J. CYP2C9 gene variants, drug dose, and bleeding risk in warfarin-treated patients: a HuGEnet systematic review and meta-analysis. *Genetic Medicine* 2005; **7**: 97–104.
29 Linder MW, Looney S, Adams JE, 3rd, *et al*. Warfarin dose adjustments based on CYP2C9 genetic polymorphisms. *Journal of Thrombosis and Thrombolysis* 2002; **14**: 227–232.
30 Scordo MG, Pengo V, Spina E *et al*. Influence of CYP2C9 and CYP2C19 genetic polymorphisms on warfarin maintenance dose and metabolic clearance. *Clinical Pharmacology and Therapeutics* 2002; **72**: 702–710.
31 Freeman BD, Zehnbauer BA, McGrath S *et al*. Cytochrome P450 polymorphisms are associated with reduced warfarin dose. *Surgery* 2000; **128**: 281–285.
32 Loebstein R, Yonath H, Peleg D *et al*. Interindividual variability in sensitivity to warfarin-Nature or nurture? *Clinical Pharmacology and Therapeutics* 2001; **70**: 159–164.
33 Furuya H, Fernandez-Salguero P, Gregory W *et al*. Genetic polymorphism of CYP2C9 and its effect on warfarin maintenance dose requirement in patients undergoing anticoagulation therapy. *Pharmacogenetics* 1995; **5**: 389–392.
34 Taube J, Halsall D, Baglin T. Influence of cytochrome P-450 CYP2C9 polymorphisms on warfarin sensitivity and risk of over-anticoagulation in patients on long-term treatment. *Blood* 2000; **96**: 1816–1819.
35 Higashi MK, Veenstra DL, Kondo LM *et al*. Association between CYP2C9 genetic variants and anticoagulation-related outcomes during warfarin therapy. *JAMA: the Journal of the American Medical Association* 2002; **287**: 1690–1698.
36 Hillman MA, Wilke RA, Caldwell MD *et al*. Relative impact of covariates in prescribing warfarin according to CYP2C9 genotype. *Pharmacogenetics* 2004; **14**: 539–547.
37 Peyvandi F, Spreafico M, Siboni SM *et al*. CYP2C9 genotypes and dose requirements during the induction phase of oral anticoagulant therapy. *Clinical Pharmacology and Therapeutics* 2004; **75**: 198–203.
38 Rost S, Fregin A, Ivaskevicius V *et al*. Mutations in VKORC1 cause warfarin resistance and multiple coagulation factor deficiency type 2. *Nature* 2004; **427**: 537–541.
39 Rieder MJ, Reiner AP, Gage BF *et al*. Effect of VKORC1 haplotypes on transcriptional regulation and warfarin dose. *New England Journal of Medicine* 2005; **352**: 2285–2293.
40 Vitamin K epoxide reductase complex, subunit 1; VKORC1. Available from: http://www.ncbi.nlm.nih.gov/entrez/dispomim.cgi?id=608547 (accessed August 27, 2007).
41 D'Andrea G, D'Ambrosio RL, Di Perna P *et al*. A polymorphism in the VKORC1 gene is associated with an interindividual variability in the dose-anticoagulant effect of warfarin. *Blood* 2005; **105**: 645–649.
42 Sconce EA, Khan TI, Wynne HA *et al*. The impact of CYP2C9 and VKORC1 genetic polymorphism and patient characteristics upon warfarin dose requirements: proposal for a new dosing regimen. *Blood* 2005; **106**: 2329–2333.
43 Wadelius M, Pirmohamed M. Pharmacogenetics of warfarin: current status and future challenges. *Pharmacogenomics Journal* 2007; **7**: 99–111.
44 Wadelius M, Chen LY, Eriksson N *et al*. Association of warfarin dose with genes involved in its action and metabolism. *Human Genetics* 2007; **121**: 23–34.
45 Krynetskiy E, McDonnell P. Building individualized medicine: prevention of adverse reactions to warfarin therapy. *Journal of Pharmacology and Experimental Therapeutics* 2007; **322**: 427–434.
46 Caldwell MD, Berg RL, Zhang KQ *et al*. Evaluation of genetic factors for warfarin dose prediction. *Clinical Medicine and Research* 2007; **5**: 8–16.

47 Caldwell MD, Awad T, Johnson JA *et al*. CYP4F2 genetic variant alters required warfarin dose. *Blood* 2008; **111**: 4106–4112.
48 Stec DE, Roman RJ, Flasch A, Rieder MJ. Functional polymorphism in human CYP4F2 decreases 20-HETE production. *Physiological Genomics* 2007; **30**: 74–81.
49 Jin R, Koop DR, Raucy JL, Lasker JM. Role of human CYP4F2 in hepatic catabolism of the proinflammatory agent leukotriene B4. *Archives of Biochemistry and Biophysics* 1998; **359**: 89–98.
50 Ma YH, Schwartzman ML, Roman RJ. Altered renal P-450 metabolism of arachidonic acid in Dahl salt-sensitive rats. *American Journal of Physiology* 1994; **267**: R579–589.
51 Sontag TJ, Parker RS. Cytochrome P450 omega-hydroxylase pathway of tocopherol catabolism. Novel mechanism of regulation of vitamin E status. *Journal of Biological Chemistry* 2002; **277**: 25290–25296.
52 Parker RS, Sontag TJ, Swanson JE, McCormick CC. Discovery, characterization, and significance of the cytochrome P450 omega-hydroxylase pathway of vitamin E catabolism. *Annals of the New York Academy of Sciences* 2004; **1031**: 13–21.
53 Watanabe M, Toyoda M, Imada I, Morimoto H. Ubiquinone and related compounds. XXVI. The urinary metabolites of phylloquinone and alpha-tocopherol. *Chemical and Pharmaceutical Bulletin* 1974; **22**: 176–182.
54 Harrington DJ, Soper R, Edwards C *et al*. Determination of the urinary aglycone metabolites of vitamin K by HPLC with redox-mode electrochemical detection. *Journal of Lipid Research* 2005; **46**: 1053–1060.
55 Shireman TI, Mahnken JD, Howard PA *et al*. Development of a contemporary bleeding risk model for elderly warfarin recipients. *Chest* 2006; **130**: 1390–1396.

Appendix

Alleles: Alternate sequences of the same *gene*, one inherited from each parent.

Association: A statistical finding that the frequency of one or more *genetic variants* is significantly different in those with a *phenotype* than in those without the *phenotype*.

Candidate gene: A *gene* in which variants could plausibly explain a given *phenotype*, such as severity of disease or variable response to drug. Candidate genes are generally identified by studying the basic biology of the phenotype in question. In addition, regions within the genome associated with a phenotype may be identified by *linkage analysis* or *genome-wide association*; in such cases, the genes within the region can then be examined to determine if any could be plausible biologic candidates for the phenotype. For example, linkage analysis implicated a region on chromosome 3 in some cases of the long QT syndrome; one of the genes in the linked region encodes the cardiac sodium channel, which then became a candidate (and in fact was ultimately shown to harbor causative mutations).

Complementary DNA (cDNA): cDNA is double-stranded *DNA* generated from single-stranded messenger *RNA*. cDNA is much more stable and easy to manipulate in the laboratory than mRNA, and so is often preferable for experimental purposes.

CNV (Copy number variation): A *DNA polymorphism* that involves the presence or absence of relatively large regions (thousands or more base pairs).

Deoxyribonucleic acid (DNA): DNA is a macromolecule consisting of two very long strands each consisting of thousands of deoxyribose sugars, phosphates, and nucleotides (cytosine, guanine, adenine, or thymine) linked to each other. Each nucleotide in one strand binds to its partner in the other (A to T and C to G) to create the familiar double helix. Some regions of DNA encode proteins, but most DNA sequences regulate protein production, or serve a structural or as yet unidentified roles.

Dominant: describes the situation in which the effects of one of a pair of *heterozygous* alleles produces a *phenotype*. Most *monogenic* cardiovascular diseases display dominant inheritance: a single copy of the abnormal allele is sufficient to confer the disease phenotype. See also: *recessive.*

Dominant negative refers to the situation in which the an abnormal allele generates a protein that results in a greater than expected loss of function (e.g. by suppressing the function of the protein generated by the normal allele).

Epigenetic: The concept that a change in gene function can be conferred by non-genetic factors and procreate over generations. Examples include chromatin remodeling or *DNA* methylation that allow or inhibit transcription of specific genes. The term was originally used to describe how stem cells could differentiate into specific cellular phenotypes (heart cell, liver cell, etc) that are then preserved as cells divide.

Exon: Refers to a region of *DNA* that after transcription and splicing is retained in messenger RNA. Exons include both coding regions that are translated into protein as well as flanking untranslated regions.

Gene: A sequence of *DNA* that encodes a protein. The coding sequence in *exons* is often separated by non-coding intervening sequences (*introns*) that are removed when pre-mRNA is spliced into *mRNA*.

Genetic code: Refers to the way in which nucleotide sequences in exons result in amino acid sequences within proteins. Each of the 21 amino acids that are used to generate proteins from mRNA is encoded by a sequence of three nucleotides, termed a codon. Because there are 4 possible nucleotides at each position, there are 64 (4^3) possible codons. Thus some amino acids are encoded by more than one codon (this is referred to as redundancy), so a genetic variant may not necessarily change the encoded be amino acid. For example, the RNA sequences "cytosine-alanine-alanine" (CAA) and "cytosine-alanine-guanine" (CAG) both encode the amino acid glutamine.

Genetic variant: A difference in *DNA* sequence when compared to a reference sequence. These are often classified as *mutations* (rare) or *polymorphisms* (common), although the distinction can be blurred.

Genotype is the genetic makeup of an individual, and may refer to the whole genome, or to specific genes or regions of genes.

Genome: The collection of all *DNA* in an organism. Only a small proportion (probably <3%) of human genomes encodes proteins; the remainder is thought to regulate gene expression or to serve as yet unidentified functions.

Genome-wide analysis seeks to identify new genetic regions involved in variable *phenotypes;* the technique compares *genotypes* at hundreds of thousands of common polymorphic sites in large numbers of patients with and without a specific *phenotype.*

Haploinsufficiency refers to the situation in which a phenotype that results from absence of a protein product of an abnormal allele (e.g. a truncated or non-functional protein).

Haplotype: A set of *genetic variants* that are inherited together. **Haplotype blocks** may include many individual *polymorphisms* with a high degree of *linkage disequilibrium;* as a result, establishing *genotype* at any single polymorphic site with such a block may establish genotypes at linked sites within the block.

Heterozygous: Two different *alleles* in a specific region of *DNA.*

Homozygous: The same *alleles* in a specific region of *DNA.*

Indel (Insertion/deleetion polymorphism): A *DNA polymorphism* in which multiple sequential nucleotides are present (insertion) or absent (deleted) in a *DNA* sequence.

Intron: A region of *DNA* that is within a gene but is removed from pre-mRNA during splicing to form the final messenger RNA from which protein is transcribed.

Linkage analysis is a technique to identify genomic regions, and ultimately single genetic variants, that associate a phenotype with a genotype within a kindred. This involves precise phenotyping, construction of extensive family trees, and asking which genetic regions are shared among those with disease.

Linkage disequilibrium: The extent to which *polymorphisms* located near each other are co-inherited. Polymorphisms that are always co-inherited are said to be in complete linkage disequilibrium.

Mitochondrial DNA: *DNA* located in mitochondria (mtDNA) encode 13 proteins in the cellular respiratory cascadee, as well as transfer and ribosomal RNA. Each mitochondrion contains hundreds or thousands of copies of the ~16,000 bp mtDNA, each as a closed loop (circular *DNA*). Mutations in mtDNA can be disease causing. Unlike nuclear *DNA,* mtDNA is inherited from the mother only.

Monogenic describes a disease in which a *mutation* in a single gene is sufficient to produce the disease phenotype. The severity of the *phenotype* may vary among mutation carriers (variable *penetrance*), a poorly-understood phenomenon generally attributed to the influence of other genetic variants on the final disease *phenotype.*

Mutation refers to rare variants, most often in coding regions, that are often associated with genetic diseases like HCM or long QT.

Non-synonymous polymorphism: A coding region *polymorphism* that alters the amino acid of the encoded protein. Because the *genetic code* is redundant, a coding region *polymorphism* can also be synonymous, i.e. it need not change the encoded amino acid.

Penetrance: The proportion of patients with a disease-associated *mutation* who actually display the disease *phenotype*. Penetrance in *monogenic* diseases is often much less than 100%.

Pharmacogenetics: The study of the relationship between individual *DNA* variants and variable drug effects.

Pharmacogenomics: The study of the relationship between *DNA* variants in a large collection of genes, up to the whole genome, and variable drug effects.

Phenotype: Measurable characteristics of an organism. These may derive from genotype, environment, or their combination. Organisms with the same phenotype can have different *genotypes*.

Polygenic diseases are those in which multiple rare and common *polymorphisms* are thought to contribute to the disease phenotype. Atherosclerosis and hypertension are examples, although rare "*monogenic*" forms (i.e. those in which a single gene variant dominates the clinical picture) have been described.

Polymorphisms are *DNA* variants that are common, often defined as >1% in a given population (although rare polymorphisms are increasingly recognized). Polymorphisms can be in coding regions (where they may be synonymous or *non-synonymous*) or, more commonly, in non-coding regions, and often vary by ethnicity. *SNPs*, *indels*, *VNTRs*, and *CNVs* are types of polymorphisms. While some genetic variants are known to alter protein abundance or function, the functional consequences of most polymorphisms are unknown.

Post-translational modification: This term refers to modification of a protein's structure after it has been translated. Examples include phosphorylation, glycosylation, or the creation of intramolecular disulfide bonds.

Recessive: Recessive disorders are those in which two copies of an abnormal *allele* are required to generate the phenotype in question (e.g. sickle cell anemia or the Jervell Lange Neilson Syndrome).

Ribonucleic acid (RNA): RNA is a polymer very similar in structure to *DNA* except it is usually a single strand, its sugar is ribose (not deoxyribose), and it uses uracil rather than thymidine. *DNA* transcription generates pre-messenger RNA which is then spliced to messenger RNA (mRNA).

SNP (Single Nucleotide Polymorphism): A change in one nucleotide (base-pair) in a *DNA* sequence. This is the commonest type of *DNA polymorphism*.

Splicing: The primary product of transcription is the pre-mRNA molecule, which then undergoes removal of intronic sequences and reconnection (splicing) of exons. Alternate patterns of exon splicing generate different forms of mRNA, termed splice variants, and thus potentially different proteins.

Transcription: The process of generating a single strand of pre-messenger RNA (pre-mRNA) from a sequence of *DNA* encoding a gene. Most gene sequences include both coding and non-coding regions. Messenger RNA is produced by removing *introns* and other non-coding sequences from pre-mRNA (*splicing*). Gene transcription is initiated by the binding of a series of proteins (transcription factors and others) to regulatory regions generally adjacent to a gene.

Translation: Messenger RNA is exported from the nucleus to the cytosol, where transfer RNAs use the mRNA template to generate protein chains, dictated by the *genetic code*.

VNTR (Variable Number of Tandem Repeats): A specific type of *DNA polymorphism* in which a short sequence (generally up to 5 nucleotides) is repeated a variable number of times, which is usually inherited. Variable repeat regions were among the first polymorphic sites to be identified in the genome and were used for early mapping studies to associate genomic regions with specific inherited diseases by linkage analysis. In some instances, tandem repeats can vary from generation to generation and can be associated with disease. For example, the number of disease-associated trinucleotide repeats increases from generation to generation in Huntingdon's Disease, and explains the increasing severity of disease as it is passed into subsequent generations ("genetic anticipation").

Index

Author Disclosure Table

Working group member	Employment	Research grant	Other research support	Speakers bureau/honoraria	Expert witness	Ownership interest	Consultant/ advisory board	Other
Alberts	Northwestern University Medical School	None	None	None	None	None	None	None
Arnett	University of Alabama at Birmingham	None	None	None	None	None	None	None
Berg	Marshfield Clinic Research Foundation	None	Agency for Healthcare Research and Quality*	None	None	CYP4F2 Provisional Patent	None	None
Caldwell	Marshfield Clinic	None	None	None	None	None	None	None
Crawford	Vanderbilt University	None	None	None	None	None	None	None
Darbar	Vanderbilt University	NIH research grant on genetics of AF+	None	None	None	None	None	None
De Jong	Academic Medical Center	None	None	None	None	None	None	None
Dekker	Catharina Hospital	None	None	None	None	None	None	None

(*Continued*)

Author Disclosure Table (Continued)

Working group member	Employment	Research grant	Other research support	Speakers bureau/honoraria	Expert witness	Ownership interest	Consultant/ advisory board	Other
Faraday	Johns Hopkins University	NIH Grants+*	None	None	None	None	None	Patent Pending – Novel antithrombotic agents and methods of use thereof*
Haines	Vanderbilt University	None	None	None	None	None	None	None
Ho	Brigham and Women's Hospital	None	None	None	None	None	None	None
Hreiche	Universite de Montreal	None	None	None	None	None	None	None
Johnson	University of Florida	None	None	None	None	None	Third Wave Technologies, Medco*	None
Khan	Maryland Endocrine	None	None	None	None	None	None	None

MacRae	Mass Generals Physicians Organization	NIH Grants+	None	None	None	None	None	None
McKenna	The Heart Hospital	British Heart Foundation+	None	None	None	None	None	None
McPherson	University Ottawa Heart Institute	None	None	Merck Schering – Canada, Astra Zeneca – Canada, Pfizer - Canada*	None	None	Astra Zeneca Canada*	None
Michaud	Universite de Montreal	None	None	None	None	None	None	None
Newton-Cheh	Massachusetts General Hospital	None	None	None	None	None	None	None
Pacanowski	University of Florida	None	None	None	None	None	None	None
Ridker	Brigham and Women's Hospital	NHLBI, Amgen, Roche Diagnostics+	None	None	None	None	None	None
Ritchie	Vanderbilt University	None	None	None	None	None	None	None
Roberts	University of Ottawa Heart Institute	CIHR*	None	None	None	None	None	None

(Continued)

Author Disclosure Table (Continued)

Working group member	Employment	Research grant	Other research support	Speakers bureau/honoraria	Expert witness	Ownership interest	Consultant/ advisory board	Other
Roden	Vanderbilt University School of Medicine	None	None	None	None	None	None	Patent License Fee – Clinical Data Inc – A genetic test for Long QT Syndrome*
Sen-Chowdhry	None	None	None	None	None	None	None	None
Shuldiner	University of Maryland	NIH Grant+	None	None	None	None	None	None
Smith	Broad Institute of Harvard and MIT	None	None	None	None	None	None	None
Stewart	University of Ottawa Heart Institute	None	None	None	None	None	None	None
Suk-Danik	Brigham and Women's Hospital	NHLBI, Amgen, Roche Diagnostics+	None	None	None	None	None	None

Syrris	University College London	None	None	None	None	None	None	None
Towbin	Baylor College of Medicine	None	None	None	None	None	None	None
Turgeon	Universite de Montreal	None	None	None	None	None	None	None
Vatta	Baylor College of Medicine	None	None	None	None	None	None	None
Wilde	Academic Medical Center	None	None	None	None	None	None	None
Zineh	University of Florida	None	None	None	None	None		None

*Modest
+Significant
This table represents the relationships of writing group members that may be perceived as actual or reasonably perceived conflicts of interest as reported on the Disclosure Questionnaire which all writing group members are required to complete and submit. A relationship is considered to be "Significant" if (a) the person receives $10,000 or more during any 12 month period, or 5% or more of the person's gross income; or (b) the person owns 5% or more of the voting stock or share of the entity, or owns $10,000 or more of the fair market value of the entity. A relationship is considered to be "Modest" if it is less than "Significant" under the preceding definition.

The AHA Clinical Series

SERIES EDITOR • ELLIOTT ANTMAN

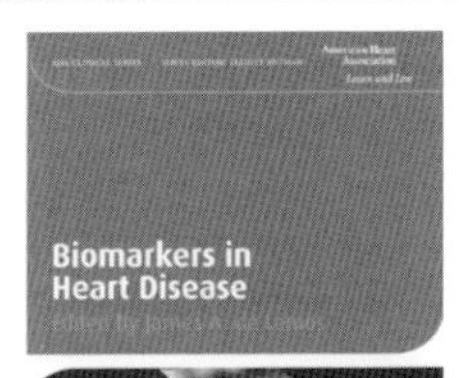

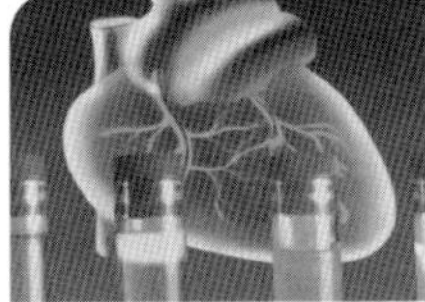

Biomarkers in Heart Disease
James A. de Lemos
9781405175715

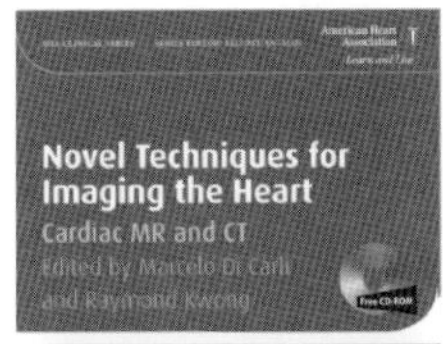

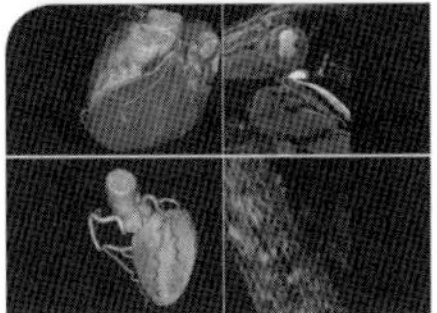

Novel Techniques for Imaging the Heart
Marcelo Di Carli & Raymond Kwong
9781405175333

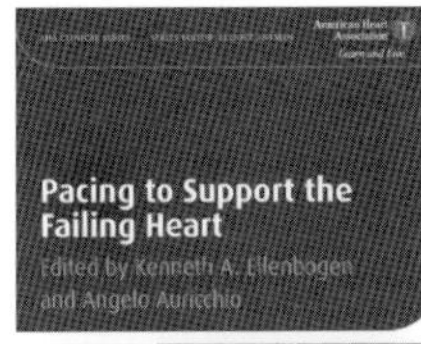

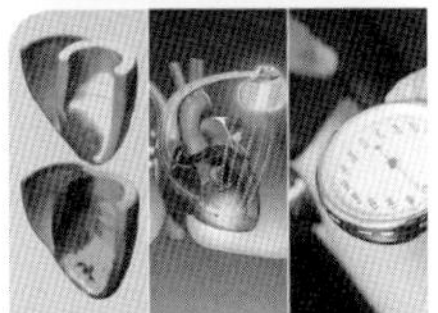

Pacing to Support the Failing Heart
Kenneth A. Ellenbogen
& Angelo Auricchio
9781405175340

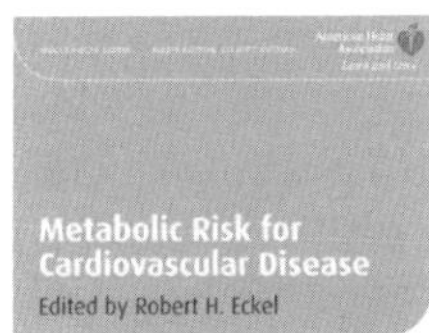

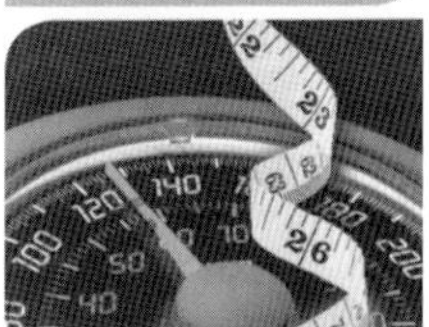

Metabolic Risk for Cardiovascular Disease
Robert H. Eckel
9781405181044

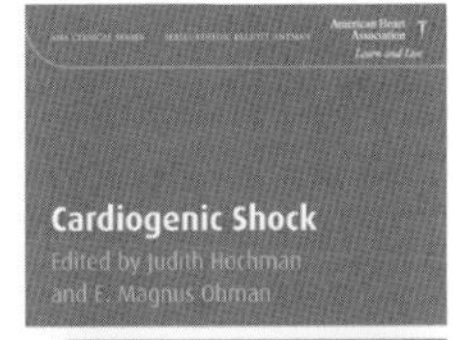

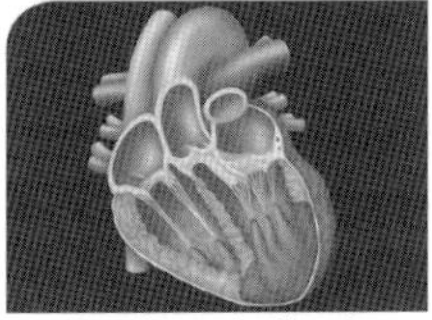

Cardiogenic Shock
Judith Hochman
& E. Magnus Ohman
9781405179263

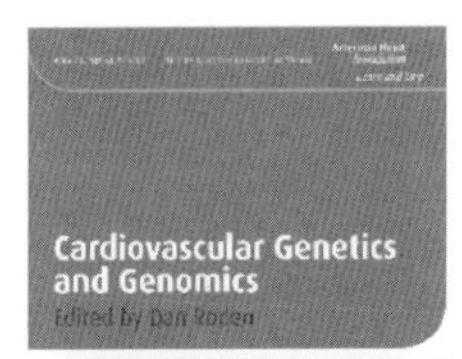

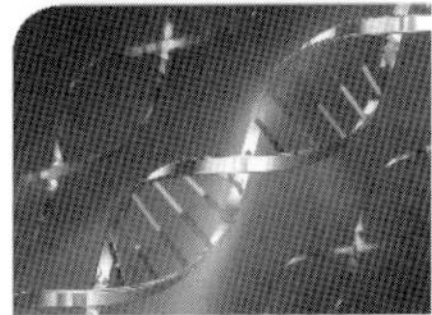

Cardiovascular Genetics and Genomics
Dan Roden
9781405175401

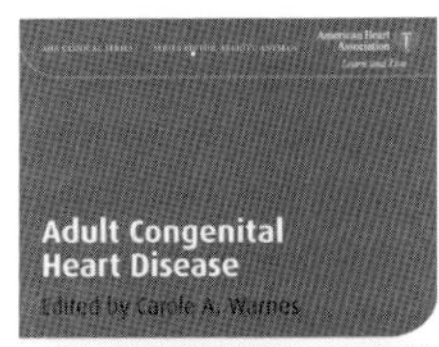

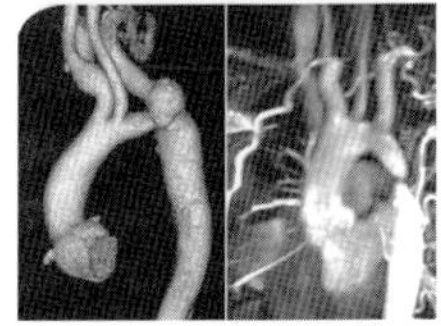

Adult Congenital Heart Disease
Carole A. Warnes
9781405178204

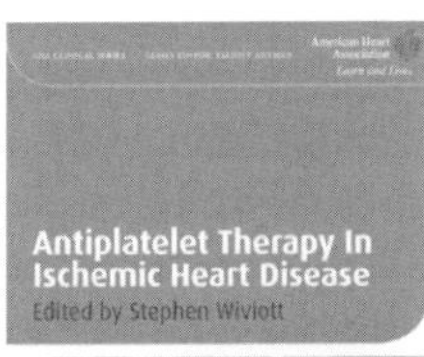

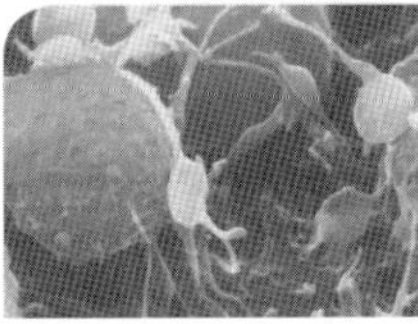

Antiplatelet Therapy In Ischemic Heart Disease
Stephen Wiviott
9781405176262

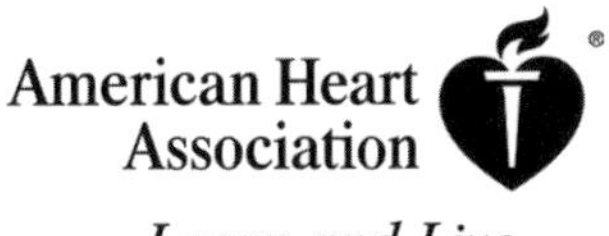

AHA/ASA Premium Professional Members

Save 20%

To join and order visit
my.americanheart.org